Handbook of Experimental Pharmacology

Volume 185/II

Wolfhard Semmler · Markus Schwaiger

Editors

Molecular Imaging II

Contributors

F. Blankenberg, R. Blasberg, A. Bogdanov, R.G. Boy, C. Bremer, R. Deckers, S.L. Deutscher, I. Dijkgraaf, M. Eisenhut, S.S. Gambhir, A. Haase, R. Haubner, A.H. Jacobs, P.M. Jakob, U. Haberkorn, A. Hagooly, K.-H. Hiller, R. Huang, F. Kiessling, L.W. Kracht, P. Mayer-Kukuck, W. Mier, J.-J. Min, C.T.W. Moonen, J. Newton, M. Querol, C. Rome, R. Rossin, M.A. Rueger, I. Serganova, H.W. Strauss, J. Tait, A.V. Thomas, J.-L. Vanderheyden, C. Waller, M.J. Welch, H.J. Wester, A. Winkeler

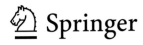 Springer

Prof. Dr. rer. nat. Dr. med. Wolfhard Semmler
Leiter der Abteilung für Medizinische Physik
in der Radiologie (E 020)
Forschungsschwerpunkt Innovative
Krebsdiagnostik und -therapie (E)
Deutsches Krebsforschungszentrum
Im Neuenheimer Feld 280
69120 Heidelberg
Germany
wolfhard.semmler@dkfz.de

Prof. Dr. med. Markus Schwaiger
Nuklearmedizinische Klinik und
Poliklinik
Klinikum rechts des Isar des
Technischen Universität München
Ismaninger Str. 22
81675 München
Germany
markus.schwaiger@tum.de

ISBN: 978-3-540-77449-5   e-ISBN: 978-3-540-77496-9

Handbook of Experimental Pharmacology ISSN 0171-2004

Library of Congress Control Number: 2007943479

Cover Design: WMXDesign GmbH, Heidelberg

Printed on acid-free paper

9 8 7 6 5 4 3 2 1

springer.com

Foreword

Bayer Schering Pharma welcomes Springer Verlag's endeavor to open its well-known Handbook of Pharmacology to the exciting field of molecular imaging and we are pleased to contribute to the printing costs of this volume.

In principle, noninvasive diagnostic imaging can be divided into morphological/anatomical imaging on the one hand, with CT/MRI the most important imaging technologies, and molecular imaging on the other. In CT/MRI procedures, contrast agents are injected at millimolar blood concentrations, while today's molecular imaging technologies such as PET/SPECT use tracers at nanomolar blood concentrations. Morphological imaging technologies such as X-ray/CT/MRI achieve very high spatial resolution. However, they share the limitation of not being able to detect lesions until the structural changes in the tissue (e.g., caused by cancer growth) are large enough to be seen by the imaging technology. Molecular imaging offers the potential of detecting the molecular and cellular changes caused by the disease process before the lesion (e.g., a tumor) is large enough to cause the kind of structural changes that can be detected by other imaging modalities. On the other hand, molecular imaging methods suffer from a rather poor level of spatial resolution, although current PET machines are better than SPECT devices.

The current diagnostic imaging revolution of fusing conventional diagnostic imaging (CT, MRT) with molecular imaging technologies (PET, SPECT) combines the strength of molecular imaging — i.e., detecting pathophysiological changes at the onset of the disease — with the strength of morphological imaging — i.e., high structural resolution. Today, already more than 95% of new PET scanners installed are PET/CT scanners. PET/CT fusion imaging is currently the fastest-growing imaging technology. And PET/MRI fusion scanners are also on the horizon. The trend toward specialized imaging centers, where all the required equipment is available in one facility, is expected to continue. The former technology-driven focus in diagnostic imaging research looks set to change into a more disease-oriented one.

Fusion imaging will make it possible to detect the occurrence of a disease earlier than is possible today. This is significant, because the likelihood of successful therapeutic interventions increases the earlier diseases are diagnosed. Furthermore, because a disease can be characterized at the molecular level, patients can be stratified for a given therapy and therapeutic responses monitored early on and in a quantitative manner. The growing pressure for selection, early therapy monitoring and justification (outcome) of a specific treatment will have a significant impact on molecular imaging procedures. Hence, molecular imaging technologies are now an integral part of both research and development (early clinical prediction of drug distribution and efficiency) at most pharmaceutical companies.

Bayer Schering Pharma (BSP) has always been a pioneer in the research and development of new imaging agents for "classic" modalities like CT and MRI. In line with this history and BSP's focus on innovation, we are now fully committed to breaking new ground in molecular imaging, especially in research and development of radio-tracers like PET imaging agents.

A strong and active partnership with academia is essential in order to be successful in the exciting new field of molecular imaging. We want to help make innovative imaging solutions invented in university research labs available to the patients. Furthermore, the low doses of "tracers" injected make it possible to perform clinical research studies under the microdosing/exploratory IND regulations. This will help molecular imaging move into the hospital and, hopefully, also generate early and fruitful collaborations between academia, clinic, regulatory authorities and the pharmaceutical industry.

Bayer Schering Pharma, Berlin   *Matthias Bräutigam and Ludger Dinkelborg*

Preface

"Molecular imaging (MI) is the in vivo characterization and measurement of biologic processes on the cellular and molecular level. In contradistinction to 'classical' diagnostic imaging, it sets forth to probe such molecular abnormalities that are the basis of disease rather than to image the end results of these molecular alterations" (Weissleder and Mahmood 2001).[a]

Imaging has witnessed a rapid growth in recent decades. This successful development was primarily driven by impressive technical advances in structural imaging; i.e., fast computer tomography (CT) and magnetic resonance imaging (MRI). In parallel, functional imaging emerged as an important step in the diagnostic and prognostic assessment of patients addressing physiological functions such as organ blood flow, cardiac pump function and neuronal activity using nuclear, magnetic resonance and ultrasonic techniques. More recently the importance of molecular targets for diagnosis and therapy has been recognized and imaging procedures introduced to visualize and quantify these target structures. Based on the hypothesis that molecular imaging provides both a research tool in the laboratory and a translational technology in the clinical arena, considerable funding efforts in the US and Europe were directed to accelerate the development of this imaging technology. In addition, the industry responded to the new demand with the introduction of dedicated imaging equipment for animal research as well as multimodality imaging (PET/CT), used to combine high-resolution imaging with the high sensitivity of tracer techniques.

Molecular imaging has been applied academically in neuroscience with emphasis on cognition, neurotransmission and neurodegeneration. Besides this established area, cardiology and oncology are currently the fastest growing applications. Vascular biology provides new targets to visualize atherosclerotic plaques, which may lead to earlier diagnosis as well as better monitoring of preventive therapies. Labeling of cells allows localization of inflammation or tumors and labeled stem-cell tracking of these cells in vivo. The noninvasive biologic characterization of tumor tissue in animals and humans opens not only exciting new research strategies but also appears

---

[a] Weissleder R, Mahmood U (2001) Molecular imaging. Radiology 219:316–333

promising for personalized management of cancer patients, which may alter the diagnostic and therapeutic processes.

Detection and characterization of lesions, especially tumors, remains challenging, and can be only achieved by using specific tracers and/or contrast media. The past decade has seen the development of specific approaches that use labeled antibodies and fragments thereof. However, in general only a relatively low target-to-background ratio has been attained due to the slow clearance of unbound antibody. Other target-specific approaches include labeled proteins, peptides, oligonucleotides, etc. Due to the low concentration of proteins, such as receptors in the target (e.g., tumors, cells), imaging requires highly sensitive probes addressing these structures. Whereas this challenge does not affect the use of positron emission tomography (PET) nor single photon emission tomography (SPECT) because of their high physical sensitivity, optical imaging methods (OT) as well as magnetic resonance imaging (MRI) have limitations: low penetration depth (OT) and inherent low physical sensitivity (MRI prevents straightforward imaging strategies for both latter modalities). PET and SPECT have been successfully used in the past for molecular imaging, employing imaging probes such as monoclonal antibodies, labeled peptides [i.e., somatostatine analogues (Octreotide)], and labeled proteins such as ^{99m}Tc-AnnexinV, etc. Specific imaging probes for OT and MR are under development. However, OT is likely to remain an experimental tool for investigations in small animals, and will be used in humans only for special indications, where close access to targets can be achieved by special imaging devices such as endoscopy or intraoperative probes. In recent years, molecular imaging with ultrasound devices has developed quickly and the visualization of targeted microbubbles offers not only identification of specific binding but also the regional delivery of therapeutics after local destruction of the bubbles by ultrasound.

Achieving disease-specific imaging requires passive, or better yet, active accumulation of specific molecules to increase the concentration of the imaging agent in the region of interest. Marker substrates as well as reporter agents can be used to visualize enzyme activity, receptor or transporter expression. The introduction of new imaging agents requires a multistep approach, involving the target selection, synthetic chemistry and preclinical testing, before clinical translation can be considered. Target identification is supported by molecular tissue analysis or by screening methods, such as phage display. Subsequently, further development requires methods to synthesize macromolecules, minibodies, nanoparticles, peptide conjugates and other conjugates, employing innovative biotechnology tools for specific imaging with high accumulation in the target area. This process involves optimization of the target affinity and pharmacokinetics before in-vivo application can be considered. Amplification of the imaging signal can be enhanced by targeted processes which involve internalization of receptors, transport mechanisms or enzymatic interaction with build-up of labeled products. (i.e., phosphorylated deoxyglucose). Reporter gene imaging provides not only high biological contrast if a protein, which does not occur naturally, is expressed after gene transfer but also leads to signal amplification if tissue-specific promoters in combination with enzymatic or transporter activity are used.

The development process usually produces numerous candidates, of which only a few pass preclinical evaluation with the promise of clinical utility. The most suitable substances have to undergo in-depth toxicological evaluation before the regulatory process for clinical use can be started. Currently, this is the major rate-limiting step in the process and requires not only the biological qualification of the compound but also the necessary financial support for the clinical testing required by the regulatory agencies.

With the increasing interest in the experimental and clinical application of molecular imaging, many institutions have created research groups or interdisciplinary centers focusing on the complex development processes of this new methodology. The aim for this textbook of molecular imaging is to provide an up-to-date review of this rapidly growing field and to discuss basic methodological aspects necessary for the interpretation of experimental and clinical results. Emphasis is placed on the interplay of imaging technology and probe development, since the physical properties of the imaging approach need to be closely linked with the biological application of the probe (i.e., nanoparticles and microbubbles). Various chemical strategies are discussed and related to the biological applications. Reporter-gene imaging is being addressed not only in experimental protocols but also first clinical applications are discussed. Finally, strategies of imaging to characterize apoptosis and angiogenesis are described and discussed in the context of possible clinical translation.

The editors thank all the authors for their contributions. We appreciate the extra effort preparing a book chapter during the already busy academic life. We hope this methodological discussion will increase the understanding of the reader with respect to established methods and generate new ideas for further improvement and for the design of new research protocols employing imaging. There is no question that this young field will further expand, stimulated by the rapid growth of biological knowledge and biomedical technologies. It is expected that the experimental work of today will become the clinical routine of tomorrow.

Heidelberg, Germany   *Wolfhard Semmler*
Munich, Germany   *Markus Schwaiger*

Contents

Contents of Companion Volume 185/I

Contributors

Francis Blankenberg
Lucile Salter Packard Children's Hospital, 725 Welch Road, Room 1673 Clinic F, Pediatric Radiology, Stanford, CA 94304, USA

Ronald Blasberg
Departments of Neurology and Radiology, Memorial Sloan-Kettering Cancer Center, 1275 York Avenue, New York, NY 10021, USA, blasberg@neuro1.mskcc.org

Alexei Bogdanov Jr
UMASS Medical School, S2-808 Department of Radiology, 55 Lake Av, No Worcester, MA 01655, USA, alexei.bogdanov@umassmed.edu

Christoph Bremer
Department of Clinical Radiology, University of Muenster, University Hospital, Münster, Germany;
Interdisciplinary Center for Clinical Research (IZKF Muenster, FG3), University of Muenster, Albert-Schweitzer-Str. 33, D-48129 Münster, Germany, bremerc@uni-muenster.de

Roel Deckers
Laboratory for Molecular and Functional Imaging: From Physiology to Therapy, ERT CNRS, Université "Victor Segalen" Bordeaux 2, Bordeaux, France

Susan L. Deutscher
Department of Biochemistry, M743 Medical Sciences Bldg., University of Missouri, Columbia, MO 65212, USA;
Harry S Truman Memorial Veterans Administration Hospital, Research Service, 800 Hospital Dr., Columbia, MO 65201-5297, USA, deutschers@missouri.edu

I. Dijkgraaf
Department of Nuclear Medicine, Technische Universität München, Ismaninger Strasse 22, 81675 München, Germany

Michael Eisenhut
Deutsches Krebsforschungszentrum, Abteilung Radiopharmazeutische Chemie, Im
Neuenheimer Feld 280, 69120 Heidelberg, Germany, m.eisenhut@dkfz.de

Sanjiv S. Gambhir
Molecular Imaging Program at Stanford, The James H Clark Center, 318
Campus Drive, East Wing, 1st Floor, Stanford, CA 94305-5427, USA,
sgambhir@stanford.edu

Regine Garcia Boy
Universitätsklinikum Heidelberg, Abteilung für Nuklearmedizin, Im Neuenheimer
Feld 400, 69120 Heidelberg, Germany, r.garcia@med.uni-heidelberg.de

Axel Haase
Physikalisches Institut, Universität Würzburg, 97074 Würzburg, Germany;
MRB Research Center of Magnetic Resonance Bavaria, 97074 Würzburg, Germany

Uwe Haberkorn
Department of Nuclear Medicine, University of Heidelberg, Im Neuenheimer Feld
400, 69120 Heidelberg, Germany, uwe_haberkorn@med.uni-heidelberg.de

Aviv Hagooly
Mallinckrodt Institute of Radiology, Washington University School of Medicine,
510 S. Kingshighway Blvd. Campus Box 8225, St. Louis, MO 63110, USA,
hagoolya@mir.wustl.edu

Roland Haubner
Universitätsklinik für Nuklearmedizin, Medizinische Universität Innsbruck,
Anichstrasse 35, A-6020 Innsbruck, Austria, roland.haubner@uibk.ac.at

Karl-Heinz Hiller
Physikalisches Institut, Universität Würzburg, 97074 Würzburg, Germany;
MRB Research Center of Magnetic Resonance Bavaria, 97074 Würzburg,
Germany, hiller@mr-bavaria.de

Ruimin Huang
Departments of Neurology and Radiology, Memorial Sloan-Kettering Cancer
Center, 1275 York Avenue, New York, NY 10021, USA

Andreas H. Jacobs
Laboratory for Gene Therapy and Molecular Imaging at the Max-Planck Institute
for Neurological Research with Klaus-Joachim-Zülch-Laboratories of the Max
Planck Society and the Faculty of Medicine of the University of Cologne, Center
for Molecular Medicine (CMMC), Departments of Neurology at the University of
Cologne and Klinikum Fulda, Germany, andreas.jacobs@nf.mpg.de

Peter M. Jakob
Physikalisches Institut, Universität Würzburg, 97074 Würzburg, Germany;
MRB Research Center of Magnetic Resonance Bavaria, 97074 Würzburg,
Germany, Peter.Jakob@physik.uni-wuerzburg.de

Fabian Kiessling
Abteilung Medizinische Physik in der Radiologie, Deutsches Krebs-forschungszentrum, Im Neuenheimer Feld 280, 69120 Heidelberg, Germany, f.kiessling@dkfz.de

Lutz W. Kracht
Laboratory for Gene Therapy and Molecular Imaging at the Max-Planck Institute for Neurological Research with Klaus-Joachim-Zülch-Laboratories of the Max Planck Society and the Faculty of Medicine of the University of Cologne, Center for Molecular Medicine (CMMC), Departments of Neurology at the University of Cologne and Klinikum Fulda, Germany

Phillipp Mayer-Kukuck
Departments of Neurology and Radiology, Memorial Sloan-Kettering Cancer Center, 1275 York Avenue, New York, NY 10021, USA

Walter Mier
Universitätsklinikum Heidelberg, Abteilung für Nuklearmedizin, Im Neuenheimer Feld 400, 69120 Heidelberg, Germany, w.mier@med.uni-heidelberg.de

Jung-Joon Min
Department of Nuclear Medicine, Chonnam National University Medical School, 160 Ilsimri, Hwasun, Jeonnam 519-809, Republic of Korea, jjmin@jnu.ac.kr

Chrit T.W. Moonen
Laboratory for Molecular and Functional Imaging: From Physiology to Therapy, ERT CNRS, Université "Victor Segalen" Bordeaux 2, Bordeaux, France, chrit.moonen@imf.u-bordeaux2.fr

Jessica Newton
Department of Biochemistry, M743 Medical Sciences Bldg., University of Missouri, Columbia, MO 65212, USA

Manuel Querol
UMASS Medical School, S2-808 Department of Radiology, 55 Lake Av, No Worcester, MA 01655, USA, manuel.querolsans@umassmed.edu

Claire Rome
Laboratory for Molecular and Functional Imaging: From Physiology to Therapy, ERT CNRS, Université "Victor Segalen" Bordeaux 2, Bordeaux, France

Raffaella Rossin
Mallinckrodt Institute of Radiology, Washington University School of Medicine, 510 S. Kingshighway Blvd. Campus Box 8225, St. Louis, MO 63110, USA, rossinr@mir.wustl.edu

Maria A. Rueger
Laboratory for Gene Therapy and Molecular Imaging at the Max-Planck Institute for Neurological Research with Klaus-Joachim-Zülch-Laboratories of the Max Planck Society and the Faculty of Medicine of the University of Cologne, Center for Molecular Medicine (CMMC), Departments of Neurology at the University of Cologne and Klinikum Fulda, Germany

Inna Serganova
Departments of Neurology and Radiology, Memorial Sloan-Kettering Cancer
Center, 1275 York Avenue, New York, NY 10021, USA

H. William Strauss
Memorial Sloan Kettering Hospital, 1275 York Ave., Room S-212, Nuclear
Medicine, New York, NY 10021, USA, straussh@mskcc.org

Jonathan Tait
Laboratory Medicine, Room NW-120, University of Washington Medical Center,
Seattle, WA 98195-7110, USA

Anne V. Thomas
Laboratory for Gene Therapy and Molecular Imaging at the Max-Planck Institute
for Neurological Research with Klaus-Joachim-Zülch-Laboratories of the Max
Planck Society and the Faculty of Medicine of the University of Cologne, Center
for Molecular Medicine (CMMC), Departments of Neurology at the University of
Cologne and Klinikum Fulda, Germany

Jean-Luc Vanderheyden
Technology and Medical Office, GE Healthcare, 3000 N. Grandview Blvd. W-427,
Waukesha, WI 53188, USA

Christiane Waller
Medizinische Klinik und Poliklinik I/Herzkreislaufzentrum, 97080 Würzburg,
Germany

Michael J. Welch
Mallinckrodt Institute of Radiology, Washington University School of Medicine,
510 S. Kingshighway Blvd. Campus Box 8225, St. Louis, MO 63110, USA,
welchm@wustl.edu

H.J. Wester
Department of Nuclear Medicine, Technische Universität München, Ismaninger
Strasse 22, 81675 München, Germany, h.j.wester@lrz.tum.de

Alexandra Winkeler
Laboratory for Gene Therapy and Molecular Imaging at the Max-Planck Institute
for Neurological Research with Klaus-Joachim-Zülch-Laboratories of the Max
Planck Society and the Faculty of Medicine of the University of Cologne, Center
for Molecular Medicine (CMMC), Departments of Neurology at the University of
Cologne and Klinikum Fulda, Germany

Glossary

Definition of the terms used in molecular imaging.

Allele The gene regarded as the carrier of either of a pair of alternative hereditary characters.

$\alpha_v\beta_3$ An integrin expressed by activated endothelial cells or tumor cells which plays an important role in angiogenesis and metastatic tumor spread ($\Rightarrow$ Integrins)

Amino acid An organic compound containing an amino and carboxyl group. Amino acids form the basis of protein synthesis.

Angiogenesis Formation of new blood vessels. May be triggered by physiological conditions, like during embryogenesis or certain pathological conditions, such as cancer, where the continuing growth of solid tumors requires nourishment from new blood vessels.

Annexin V A protein in blood which binds to phosphatidyl serine (PS) binding sites exposed on the cell surface by cells undergoing programmed cell death. $\Rightarrow$ Apoptosis.

Antibody A protein with a particular type of structure that binds to antigens in a target-specific manner.

Antigen Any substance which differs from substances normally present in the body, and can induce an immune response.

Antiangiogenesis The inhibition of new blood vessel growth and/or destruction of preformed blood vessels.

Antisense A strategy to block the synthesis of certain proteins by interacting with their messenger RNA (mRNA). A gene whose messenger RNA (mRNA) is complementary to the RNA of the target protein is inserted in the cell genome. The protein synthesis is blocked by interaction of the antisense mRNA and the protein-encoding RNA.

Apoptosis Programmed cell death. A process programmed into all cells as part of the normal life cycle of the cell. It allows the body to dispose of damaged, unwanted or superfluous cells.

Aptamer RNA or DNA-based ligand.

Asialoglycoproteins Endogenous glycoproteins from which sialic acid has been removed by the action of sialidases. They bind tightly to their cell surface receptor, which is located on hepatocyte plasma membranes. After internalization by adsorptive endocytosis, they are delivered to lysosomes for degradation.

Attenuation correction (AC) Methodology which corrects images for the differential absorption of photons in tissues with different densities.

Avidin A biotin-binding protein (68 kDa) obtained from egg white. Binding is so strong as to be effectively irreversible.

Bioinformatics The science of managing and analyzing biological data using advanced computing techniques. Especially important in analyzing genomic research data.

Biotechnology A set of biological techniques developed through basic research and now applied to research and product development. In particular, biotechnology refers to the industrial use of recombinant DNA, cell fusion, and new bioprocessing techniques.

Biotin A prosthetic group for carboxylase enzyme. Important in fatty acid biosynthesis and catabolism, biotin has found widespread use as a covalent label for macromolecules, which may then be detected by high-affinity binding of labeled avidin or streptavidin. Biotin is an essential growth factor for many cells.

Cancer Diseases in which abnormal cells divide and grow unchecked. Cancer can spread from its original site to other parts of the body and is often fatal.

Carrier An individual who carries the abnormal gene for a specific condition but has no symptoms.

Cavitation The sudden formation and collapse of low-pressure bubbles in liquids as a result of mechanical forces.

cDNA ⇒ Complementary DNA.

Cell The basic structural unit of all living organisms and the smallest structural unit of living tissue capable of functioning as an independent entity. It is surrounded by a membrane and contains a nucleus which carries genetic material.

Chromosome A rod-like structure present in the nucleus of all body cells (with the exception of the red blood cells) which stores genetic information. Normally, humans have 23 pairs, giving a total of 46 chromosomes.

Coincidence detection A process used to detect emissions from positron-emitting radioisotopes. The technology utilizes opposing detectors that simultaneously detect two 511 keV photons which are emitted at an angle of 180 degrees from one another as a result of the annihilation of the positron when it combines with an electron.

Complementary DNA (cDNA) DNA synthesized in the laboratory from a messenger RNA template by the action of RNA-dependent DNA polymerase.

Cytogenetics The study of the structure and physical appearance of chromosome material. It includes routine analysis of G-banded chromosomes, other cytogenetic banding techniques, as well as molecular cytogenetics such as fluorescent in situ hybridization (FISH) and comparative genomic hybridization (CGH).

Deoxyglucose $\Rightarrow$ 18 F-deoxyglucose.

DNA Deoxyribonucleic acid: the molecule or 'building block' that encodes genetic information.

DNA repair genes Genes encoding proteins that correct errors in DNA sequencing.

Enzyme A protein that acts as a catalyst to speed the rate at which a biochemical reaction proceeds.

Epistasis A gene that interferes with or prevents the expression of another gene located at a different locus.

Epitope The specific binding site for an antibody.

Expression $\Rightarrow$ Gene expression.

^{18}**F-deoxyglucose** The predominant PET imaging agent used in oncology. The deoxyglucose is 'trapped' in cells which have increased metabolic activity as a result of phosphorylation. The process results in an accumulation of fluorine-18 (^{18}F) in the cells, allowing the location of the cells and intensity of tumor metabolism to be determined using PET imaging.

Fluorine-18 (^{18}F) A positron-emitting radioisotope used to label deoxyglucose or other molecular probes for use as radiopharmaceuticals.

F(ab) fragment The shape of an antibody resembles the letter 'Y'. Antigen binding properties are on both short arms. Digestion by various enzymes yields different fragments. Fragments with one binding site are called F(ab).

F(ab')$_2$ fragment Antibody fragment with two binding sites ($\Rightarrow$ also F(ab) fragment).

Fc fragment (Crystallizable) antibody fragment which has no binding properties ($\Rightarrow$ also F(ab) fragment). The Fc fragment is used by the body's immune system to clear the antibody from the circulation.

Fibrin Fibrous protein that forms the meshwork necessary for forming of blood clots.

Fibroblast growth factor Acidic fibroblast growth factor (alpha-FGF, HBGF 1) and basic FGF (beta-FGF, HBGF-2) are the two founder members of a family of structurally related growth factors for mesodermal or neuroectodermal cells.

Fingerprinting In genetics, the identification of multiple specific alleles on a person's DNA to produce a unique identifier for that person.

Gadolinium A paramagnetic ion which changes the relaxivity of adjacent protons. It affects signal intensity in MR images ($\Rightarrow$ garamagnetism).

Ganciclovir An antiviral agent which is phosphorylated by thymidine kinase. As a phosphorylated substance it stops cell division by inhibiting DNA synthesis.

Gene The fundamental physical and functional unit of heredity. A gene is an ordered sequence of nucleotides located in a particular position on a particular chromosome that encodes a specific functional product (i.e., a protein or RNA molecule). The totality of genes present in an organism determines its characteristics.

Gene expression The process by which a gene's coded information is converted into the structures present and operating in the cell. Expressed genes include those that are transcribed into mRNAs and then translated into proteins, and those that are transcribed into RNAs but not translated into proteins (e.g., transfer and ribosomal RNAs).

Gene mapping Determination of the relative positions of genes on a DNA molecule (chromosome or plasmid) and of the distance, in linkage units or physical units, between them.

Gene prediction Predictions of possible genes made by a computer program based on how well a stretch of DNA sequence matches known gene sequences.

Gene sequence (full) The complete order of bases in a gene. This order determines which protein a gene will produce.

Gene, suicide $\Rightarrow$ Suicide gene.

Gene therapy An experimental procedure aimed at replacing, manipulating, or supplementing nonfunctional or misfunctioning genes with therapeutic genes.

Genetic code The sequence of nucleotides, coded in triplets (codons) along the mRNA, that determines the sequence of amino acids in protein synthesis. A gene's DNA sequence can be used to predict the mRNA sequence, and the genetic code can, in turn, be used to predict the amino acid sequence.

Genetic marker A gene or other identifiable portion of DNA whose inheritance can be followed.

Genetic susceptibility Susceptibility to a genetic disease. May or may not result in actual development of the disease.

Genome All the genetic material in the chromosomes of a particular organism; its size is generally given as its total number of base pairs.

Genomics The science aimed at sequencing and mapping the genetic code of a given organism.

Genotype The genetic constitution of an organism, as distinguished from its physical appearance (its phenotype).

ICAM Intercellular adhesion molecules: glycoproteins that are present on a wide range of human cells, essential to the mechanism by which cells recognize each other, and thus important in inflammatory responses.

Indium-111 (^{111}In) A single-photon-emitting radioisotope used to label various molecular probes for SPECT imaging.

Integrins A specific group of transmembrane proteins that act as receptor proteins. Different integrins consist of different numbers of alpha and beta subunits. Over 20 different integrin receptors are known.

Lectin Sugar-binding proteins which are highly specific for their sugar moieties. They bind to glycoproteins on the cell surface or to soluble gylcoproteins and play a role in biological recognition phenomena involving cells and proteins, e.g., during the immune response.

Liposome A spherical particle in an aqueous medium, formed by a lipid bilayer enclosing an aqueous compartment.

Locus The relative position of a gene on a chromosome.

Lysosome A minute intracellular body involved in intracellular digestion.

Messenger RNA (mRNA) RNA that serves as a template for protein synthesis.

Microarray Sets of miniaturized chemical reaction areas that may also be used to test DNA fragments, antibodies, or proteins.

Micronuclei Chromosome fragments that are not incorporated into the nucleus at cell division.

MID Molecular imaging and diagnostics.

Molecular biology The study of the structure, function, and makeup of biologically important molecules.

Molecular genetics The study of macromolecules important in biological inheritance.

Molecular medicine The treatment of injury or disease at the molecular level. Examples include the use of DNA-based diagnostic tests or medicine derived from a DNA sequence. It includes molecular diagnostics, molecular imaging and molecular therapy.

Monoclonal antibodies Antibodies made in cell cultures; these antibodies are all identical.

Monosaccharide A simple sugar that cannot be decomposed by hydrolysis.

Nucleic acid A nucleotide polymer. There are two types: DNA and RNA.

Nucleotide A subunit of DNA or RNA consisting of a nitrogenous molecule, a phosphate molecule, and a sugar molecule. Thousands of nucleotides are linked to form a DNA or RNA molecule.

Oligonucleotides Polymers made up of a few (2-20) nucleotides. In molecular genetics, they refer to a short sequence synthesized to match a region where a mutation is known to occur, and then used as a probe (oligonucleotide probes).

Operon Combination of a set of structural genes and the DNA sequences which control the expression of these genes.

Oncogene A gene, one or more forms of which is associated with cancer. Many oncogenes are directly or indirectly involved in controlling the rate of cell growth.

Paramagnetism Magnetism which occurs in paramagnetic material (e.g. $\Rightarrow$ gadolinium), but only in the presence of an externally applied magnetic field. Even in the presence of the field there is only a small induced magnetization because only a small fraction of the spins will be orientated by the field. This fraction is proportional to the field strength. The attraction experienced by ferromagnets is nonlinear and much stronger.

Peptide A short chain of amino acids. Most peptides act as chemical messengers, i.e., they bind to specific receptors.

Peptidomimetics Engineered compounds that have similar binding characteristics to those of naturally occurring proteins. The advantages are increased stability and prolonged presence in the bloodstream.

Perfluorocarbon A compound containing carbon and fluorine only.

PESDA Perfluorocarbon exposed sonicated dextrose albumin microbubbles.

PET Positron emission tomography. An imaging modality which utilizes opposing sets of detectors to record simultaneous emissions from a positron-emitting radioisotope throughout $360°$. The image data are processed using reconstruction algorithms to create tomographic image sets of the distribution of the radioisotope in the patient.

PET/CT A combination technology which creates tomographic image sets of the metabolic activity from PET and the anatomical tomographic image sets from CT. CT $\Rightarrow$ computed tomography: An imaging modality employing a rotating x-ray tube and a detector as well producing numbers of projection imagings during its rotation around the object of interest. Specific reconstruction algorithms are used to generate three-dimensional image of the inside of an object. The two images sets are fused to form a single image, which is used to assign the PET abnormalities to specific anatomical locations.

Phage A virus for which the natural host is a bacterial cell.

Phagocytosis Endocytosis of particulate material, such as microorganisms or cell fragments. The material is taken into the cell in membrane-bound vesicles (phagosomes) that originate as pinched-off invaginations of the plasma membrane. Phagosomes fuse with lysosomes, forming phagolysosomes, in which the engulfed material is killed and digested.

Pharmacodynamics The study of what a drug does to the body and of its mode of action.

Pharmacogenomics The influence of genetic variations on drug response in patients. This is performed by correlating gene expression or single-nucleotide polymorphisms with a drug's efficacy or toxicity during therapy.

Pharmacokinetics The determination of the fate of substances administered externally to a living organism, e.g., the metabolism and half-life of drugs.

Phenotype The physical characteristics of an organism or the presence of a disease that may or may not be genetic.

Phosphorylation A metabolic process in which a phosphate group is introduced into an organic molecule.

Plasmid Autonomously replicating extrachromosomal circular DNA molecules.

Polymerase An enzyme that catalyzes polymerization, especially of nucleotides.

Polysaccharides Any of a class of carbohydrates, such as starch and cellulose, consisting of a number of monosaccharides joined by glycosidic bonds. Polysaccharides can be decomposed into the component monosaccharides by hydrolysis.

Polypeptide A peptide containing more than two amino acids.

Probe Single-stranded DNA or RNA molecules of specific base sequence, labeled either radioactively or immunologically, that are used to detect the complementary base sequence by hybridization.

Promoter A specific DNA sequence to which RNA polymerase binds in order to 'transcribe' the adjacent DNA sequence and produce an RNA copy. The action of RNA polymerase is the first step in the translation of genes, via mRNA, into proteins.

Protein A large molecule comprising one or more chains of amino acids in a specific order that is determined by the base sequence of nucleotides in the gene that codes for the protein. Proteins are required for the structure, function, and regulation of the body's cells, tissues, and organs. Each protein has unique functions. Examples are hormones, enzymes, and antibodies.

Proteomics The global analysis of gene expression in order to identify, quantify, and characterize proteins.

Receptor A molecular structure within a cell or on the cell surface that selectively binds a specific substance having a specific physiological effect.

Rhenium-188 (^{188}Re) A beta-emitting radioisotope used to label various molecular probes for targeted radiotherapy applications.

Reporter gene imaging Imaging of genetic or enzymatic products/events initiated by molecular therapies which have assigned specific reporter genes to express specific targets.

Ribosomal RNA (rRNA) A class of RNA found in the ribosomes of cells.

RNA Ribonucleic acid: a chemical found in the nucleus and cytoplasm of cells; it plays an important role in protein synthesis and other chemical activities of the cell. The structure of RNA is similar to that of DNA. There are several classes of RNA molecules, including messenger RNA, transfer RNA, ribosomal RNA, and other small RNAs, each serving a different purpose.

Selectins A family of cell adhesion molecules consisting of a lectin-like domain, an epidermal growth factor-like domain, and a variable number of domains that encode proteins homologous to complement-binding proteins. Selectins mediate the binding of leukocytes to the vascular endothelium.

Sequencing Determination of the order of nucleotides (base sequences) in a DNA or RNA molecule or the order of amino acids in a protein.

Sonothrombolysis Dissolving a thrombus using ultrasound, either alone or in conjunction with microbubbles.

SPECT Single photon emission computerized tomography: an imaging modality in which a detector is rotated about the patient, recording photon emissions throughout 360°. Reconstruction algorithms are used to convert the data into a set of tomographic images.

Stem cell Undifferentiated, primitive cells in the bone marrow that have the ability both to multiply and to differentiate into specific cells for the formation of specific tissues (hematopoetic, mesenchymal and neuronal stem cells).

Streptavidin A biotin-binding protein obtained from bacteria.

Structural genomics The study to determine the 3D structures of large numbers of proteins using both experimental techniques and computer simulation.

Suicide gene A protein-coding sequence that produces an enzyme capable of converting a nontoxic compound to a cytotoxic compound, used in cancer therapy.

Technetium-99m (^{99m}Tc) A single-photon-emitting radioisotope used to label various molecular probes for scintigraphic imaging, including SPECT imaging.

Theragnostics The application of MID for therapy guidance using genomic, proteomic and metabolomic data for predicting and assessing drug response.

Thymidine kinase (tk) The gene coding for the tk from the herpes simplex virus (HSV-tk) can be used as a 'suicide gene' or a reporter gene ($\Rightarrow$ Reporter gene imaging) in cancer therapy. $\Rightarrow$ also Ganciclovir.

Tissue factor An integral membrane glycoprotein of around 250 residues that initiates blood clotting after binding factors VII or VIIa.

Tracer principle The use of molecular probes labelled with radioisotopes to allow for nuclear imaging devices to detect the presence and location of the targeted structures by specific binding (e.g., to receptors, proteins,...) or trapping in cells.

Transfection The introduction of DNA into a recipient cell and its subsequent integration into the recipient cell's chromosomal DNA.

Transfer RNA Small RNA molecules with a function in translation. They carry specific amino acids to specified sites.

Transgene A gene transferred from one organism to another.

Translation The process by which polypeptide chains are synthesized, forming the structural elements of proteins.

Translational research Applying results obtained by basic research to answer scientific questions concerning human disease processes.

USPIO Ultrasmall particles of iron oxide. These particles have a high magnetic moment causing strong local susceptibility and field inhomogeneities, with strong effects in T2- and T2*-weighted MR imaging.

VEGF Vascular endothelial growth factor. VEGF is a protein secreted by a variety of tissues, when stimulated by triggers like hypoxia. VEGF stimulates endothelial cell growth, angiogenesis, and capillary permeability.

Virus A noncellular biological entity that can only reproduce within a host cell. Viruses consist of nucleic acid (DNA or RNA) covered by protein; some animal viruses are also surrounded by membrane. Inside the infected cell, the virus uses the synthetic capability of the host to produce progeny viruses.

Part III
Amplification Strategies

Optical Methods

Christoph Bremer

Abstract Molecular imaging requires the highest possible signal-to-noise ratios (SNRs) at the target of interest. In order to maximize the SNR for optical imaging techniques, various strategies have been developed to design fluorescent probes that can be activated, for example, by proteolytic degradation. Generally speaking, these probes are quenched in their native state—e.g., by fluorescence resonance energy transfer (FRET)—and dequenched after cleavage or hybridization, which is associated with a strong fluorescence signal increase.

Different strategies of fluorescence signal amplification ranging from large and small protease-sensing molecules to oligonucleotide-sensing and nanoparticle-based probes are presented in this chapter.

1 Introduction

Molecular imaging techniques require maximal signal-to-noise yields in order to noninvasively resolve specific molecular targets in vivo. Different, mainly enzyme-based signal amplification strategies have been described, which aim at

Christoph Bremer

Department of Clinical Radiology, University of Münster, University Hospital Münster, Germany

Interdisciplinary Center for Clinical Research (IZKF Münster, FG3), University of Münster, Albert-Schweitzer-Str. 33, 48129 Münster, Germany
bremerc@uni-muenster.de

W. Semmler and M. Schwaiger (eds.), *Molecular Imaging II.*
Handbook of Experimental Pharmacology 185/II.
© Springer-Verlag Berlin Heidelberg 2008

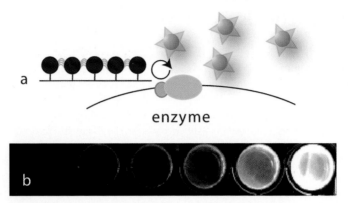

Fig. 1 a, b First generation of large protease sensing probes. The first class of proteolytically activatable optical probes is depicted. These probes consist of a poly-L-lysine backbone shielded by multiple methoxy-polyethylene glycol sidechains. Approximately 12–14 fluorochromes are attached to the backbone, resulting in a FRET-based signal quench in the native state of the molecule. Proteolytic cleavage of the backbone results in **a** a release of the fluorochromes, followed by **b** a strong fluorescence signal increase. (Modified from Bremer et al. 2003)

(1) maximizing the fluorescence signal yield after target interaction and (2) reducing the unspecific background signal of circulating probes. In recent years, various activatable or 'smart' probes have been developed for molecular imaging. Typically, they show a strong fluorescence signal increase after interaction with an enzyme (e.g., a protease). The underlying principle is that the native probe is 'quenched', a phenomenon which has been known for a long time; e.g., in fluorescence microscopy. Enzymatic conversion results in dequenching of the probe accompanied by a strong increase in the fluorescence signal (Fig. 1). Quenching can result from the transfer of energy to other acceptor molecules residing physically close to the excited fluorochromes (e.g., a second acceptor fluorochrome), a phenomenon known as fluorescence resonance energy transfer (FRET). Quenching can, moreover, occur by competing processes such as temperature, high oxygen concentrations, molecular aggregation in the presence of salts and halogen compounds or interaction with metals.

2 Large Protease-sensing Probes

For molecular imaging applications, activatable probes ideally undergo a status of virtually zero signal in their native state to a strong fluorescence signal after target interaction. A class of 'smart' optical contrast agents, which undergoes conformational changes after cleavage by various enzymes, was first described by Weissleder et al. (1999) (Fig. 1). The first autoquenched fluorescent probe was developed in 1999. This was converted from a non-fluorescence to fluorescence state by proteolytic activation (Weissleder et al. 1999). This type of molecular contrast agent consists of a long circulating carrier molecule (poly-lysine backbone) shielded by multiple methoxy-polythylene-glycol side chains (PLL-MPEG). The molecular weight of these probes ranges around 450–500 kDa. Between 12 and 14 cyanine dyes (Cy 5.5) are loaded onto this carrier molecule in close proximity to each other, resulting in a FRET-based signal quench (see above; Weissleder et al. 1999). Thus, in its native state, the molecule exhibits very little to no fluorescence, whereas after enzymatic cleavage a strong fluorescence signal increase can be detected (dequenching; Fig. 1). Inhibition experiments revealed that this first generation of protease-sensing optical probe is activated mainly by lysosomal cysteine or serine proteases, such as cathepsin-B (Weissleder et al. 1999). However, the selectivity of this smart optical probe can be tailored to other enzymes by insertion of specific peptide stalks between the carrier and the fluorochromes. Using this approach, smart optical probes have been developed for targeting—e.g., matrix-metalloproteinase-2, cathepsin-D, thrombin or caspases (Tung et al. 2000, 2004; Bremer et al. 2002; Jaffer et al. 2004; Messerli et al. 2004; Kim et al. 2005). In order to impart MMP-2 selectivity, for example, a peptide stalk with the sequence -Gly-Pro-Leu-Gly-Val-Arg-Gly-Lys- was inserted between the backbone and the fluorochrome. This peptide sequence is recognized by MMP-2 with a high affinity, resulting in an efficient dequenching of the completely assembled MMP-2 probe by the purified enzyme (Fig. 2). A control probe, which was synthesized using a scrambled peptide sequence (-Gly-Val-Arg-Leu-Gly-Pro-Gly-Lys-), remained quenched after incubation with the purified enzyme (Fig. 2).

Proteases are known to be key players in a whole variety of pathologies, ranging from carcinogenesis to inflammatory and cardiovascular diseases (Edwards and Murphy 1998). From the oncological literature it is known that various proteases, such as cathepsins and matrix-metalloproteinases, are involved in a cascade of enzymes, which finally leads to digestion of the extracellular matrix and, thus, local as well as metastatic tumor cell infiltration (Edwards and Murphy 1998; Aparicio et al. 1999; Folkman 1999; Herszenyi et al. 1999; Fang et al. 2000; Koblinski et al. 2000). Indeed, clinical data suggest that the tumoral protease burden correlates with clinical outcome. Thus, the activatable probes outlined above have been applied for a variety of different oncological models, including xenograft and spontaneous tumor models (Figs. 2, 3). A cathepsin-sensing probe could be applied successfully to detect micronodules of tumor xenografts and spontaneous tumors using fluorescence reflectance imaging (FRI) or fluorescence-mediated tomography (FMT). The response to protease inhibitor treatment could be monitored early and noninvasively using a MMP sensitive probe (Bremer et al. 2005). Other experimental data suggest that a noninvasive tumor grading (aggressive versus nonaggressive phenotype) may be facilitated using these probes (Bremer et al. 2002).

Since proteases are ubiquitously expressed, the aforementioned probes could also be successfully applied for imaging of inflammatory responses; e.g., in an experimental arthritis model. Interestingly, treatment effects (e.g., methotrexate application) could be monitored sensitively using this approach (Wunder et al. 2004; Fig. 4). Successful treatment of arthritis resulted in a clear reduction of the joint associated fluorescence (Wunder et al. 2004). In a cardiovascular plaque model

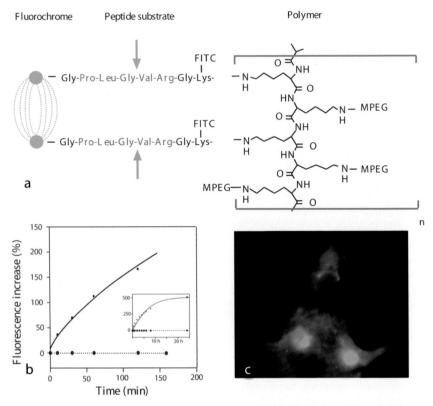

Fig. 2 a-c Second generation of large protease sensing probes: MMP imaging. A modification of the first generation of 'smart' optical probes is shown. **a** In order to impart specificity of the probe for matrix metalloproteinases, the fluorochromes were conjugated to the backbone through peptide stalks, which are cleaved with a high affinity by MMP-2. **b** Incubation with the purified enzymes showed a strong fluorescence signal increase for the MMP probe, while the probe containing a scrambled peptide sequence remained quenched. **c** Tumor xenografts overexpressing MMP-2 could clearly be visualized using this approach. (From Bremer et al. 2002)

(ApoE mice), strong probe activation within the atherosclerotic plaques most likely representing inflammatory plaque reactions could be successfully visualized using this approach (Chen et al. 2002).

3 Small Protease-sensing Probes

Smaller molecules that also undergo an enzymatic conversion have more recently been described. They can be designed by flanking an enzyme substrate with two fluorophores or a fluorophore and a spectrally matched quencher molecule, which absorbs the energy of the fluorochrome via FRET without the emission of photons (Fig. 5).

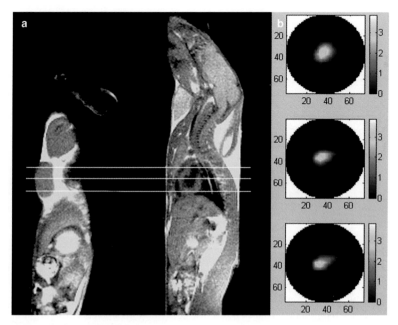

Fig. 3 a, b Application of a cathepsin-sensing probe for in vivo tumor detection. Fluorescence mediated tomography (FMT) of spontaneous mammary cancer after injection of a cathepsin sensing optical probe. **a** FMT images were acquired at the levels illustrated in the corresponding sagittal MR images. **b** After injection of the optical probe strong tissue fluorescence could be reconstructed in the tumor region as seen in the corresponding axial FMT slice. (From Bremer et al. 2005)

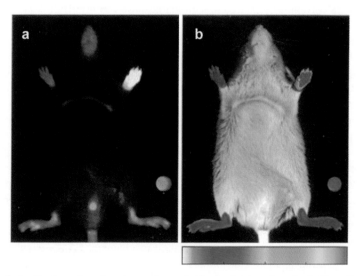

Fig. 4 a, b Application of a cathepsin-sensing probe for in vivo imaging of arthritis. **a** Raw NIRF image of a mouse with collagen-induced arthritis in the right for paw, obtained 24 h after probe injection. Note the high fluorescence intensity in the affected extremity. **b** Color-coded NIRF image of **a** superimposed on white-light image. Cy 5.5 dye (16 nmol/ml), seen above the right hind paw, was used for standardization. (Wunder et al. 2004)

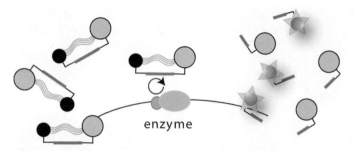

Fig. 5 Small protease-sensing probes. Small protease-sensing probes are designed by flanking an enzyme substrate (*red bar*) with two fluorophores or a fluorophore and a spectrally matched quencher molecule (*gray dot*), which absorbs the energy of the fluorochrome via FRET without the emission of photons. Enzymatic cleavage of the probes results in a significant dequenching effect, followed by a fluorescence signal increase

The coupling of a quencher to a fluorophore via a caspase-cleavable nonapeptide, for example, can be exploited to detect caspase activity (a marker of cellular apoptosis) in vitro (Pham et al. 2002). A similar design was proposed for imaging MMP activity using a different peptide bridge, which is cleaved with a high affinity by MMPs (Pham et al. 2004). Here an absorber molecule (NIRQ820) was linked to Cy 5.5 via a MMP-7 substrate. Incubation of the probe with the purified enzyme resulted in a sevenfold signal increase after dequenching, while MMP-9, for example, did not result in dequenching of the probe, which supports the selectivity of this system. Bullok and co-workers recently presented a small, membrane-permeable probe that is capable of sensing intracellular caspase activity (Bullok and Piwnica-Worms 2005). The molecule consists of a Tat-peptide-based permeation sequence and a caspase recognition sequence (DEVD) flanked by a fluorochrome (Alexa Fluor 647) and a quencher (QSY 21) (Bullok and Piwnica-Worms 2005). Efficient quenching was achieved in the native state of the molecule, while incubation with the effector caspases (especially caspases 3 and 7) resulted in a significant dequenching of the probe. Cell experiments demonstrated a successful permeation of the probe into the cell so that caspase activity could be visualized by a clear fluorescence signal (Bullok and Piwnica-Worms 2005).

Law et al. (2005) recently developed a small FRET-based probe that recognized protein kinase A (PKA). The probe consists of a specific binding peptide sequence (LRRRRFAFC) conjugated with two fluorophores (FAMS, TAMRA). In the absence of PKA, the two fluorophores associate by hydrophobic interactions, forming an intramolecular ground-state dimer; this results in fluorescein quenching (>93%). Upon PKA addition, the reporter reacts with the sulfhydryl functionality at Cys199 through a disulfide-exchange mechanism. FAMS is subsequently released, resulting in significant fluorescence amplification (Law et al. 2005). The remaining peptide sequence, which acts as an inhibitor, is attached covalently to the enzyme.

While the in vitro results of these small protease-sensing probes are promising, in vivo applications may be more difficult since rapid clearance of the probes may counteract sufficient probe accumulation at the target of interest.

4 Oligonucleotide-sensing Probes

A number of different oligonucleotide-based small, activatable optical probes have been described which were designed to monitor gene expression. As outlined in 4.1.2, these probes are quenched in their native state by either dimerization of fluorophores or by interaction with a specific quencher molecule. Tyagi et al. (2000) designed a probe that contains a harvester fluorophore that absorbs strongly in the wavelength range of the monochromatic light source, an emitter fluorophore of the desired emission color, and a nonfluorescent quencher (Fig. 6). In the absence of complementary nucleic acid targets, the probes are dark, whereas in the presence of targets, they fluoresce, though not in the emission range of the harvester fluorophore that absorbs the light, but rather in the emission range of the emitter fluorophore (Tyagi et al. 2000). This shift in emission spectrum is due to the transfer of the absorbed energy from the harvester fluorophore to the emitter fluorophore by fluorescence resonance energy transfer, and it only takes place in probes that are bound to targets (i.e., hybridized to the target oligonucleotides).

Metelev et al. (2004) proposed a similar molecule that consists of a hairpin oligonucleotide flanked by two cyanine dyes (e.g., Cy 5.5), which upon hybridization with the target oligonucleotide sequence (here: NF-κB) shows a strong de-quenching effect. These types of probes can be applied for in vitro gene analysis or, ultimately, potentially for in vivo genotyping. However, delivery barriers for in vivo applications are significant so that up to date true in vivo applications have not yet been described.

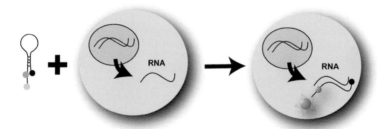

Fig. 6 Oligonucleotide-sensing probes. These consist of an oligonucleotide coupled to two fluorochromes or a harvester fluorochrome, an emitter fluorochrome and a nonfluorescent quencher. In the absence of complementary nucleic acid targets, the probes are dark, due to their hairpin configuration with approximation of the quencher (or the second fluorophor) to the fluorochrome (*left*). In the presence of targets, however, the probe unfolds and hybridizes with the oligonucleotide, resulting in spatial separation of the fluorochromes from the quencher/second fluorophor so that a fluorescent signal can be detected (*right*). (From Bremer et al. 2003)

5 Nanoparticle-based Probes

Fluorophores can interact with nanoparticles, such as superparamagnetic iron oxides, resulting in a signal quench of the probe (Fig. 7). Josephson et al. (2002) recently described a hydrid iron oxide-based nanoparticle that was conjugated with a fluorochrome (Cy 5.5). The surface of the nanoparticles was covered with aminated cross-linked dextran, which allowed covalent binding of Cy 5.5 via protease-sensitive (or protease-resistant) peptides. Interestingly, the authors found that even nanoparticles that were, on average, labeled with only 0.14 Cy 5.5/particle showed significant dequenching effects, suggesting that interaction between the iron oxide nanoparticle and the fluorochrome contributes to the quenching effect. Loading the nanoparticle with multiple fluorochromes (up to 1.19/particle) significantly increased the quenching/dequenching mechanism (Josephson et al. 2002). The quenching of fluorescence in proximity to the magnetic nanoparticle may be due to nonradiative energy transfer between the dye and the iron oxide or due to collisions between Cy 5.5 and the nanoparticle. Josephson et al. (2002) could successfully apply this probe for imaging lymph nodes in a mouse model by both MRI as well as near infrared fluorescence reflectance imaging (FRI). Modifications of this multivalent magneto-optical probe were presented by Schellenberger et al. (2004) who were able to attach Annexin V to the nanoparticle and therefore target apoptotic cells using these probes. A similar phenomenon was also described by Dubertret et al. (2001), who demonstrated that colloidal gold particles can efficiently quench fluorochromes.

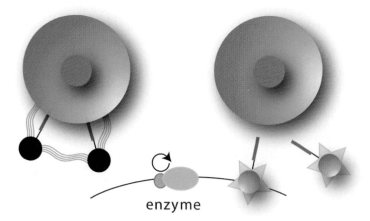

Fig. 7 Nanoparticle-based probes. Functionalized nanoparticles [e.g., aminated superparamagnetic iron oxides (SPIOs)] can be linked to fluorochromes via a peptide spacer. Quenching will occur based on interactions of the fluorochrome with the iron core and/or FRET-based quenching with neighboring fluorochromes. Enzymatic release of the fluorochromes results in a significant increase of the fluorescence signal. These multivalent probes can be applied for multimodal imaging; e.g., with MRI and optical techniques. In a clinical scenario, noninvasive MR-based probe localization could be combined with high-resolution, real-time fluorescence imaging of the probe; e.g., in an intraoperative setting

Multimodal probes may well have a clinical perspective since they may be applied, for example, preoperatively for noninvasive detection of the SPIO distribution by MRI and finally for intraoperative guidance using simple fluorescence reflectance imaging techniques (Kircher et al. 2003).

6 Other Amplification Mechanisms

In order to detect ß-galactosidase activity, Tung et al. (2004) employed a fluorogenic substrate that undergoes a significant wavelength shift after conversion by the enzyme. While the initial substrate (DDAOG) is excited at 465 nm and fluoresces at 608 nm, enzymatic cleavage by ß-galactosidase results in a release of another flourogenic substrate (DDAO), which is excited at 646 nm and fluoresces at 659 nm. Thus, the cleavage product has far-red fluorescence properties that can be imaged by FRI. Moreover, significantly, the wavelength shift (approximately 50 nm) allows detection of the cleaved substrate without background signal from the intact probe (Tung et al. 2004).

Another elegant way to amplify the optical signal in the target tissue was described by Jiang et al. (2004), who designed an imaging agent that consists of polyarginine-based cell-penetrating peptides (CPP), which are fused through a cleavable linker to an inhibitory domain consisting of negatively charged residues. Cleavage of the linker, typically by a protease, releases the CPP portion and its attached cargo (e.g., a fluorochrome) to bind and enter cells. In cell culture and in vivo, protease activities (e.g., MMP-2 and -9) were successfully visualized, showing in vivo contrast ratios of 2–3 and a 3.1-fold increase in standard uptake values for tumors relative to normal tissue or control peptides with scrambled linkers. Thus, these cell-permeating probes may be another suitable way of amplifying the fluorescence signal for molecular optical imaging.

References

Aparicio T, Kermorgant S, Dessirier V, Lewin MJ, Lehy T (1999) Matrix metalloproteinase inhibition prevents colon cancer peritoneal carcinomatosis development and prolongs survival in rats. Carcinogenesis 20:1445–1451

Bremer C, Ntziachristos V, Weissleder R (2003) Optical-based molecular imaging: contrast agents and potential medical applications. Eur Radiol 13:231–243

Bremer C, Ntziachristos V, Weitkamp B, Theilmeier G, Heindel W, Weissleder R (2005) Optical imaging of spontaneous breast tumors using protease sensing 'smart' optical probes. Invest Radiol 40:321–327

Bremer C, Tung CH, Bogdanov A Jr, Weissleder R (2002) Imaging of differential protease expression in breast cancers for detection of aggressive tumor phenotypes. Radiology 222:814–818

Bremer C, Tung CH, Weissleder R (2002) Molecular imaging of MMP expression and therapeutic MMP inhibition. Acad Radiol 9(Suppl 2):S314–S315

Bullok K, Piwnica-Worms D (2005) Synthesis and characterization of a small, membrane-permeant, caspase-activatable far-red fluorescent peptide for imaging apoptosis. J Med Chem 48:5404–5407

Chen J, Tung CH, Mahmood U, Ntziachristos V, Gyurko R, Fishman MC, Huang PL, Weissleder R (2002) In vivo imaging of proteolytic activity in atherosclerosis. Circulation 105:2766–2771

Dubertret B, Calame M, Libchaber AJ (2001) Single-mismatch detection using gold-quenched fluorescent oligonucleotides. Nat Biotechnol 19:365–370

Edwards DR, Murphy G (1998) Cancer. Proteases–invasion and more. Nature 394:527–528

Fang J, Shing Y, Wiederschain D, Yan L, Butterfield C, Jackson G, Harper J, Tamvakopoulos G, Moses MA (2000) Matrix metalloproteinase-2 is required for the switch to the angiogenic phenotype in a tumor model. Proc Natl Acad Sci USA 97:3884–3889

Folkman J (1999) Angiogenic zip code. Nat Biotechnol 17:749

Herszenyi L, Plebani M, Carraro P, De Paoli M, Roveroni G, Cardin R, Tulassay Z, Naccarato R, Farinati F (1999) The role of cysteine and serine proteases in colorectal carcinoma. Cancer 86:1135–1142

Jaffer FA, Tung CH, Wykrzykowska JJ, Ho NH, Houng AK, Reed GL, Weissleder R (2004) Molecular imaging of factor XIIIa activity in thrombosis using a novel, near-infrared fluorescent contrast agent that covalently links to thrombi. Circulation 110:170–176

Jiang T, Olson ES, Nguyen QT, Roy M, Jennings PA, Tsien RY (2004) Tumor imaging by means of proteolytic activation of cell-penetrating peptides. Proc Natl Acad Sci USA 101:17867–17872

Josephson L, Kircher MF, Mahmood U, Tang Y, Weissleder R (2002) Near-infrared fluorescent nanoparticles as combined MR/optical imaging probes. Bioconjug Chem 13:554–560

Kim DE, Schellingerhout D, Jaffer FA, Weissleder R, Tung CH (2005) Near-infrared fluorescent imaging of cerebral thrombi and blood-brain barrier disruption in a mouse model of cerebral venous sinus thrombosis. J Cereb Blood Flow Metab 25:226–233

Kircher MF, Mahmood U, King RS, Weissleder R, Josephson L (2003) A multimodal nanoparticle for preoperative magnetic resonance imaging and intraoperative optical brain tumor delineation. Cancer Res 63:8122–8125

Koblinski JE, Ahram M, Sloane BF (2000) Unraveling the role of proteases in cancer. Clin Chim Acta 291:113–135

Law B, Weissleder R, Tung CH (2005) Mechanism-based fluorescent reporter for protein kinase A detection. Chembiochem 6:1361–1367

Messerli SM, Prabhakar S, Tang Y, Shah K, Cortes ML, Murthy V, Weissleder R, Breakefield XO, Tung CH (2004) A novel method for imaging apoptosis using a caspase-1 near-infrared fluorescent probe. Neoplasia 6:95–105

Metelev V, Weissleder R, Bogdanov A, Jr. (2004) Synthesis and properties of fluorescent NF-kappa B-recognizing hairpin oligodeoxyribonucleotide decoys. Bioconjug Chem 15:1481–1487

Pham W, Choi Y, Weissleder R, Tung CH (2004) Developing a peptide-based near-infrared molecular probe for protease sensing. Bioconjug Chem 15:1403–1407

Pham W, Weissleder R, Tung CH (2002) An azulene dimer as a near-infrared quencher. Angew Chem Int Ed Engl 41:3659–3662, 3519

Schellenberger EA, Sosnovik D, Weissleder R, Josephson L (2004) Magneto/optical annexin V, a multimodal protein. Bioconjug Chem 15:1062–1067

Tung CH, Mahmood U, Bredow S, Weissleder R (2000) In vivo imaging of proteolytic enzyme activity using a novel molecular reporter. Cancer Res 60:4953–4958

Tung CH, Zeng Q, Shah K, Kim DE, Schellingerhout D, Weissleder R (2004) In vivo imaging of beta-galactosidase activity using far red fluorescent switch. Cancer Res 64:1579–1583

Tyagi S, Marras SA, Kramer FR (2000) Wavelength-shifting molecular beacons. Nat Biotechnol 18:1191–1196

Weissleder R, Tung CH, Mahmood U, Bogdanov A Jr. (1999) In vivo imaging of tumors with protease-activated near-infrared fluorescent probes. Nat Biotechnol 17:375–378

Wunder A, Tung CH, Muller-Ladner U, Weissleder R, Mahmood U (2004) In vivo imaging of protease activity in arthritis: a novel approach for monitoring treatment response. Arthritis Rheum 50:2459–2465

PET and SPECT

Uwe Haberkorn

Abstract Assessment of gene function following the completion of human genome sequencing may be done using radionuclide imaging procedures. These procedures are needed for the evaluation of genetically manipulated animals or newly designed biomolecules which require a thorough understanding of physiology, biochemistry and pharmacology. The experimental approaches will involve many new technologies, including in-vivo imaging with SPECT and PET. Nuclear medicine procedures may be applied for the determination of gene function and regulation using established and new tracers or using in-vivo reporter genes, such as genes encoding enzymes, receptors, antigens or transporters. Visualization of in-vivo reporter gene expression can be done using radiolabeled substrates, antibodies or ligands. Combinations of specific promoters and in-vivo reporter genes may deliver information about the regulation of the corresponding genes. Furthermore, protein-protein interactions and the activation of signal transduction pathways may be visualized noninvasively. The role of radiolabeled antisense molecules for the analysis of mRNA content has to be investigated. However, possible applications are therapeutic interventions using triplex oligonucleotides with therapeutic isotopes, which can be brought near to specific DNA sequences to induce DNA strand breaks at selected loci.

Uwe Haberkorn
Department of Nuclear Medicine, University of Heidelberg, Im Neuenheimer Feld 400, 69120 Heidelberg
uwe_haberkorn@med.uni-heidelberg.de

W. Semmler and M. Schwaiger (eds.), *Molecular Imaging II.*
Handbook of Experimental Pharmacology 185/II.
© Springer-Verlag Berlin Heidelberg 2008

After the identification of new genes, functional information is required to investigate the role of these genes in living organisms. This can be done by analysis of gene expression, protein-protein interaction or the biodistribution of new molecules and may result in new diagnostic and therapeutic procedures, which include visualization of and interference with gene transcription, and the development of new biomolecules to be used for diagnosis and treatment. Furthermore, the characterization of tumor cell-specific properties allows the design of new treatment modalities, such as gene therapy, which circumvent resistance mechanisms towards conventional chemotherapeutic drugs.

1 Visualization of Gene Transfer

For the clinical application of gene therapy, noninvasive tools are needed to evaluate the efficiency of gene transfer. This includes the evaluation of infection efficiency as well as the verification of successful gene transfer in terms of gene transcription. This information can be obtained by imaging methods and is useful for therapy planning, follow-up studies on treated tumors and as an indicator of prognosis.

1.1 Assessment of Viral Vector Biodistribution

An understanding of the biodistribution of vectors carrying therapeutic genes to their targets would be helpful to develop strategies for the target-specific delivery of these therapeutic agents. Schellingerhout et al. (1998) used enveloped viral particles labeled with ^{111}In, allowing the viruses to be traced in vivo by scintigraphic imaging. The labeling procedure did not significantly reduce the infectivity of the herpes simplex virus without a significant release of the radionuclide within 12 h after labeling. Sequential imaging of animals, after intravenous administration of the ^{111}In-labeled virus, showed a fast accumulation in the liver and a redistribution from the blood pool to liver and spleen. Also, the recombinant adenovirus serotype 5 knob (Ad5K) was radiolabeled with [99m]Tc (Zinn et al. 1998) and retained specific, high-affinity binding to U293 cells, which shows that the radiolabeling process had no effect on receptor binding. In-vivo dynamic scintigraphy revealed extensive liver binding, with 100% extraction efficiency. The scintigraphically determined liver uptake corresponded to the results of a biodistribution study where tissues were removed and counted.

1.2 Suicide-gene Therapy

The transfer and expression of suicide genes into malignant tumor cells represents an attractive approach for human gene therapy. Suicide genes typically code for non-mammalian enzymes which convert nontoxic prodrugs into highly toxic metabolites. Therefore, systemic application of the nontoxic prodrug results in the production of the active drug at the tumor site. Although a broad range of suicide principles has been described, two suicide systems are applied in most studies: the cytosine deaminase (CD) and herpes simplex virus thymidine kinase (HSVtk).

Cytosine deaminase, which is expressed in yeasts and bacteria, but not in mammalian organisms converts the antifungal agent 5-fluorocytosine (5-FC) to the highly toxic 5-fluorouracil (5-FU). In mammalian cells no anabolic pathway is known which leads to incorporation of 5-FC into the nucleic acid fraction. Therefore, pharmacological effects are moderate and allow the application of high therapeutic doses. The toxic effect of 5-FU is exerted by interfering with DNA and protein synthesis due to substitution of uracil by 5-FU in RNA and inhibition of thymidilate synthetase by 5-fluorodeoxy-uridine monophosphate resulting in impaired DNA biosynthesis.

Gene therapy with the herpes simplex virus thymidine kinase as a suicide gene has been performed in a variety of tumor models in vitro as well as in vivo. In contrast to human thymidine kinase, HSVtk is less specific and also phosphorylates nucleoside analogues such as acyclovir and ganciclovir (GCV) to their monophosphate metabolites. These monophosphates are subsequently phosphorylated by cellular kinases to the di- and triphosphates. After integration of the triphosphate metabolites into DNA, chain termination occurs, followed by cell death. Encouraging results have been obtained initially for suicide systems both in vitro and in vivo. However, although not all of the tumor cells have to be infected to obtain a sufficient therapeutic response, the in-vivo infection efficiency of currently used viral vectors is low and repeated injections of the recombinant retroviruses may be necessary to reach a therapeutic level of enzyme activity in the tumor. Therefore, a prerequisite for gene therapy using a suicide system is monitoring of suicide gene expression in the tumor, for two reasons: to decide if repeated gene transductions of the tumor are necessary and to find a therapeutic window of maximum gene expression and consecutive prodrug administration (Haberkorn et al. 1996). Since specific substrates of these enzymes can be labeled with radioactive isotopes, nuclear medicine techniques may be applied to assess the enzyme activity in vivo.

1.2.1 Determination of Suicide-gene Activity by the Uptake of Specific Substrates

The principle of in vivo HSVtk imaging was first demonstrated by Saito et al. (1982) for the visualization of HSV encephalitis. Recently, in-vivo studies have been done by several groups using different tracers (Haberkorn et al. 1997, 1998; Germann et al. 1998; Haberkorn 1999; Mahony et al. 1988; Gati et al. 1984; Gambir et al. 1999; Alauddin et al. 1999; Wiebe et al. 1997, 1999; Tjuvajev et al. 1995, 1998; de Vries et al. 2000; Hustinx et al. 2001; Iwashina et al. 2001; Haubner). In vitro the uptake of specific substrates, such as GCV, FIAU and FFUdR, showed a time-dependent increase in HSVtk-expressing cells and a plateau in control cells. The HPLC analysis revealed unmetabolized GCV in control cells and a time-dependent shift of GCV to its phosphorylated metabolite in HSVtk-expressing cells (Haberkorn et al. 1997). Furthermore, the ganciclovir, FFUdR and the FIAU uptake were highly correlated to the percentage of HSVtk-expressing cells and to the growth inhibition as measured in bystander experiments (Haberkorn et al. 1997; Germann et al. 1998; Haberkorn 1999). To further elucidate the transport mechanism of ganciclovir, inhibition/competition experiments were performed. The nucleoside transport in mammalian cells is known to be heterogeneous with two classes of nucleoside transporters: the equilibrative, facilitated diffusion systems and the concentrative, sodium-dependent systems. In these experiments, competition for all concentrative nucleoside transport systems and inhibition of the ganciclovir transport by the equilibrative transport systems was observed, whereas the pyrimidine nucleobase system showed no contribution to the ganciclovir uptake (Haberkorn et al. 1997, 1998). In human erythrocytes, acyclovir has been shown to be transported mainly by the purine nucleobase carrier (Mahony et al. 1988). Due to a hydroxymethyl group on its side chain, ganciclovir has a stronger similarity to nucleosides and, therefore, may be transported also by a nucleoside transporter. Moreover, the $3'$-hydroxyl moiety of nucleosides was shown to be important for their interaction with the nucleoside transporter (Gati et al. 1984). In rat hepatoma cells as well as in human mammary carcinoma cells, the GCV uptake was shown to be much lower than the thymidine uptake (Haberkorn et al. 1997, 1998). Therefore, in addition to the low infection efficiency of the current viral delivery systems, slow transport of the substrate and also its slow conversion into the phosphorylated metabolite is limiting for the therapeutic success of the HSVtk/GCV system. Cotransfection with nucleoside transporters or the use of other substrates for HSVtk with higher affinities for nucleoside transport and phosphorylation by HSVtk may improve therapy outcome.

Gambhir et al. (1999) used 8-[^{18}F]fluoroganciclovir (FGCV) for the imaging of adenovirus-directed hepatic expression of the HSVtk gene in living mice. There was a significant positive correlation between the percent injected dose of FGCV retained per gram of liver and the levels of hepatic HSVtk gene expression. Over a similar range of HSVtk expression in vivo, the percent injected dose retained per gram of liver was 0–23% for ganciclovir and 0–3% for FGCV. Alauddin et al. (1999) used 9-(4-[^{18}F]-fluoro-3-hydroxymethylbutyl)-guanine ([^{18}F]FHBG) and 9-[(3-^{18}F-fluoro-1-hydroxy-2-propoxy)methyl]-guanine ([^{18}F]-FHPG) for combined in-vitro/in-vivo studies of HT-29 human colon cancer cells transduced with a retroviral vector and also found a significant higher uptake in HSVtk-expressing cells compared with the controls. In-vivo studies in tumor-bearing nude mice demonstrated that the tumor uptake of the radiotracer is three- and sixfold higher at 2 and 5 h, respectively, in transduced cells compared with the control cells. Others used radioiodinated nucleoside analogues such as (E)-5-(2-iodovinyl)-$2'$-fluoro-$2'$-deoxyuridine (IVFRU) and 5-iodo-$2'$-fluoro-$2'$deoxy-1-b-D-arabinofuranosyluracil (FIAU) to visualize HSVtk expression (Wiebe et al. 1997; Tjuvajev et al. 1995, 1998; Haubner et al. 2000). Autoradiography, SPECT and PET images after injection of [^{131}I] or [^{124}I] labeled FIAU revealed highly specific localization of the tracer to areas of HSVtk gene expression in brain and mammary tumors (Tjuvajev et al. 1995, 1998). The amount of tracer uptake in the tumors was correlated to the in-vitro ganciclovir sensitivity of the cell lines which were transplanted in these animals

(14, 15). Haubner et al. (20) studied the early kinetics of ^{123}I-FIAU in the CMS-5 fibrosarcoma model. Biodistribution studies at 30 min post infection showed tumor/blood and tumor/muscle ratios of 3.8 and 7.2 in HSVtk-expressing tumors, and 0.6 and 1.2 in wild-type tumors. The tracer showed a bi-exponential clearance with an initial half-life of 0.6 h, followed by a half-life of 4.6 h and the highest activity accumulation in HSVtk-expressing tumors observed at 1 h post infection. Scintigraphy demonstrated specific tracer accumulation as early as 0.5 h post infection, with an increase in contrast over time, suggesting that sufficient tumor/background ratios for in vivo imaging of HSVtk expression with [^{123}I]FIAU are reached as early as 1 h post infection . Similar results were reported for IVFRU by Wiebe et al.(1997, 1999). Due to low nontarget tissue uptake, unambiguous imaging of HSVtk-expressing tumors in mice is possible with labeled IVFRU. The advantage of iodinated tracers like FIAU may be that delayed imaging is possible. Since the use of ^{18}F-labeled compounds restricts imaging to time periods early after administration of the tracer, these iodinated compounds may prove to be more sensitive in vivo. However, quantification with iodine isotopes may be a problem either with ^{131}I, a γ and β^- emitter with high radiation dose, or with the corresponding positron emitter [124]I, which shows only 23% β^+ radiation with high energy particles, multiple γ rays of high energy and leads to a high radiation dose.

To improve the detection of lower levels of PET reporter gene expression, a mutant herpes simplex virus type 1 thymidine kinase (HSV1-sr39tk) was used as a PET reporter gene (Gambir et al. 2000). After successful transfer of this mutant gene the accumulation of the specific substrates [8-^{3}H]penciclovir ([8-^{3}H]PCV) and 8-[^{18}F]fluoropenciclovir (FPCV) in C6 rat glioma cells was increased twofold when compared with wild type HSVtk-expressing tumor cells, leading to an increased imaging sensitivity.

In human glioblastoma cells, cytosine deaminase (CD) was evaluated. After stable transfection with the *E. coli CD* gene, ^{3}H-5-FU was produced in CD-expressing cells, whereas in the control cells only ^{3}H-5-FC was detected (Haberkorn et al. 1996). Moreover, significant amounts of 5-FU were found in the medium of cultured cells, which may account for the bystander effect observed in previous experiments. However, uptake studies revealed a moderate and nonsaturable accumulation of radioactivity in the tumor cells, suggesting that 5-FC enters the cells only via diffusion (Haberkorn et al. 1996). Although a significant difference in 5-FC uptake was seen between CD-positive cells and controls after 48 h incubation, no difference was observed after 2 h incubation. Furthermore, a rapid efflux could be demonstrated. Therefore, 5-FC transport may be a limiting factor for this therapeutic procedure and quantitation with PET has to rely rather on dynamic studies and modeling, including HPLC analysis of the plasma, than on nonmodeling approaches (Haberkorn et al. 1996). To evaluate the 5-FC uptake in vivo, a rat prostate adenocarcinoma cell line was transfected with a retroviral vector bearing the *E. coli CD* gene. The cells were found to be sensitive to 5-FC exposure, but lost this sensitivity with time. This may be due to inactivation of the viral promoter (CMV) used in this vector. In-vivo studies with PET and [18]FC showed no preferential accumulation of the tracer in CD-expressing tumors, although HPLC analysis revealed a production of 5-fluorouracil, which was detectable in tumor lysates as well as in the blood of the animals (Haberkorn 1997). Therefore, a considerable efflux of the enzyme product, ^{18}FU, occurs which may also impair imaging results.

Finally, the coupling of two genes as a therapeutic gene together with a reporter gene by use of bicistronic vectors (involving the internal ribosomal entry site (IRES) of picornaviruses) may be useful for the evaluation of gene transfer. By the measurement of the PET reporter gene, the assessment of another, therapeutic, gene — e.g., a cytokine — would be possible. Problems may arise from low levels of gene expression which may be influenced by the number of infected cells and also by attenuation of the gene downstream of the IRES.

1.3 Imaging Using Non-suicide Reporter Genes

Reporter genes (e.g., β-galactosidase, chloramphenicol acetyltransferase, green fluorescent protein and luciferase) play critical roles in investigating mechanisms of gene expression in transgenic animals and in developing gene delivery systems for gene therapy. However, measuring expression of these reporter genes requires biopsy or killing of the animals. In-vivo reporter genes allow the measurement of gene expression in living animals (Table 1, Fig. 1). In this respect, the HSVtk gene has been shown to be useful as a noninvasive marker (Haberkorn et al. 1997,

Table 1 Genes and radio-isotope imaging methods used for the monitoring of successful gene transfer

Gene	Principle	Imaging method	Tracer/ contrast agent
Enzymes			
CD	Enzyme activity	MRS, PET	5-fluorocytosine
HSVtk	Therapeutic effects	MRI, MRS, PET, SPECT	FDG, HMPAO, misonidazole
HSVtk	Enzyme activity	SPECT, PET	Specific substrates
HSVtk mutant	Enzyme activity	PET	Specific substrates
Tyrosinase	Metal scavenger	MRI, SPECT, scintigraphy	^{111}In
Non-suicide reporter genes			
SSTR2	Receptor expression	SPECT, scintigraphy	Radiolabeled ligand
D2R	Receptor expression	PET	Radiolabeled ligand
Transferrin receptor	Receptor expression	MRI	Radiolabeled ligand
CEA antigen	Antigen expression	Scintigraphy	Radiolabeled antibody
Modified green fluorescence protein	Transchelation	SPECT, scintigraphy	^{99m}Tc-glucoheptonate
Human sodium iodide transporter	Transport activity, therapy	Scintigraphy	^{99m}Tc, ^{123}I, ^{131}I
Human norepinephrine transporter	Transport activity, therapy	Scintigraphy	^{123}I-MIBG, ^{131}I-MIBG

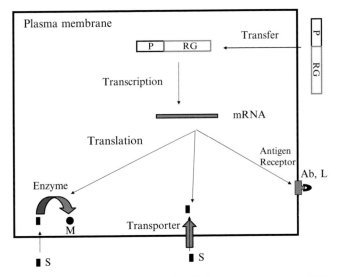

Fig. 1 Gene transfer and imaging of gene expression. As in-vivo reporter genes (*RG*) enzymes, receptors, antigens and transporters can be used. After transfection and integration (for example using retroviral vectors) a foreign protein is expressed in cells or tissues with corresponding changes in biological properties. A newly induced enzyme activity can be visualized by the accumulation of metabolites (*M*) of radioactively labeled specific substrates (*S*), receptors by the binding and/or internalization of ligands (*L*), antigens by the binding of antibodies (*Ab*) and transporters by the uptake of their substrates. These genes can be combined with specific promoters (*P*) and may be used for the characterization of gene regulation, signal transduction and other biological phenomena

1998; Germann et al. 1998; Haberkorn 1999; Mahony et al. 1988; Gati et al. 1984; Gambhir et al. 1999; Alauddin et al. 1999; Wiebe et al. 1997, 1999; Tjuvajev et al. 1995, 1998; de Vries et al. 2000; Hustinx et al. 2001; Iwashina et al. 2001; Haubner). However, receptor genes have also been used as reporter genes (MacLaren et al. 1999; Zinn et al. 2000). The dopamine D2 receptor gene represents an endogenous gene, which is not likely to invoke an immune response. Furthermore, the corresponding tracer 3-(2'-[^{18}F]-fluoroethyl)spiperone (FESP) rapidly crosses the blood-brain-barrier, can be produced at high specific activity and is currently used in patients. As a SPECT tracer [^{123}I]-iodobenzamine is available. MacLaren et al. (MacLaren et al. 1999) used this system in nude mice with an adenoviral-directed hepatic gene delivery system and also in stably transfected tumor cells which were transplanted in animals. The tracer uptake in these animals was proportional to in-vitro data of hepatic FESP accumulation, dopamine receptor ligand binding and the D2 receptor mRNA. Also, tumors modified to express the D2 receptor retained significantly more FESP than wild-type tumors. Using a replication-incompetent adenoviral vector encoding the human type 2 somatostatin receptor, Zinn et al. (Zinn et al. 2000) modified non-small cell lung tumors and imaged the expression of the hSSTr2 gene using a radiolabeled, somatostatin-avid peptide (P829), that was radiolabeled to high specific activity with ^{99m}Tc or ^{188}Re. In the genetically modified tumors a five- to tenfold greater accumulation of both radiolabeled P829 peptides compared with the control tumors was observed. Both isotopes are generator-produced, which confers advantages concerning the availability, costs, and imaging with widespread existing, high-resolution modalities. Furthermore, the [188]Re-labeled peptide offers the additional advantage of β decay, which may be used for therapy.

Specific imaging can also be obtained by radiolabeled antibodies. To overcome the limitation of low expression of human tumor-associated antigens on target cells a human glioma cell line was modified to express high levels of human carcinoembryonic antigen using an adenoviral vector (Raben et al. 1996). In these cells, high binding of an ^{131}I-labeled CEA antibody was observed in vitro as well as by scintigraphic imaging.

Another approach is based on the in-vivo transchelation of oxotechnetate to a polypeptide motif from a biocompatible complex with a higher dissociation constant than that of a dicglycilcysteine complex. It has been shown that synthetic peptides and recombinant proteins like the modified green fluorescence protein (gfp) can bind oxotechnetate with high efficiency (Bogdanov et al. 1997, 1998). In these experiments, rats were injected i.m. with synthetic peptides bearing a GGC motif. One hour later, ^{99m}Tc-glucoheptonate was applied i.v. and the accumulation was measured by scintigraphy. The peptides with three metal-binding GGC motifs showed a threefold higher accumulation compared with the controls. This principle can also be applied to recombinant proteins which appear at the plasma membrane (Simonova et al. 1999). These genes can be cloned into bicistronic vectors, which allow for the co-expression of therapeutic genes and in-vivo reporter genes. Thereafter, radionuclide imaging may be used to detect gene expression.

Tyrosinase catalyzes the hydroxilation of tyrosine to DOPA and the oxidation of DOPA to DOPAquinone, which, after cyclization and polymerization, results in melanin production. Melanins are scavengers of metal ions, such as iron and indium, through ionic binding. Tyrosinase transfer leads to the production of melanins in a variety of cells. This may be used for imaging with NMR or with ^{111}In and a gamma camera. Cells transfected with the tyrosinase gene stained positively for melanin and had a higher ^{111}In binding capacity than the wild-type cells (Weissleder et al. 1997). In transfection experiments, a dependence of tracer accumulation on the amount of the vector used could be observed. The problems of this approach are possible low tyrosinase induction with low amounts of melanin and the cytotoxicity of melanin. These problems may be encountered by the construction of chimeric tyrosinase proteins and by positioning of the enzyme at the outer side of the membrane.

2 Protein-protein Interaction

Protein interaction analysis delivers information about the possible biological role of genes with unknown function by connecting them to other, better-characterized proteins. Furthermore, it detects novel interactions between proteins that are known to be involved in a common biological process and also novel functions of previously characterized proteins.

Protein interactions have been deduced by purely computational methods or using large-scale approaches. Ideally, the characterization of protein interactions should be based on experimentally determined interactions between proteins that are known to be present at the same time and in the same compartment. With the increasing availability of intrinsically fluorescent proteins that can be genetically fused to a wide variety of proteins, their application as fluorescent biosensors has extended to dynamic imaging studies of cellular biochemistry, even at the level of organelles or compartments participating in specific processes. Fluorescence imaging allows the determination of cell-to-cell variation, the extent of variation in cellular responses and the mapping of processes in multicellular tissues. In addition, procedures for noninvasive dynamic in-vivo monitoring are needed to show whether the protein interactions also work in the complex environment of a living organism, such as mouse, rat or human, where external stimuli may affect and trigger cells or organ function. The yeast two-hybrid technique has been adapted for in-vivo detection of luciferase expression using a cooled charge coupled device (CCD) camera (Ray et al. 2002). GAL4 and VP16 proteins were expressed separately and associated by the interaction of MyoD and Id, two proteins of the helix-loop-helix family of nuclear proteins which are involved in myogenic differentiation (Fig. 2). In this experimental setting, association of GAL4 and VP16 resulted in expression of firefly luciferase, which was under the control of multiple copies of GAL4 binding sites and a minimal promoter.

Drawbacks of the cooled CCD camera are mainly its limitation to small animals with different efficiencies of light transmission for different organs, lack of detailed tomographic information and lack of an equivalent imaging modality applicable to human studies (Wu et al. 2001). Therefore, another approach based on

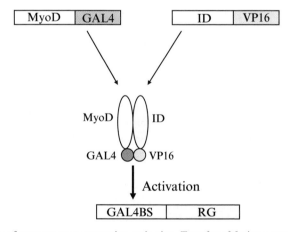

Fig. 2 Principle of reporter-gene expression activation. Transfer of fusion genes of *MyoD/GAL4* and *ID/VP16* results in the expression of the corresponding fusion proteins. Interaction of MyoD and ID leads to association of GAL4 and VP16, which together activate GAL4 binding sites (*GAL4BS*) to induce transcription of the reporter gene

the two-hybrid system used a fusion of a mutated HSVtk gene and the green fluorescent protein gene for in-vivo detection of the interaction between p53 and the large T antigen of simian virus 40 by optical imaging and positron emission tomography (PET). Interaction of both proteins resulted in association of GAL4, VP16 and reporter gene expression, which was visualized after administration of a ^{18}F-labeled, specific substrate for HSVtk (Luker et al. 2002).

Current approaches are based on intracistronic complementation and reconstitution by protein splicing. Complementation does not require the formation of a mature protein. Both parts of the reporter protein are active when closely approximated. The complementation strategy can be exploited for a wide range of studies directed at determining whether proteins derived from two active genes are coincident or colocalized within cells. Other applications include transgenic animals expressing complementary *lacZ* mutants from two promoters of interest, which should identify cell lines in which the products of both genes coincide spatially and temporally. Reconstitution is based on protein splicing in trans, which requires the reassociation of an N-terminal and C-terminal fragment of an intein, each fused to split N- and C-terminal halves of an extein, such as a reporter gene like enhanced green fluorescent protein (EGFP) or luciferase. Reassociated intein fragments form a functional protein-splicing active center, which mediates the formation of a peptide bond between the exteins, coupled to the excision of the N- and C-inteins. Newer strategies fuse the intein segments to interacting proteins, which results in initiation of protein splicing in trans by protein-protein interaction. The feasibility of imaging interaction of MyoD and Id based on both a complementation and a reconstitution strategy has been demonstrated using a CCD camera and split reporter constructs of firefly luciferase (Paulmurugan et al. 2002). After cotransfection of two plasmids, the complementation as well as the reconstitution strategy achieved activities between 40 and 60% of the activity obtained after transfection of a plasmid bearing the full length reporter gene. A cooled CCD camera was applied for visualization of luciferase activity in nude mice. This strategy presents a promising tool for the in-vivo evaluation of protein function and intracellular networks and may be extended to approaches involving combinations of reporter genes and radionuclides. However, MyoD and Id are strong interacting proteins. There may be a weaker in-vivo signal when systems with a weaker interaction are used.

Protein interactions occur not only as physical interactions but also as functional interactions. These may be studied by analysis of promoters or promoter modules or using combinations of specific promoters and reporter genes (Haberkorn et al. 2002, 2003).

Tissue-specific transcriptional regulation is often mediated by a set of transcription factors whose combination is unique to specific cell types. The vast majority of genes expressed in a cell-type-specific manner are regulated by promoters containing a variety of recognition sequences for tissue-specific and ubiquitous transcription factors. It is the precise functional interaction between these various regulating proteins and the regulatory DNA sequences which enables individual cell types to play their role within an organism. To date, three transcription factors that specifically regulate thyroid-specific gene expression have been identified: thyroid transcription factor-1 (TTF-1) is a homeodomain-containing protein expressed in embryonic diencephalon, thyroid and lung. Thyroid transcription factor-2 (TTF-2), a forkhead domain containing protein is expressed in the pituitary gland and thyroid, and Pax8, which belongs to the Pax family of paired-domain-containing genes, is expressed in the kidney, the developing excretory system and in the thyroid. None of these transcription factors is expressed exclusively in the thyroid, but their combination is unique to this organ and is likely to be responsible for differentiation of thyrocytes. TTF-1 and pax-8 directly interact and synergistically activate thyroid-specific transcription and, therefore, represent a promising model system for the visualization of functional protein-protein interaction. Therefore, these genes were transfected into hepatoma cells to measure functional protein-protein interaction expressed as activation of reporter gene constructs bearing combinations of the human thyroglobulin (hTg), human thyroperoxidase (hTPO) or the sodium iodide symporter (NIS) promoter/enhancer elements with the luciferase gene (Altmann et al. 2005). Low transcriptional activation of these constructs was observed in cells expressing either hPax8 or dTTF-1 alone. In contrast, the hTg, hTPO and, to a lesser extent, the rNIS regulatory regions were significantly activated in cell lines expressing both transcription factors. Imaging the transcriptional activation of the thyroid-specific regulatory regions by Pax8 and TTF-1 was possible in nude mice implanted with MHhPax8dTTF-1 cells using a cooled charge-coupled device (CCD) camera. Na^{125}I uptake experiments and RT-PCR showed no effect of hPax8 and dTTF-1 on endogenous thyroid-specific gene expression in genetically modified cells, even in the absence of the histone deacetylase inhibitor trichostatin A. A possible explanation is that the endogenous thyroid-specific regulatory regions may be inaccessible to Pax8 and TTF-1. The appropriate regulation of gene expression requires the interplay of complexes that remodel chromatin structure and thereby regulate the accessibility of individual genes to sequence-specific transcription factors and the basal transcription machinery.

For the examination of whole organisms, in-vivo reporter systems are promising. These in-vivo reporters may be used for the characterization of promoter regulation involved in signal transduction, gene regulation during changes of the physiological environment and gene regulation during pharmacological intervention. This may be done by combining specific promoter elements with an in-vivo reporter gene. However, specific promoters are usually weak. This problem was addressed using a two-step amplification system (Fig. 3) for optical imaging of luciferase and PET imaging of HSVtk expression (Iyer et al. 2001). In that study, tissue-specific reporter gene expression driven by the prostate-specific antigen promoter was enhanced by the transfer of a plasmid bearing a GAL4-VP16 fusion protein under the control of the prostate specific antigen (PSA) promoter, together with a second plasmid bearing multiple GAL4 responsive elements and the reporter gene. Optical imaging revealed a fivefold signal enhancement in nude mice. Another strategy may be the use of multiple specific enhancer elements upstream of their corresponding promoter.

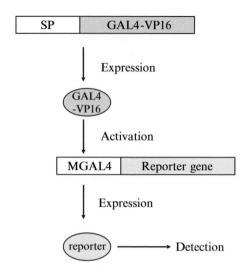

Fig. 3 Enhancement of tissue-specific reporter-gene expression. A specific promoter (*SP*) drives the expression of a GAL4-VP16 fusion protein. This fusion protein activates the reporter gene, which is under the control of multiple GAL4 responsive elements (*MGAL4*). The resulting protein can then be detected

3 Enhancement of Iodide Uptake in Malignant Tumors

Currently used viral vectors for gene therapy of cancer have a low infection efficiency, leading to moderate or low therapy effects. This problem could be solved using an approach which leads to accumulation of radioactive isotopes with β emission. In this case, isotope trapping centers in the tumor could create a crossfiring of β particles, thereby efficiently killing transduced and nontransduced tumor cells. To date, transfer of genes for sodium iodide or norepinephrine transporters or the thyroid peroxidase has been tried.

The first step in the complex process of iodide trapping in the thyroid is the active transport of iodide together with sodium ions into the cell, which is mediated by the sodium-iodide symporter. This process, against an electrochemical gradient requires energy, is coupled to the action of Na^+/K^+-ATPase and is also stimulated by TSH. Since the cloning of the human and rat cDNA sequences, several experimental studies have been performed which investigated the recombinant expression of the human sodium iodide symporter (hNIS) gene in malignant tumors by viral transfer of the hNIS gene under the control of different promoter elements (Haberkorn et al. 2001b, 2003; Mandell et al. 1999; Cho et al. 2000; Boland et al. 2000; Spitzweg et al. 1999, 2000, 2001; La Perle et al. 2002; Nakamoto et al. 2000; Shimura et al. 1997; Sieger et al. 2003; Smit et al. 2000, 2002). Although all of them reported high initial uptake in the genetically modified tumors (Fig. 4), differing results have been obtained concerning the efficiency of radioiodine treatment based on NIS gene transfer, with generally very high doses given to tumor-bearing mice.

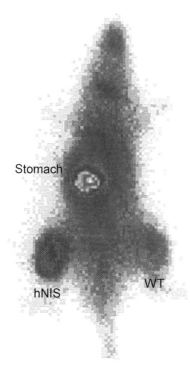

Stomach

hNIS

WT

Fig. 4 Scintigraphic image of a tumor-bearing male adult Copenhagen rat subcutaneously trans-planted with hNIS-expressing (*hNIS*) or wild-type rat prostate adenocarcinoma cells (*WT*) at 30 min after injection of $^{131}I^-$

In vitro a rapid efflux of iodide occurred with 80% of the radioactivity released into the medium after 20 min. Since the effectiveness of radioiodine therapy depends not only on the type and amount but also on the biological half-life of the isotope in the tumor, a therapeutically useful absorbed dose seems unlikely for that type of experiment. A significant efflux was also seen in vivo when doses were applied which are commonly administered to patients: only $0.4 \pm 0.2(1,200\,\text{MBq/m}^2)$ and $0.24 \pm 0.02\%(2,400\,\text{MBq/m}^2)$ of the injected dose per gram in the hNIS-expressing tumors were observed at 24 h after tracer administration (Haberkorn et al. 2001b, 2003). Similarly, Nakamoto et al. (2000) found less than 1% of the injected radioactivity at 24 h after ^{131}I administration in modified MCF7 mammary carcinomas, although initially a high uptake was seen. This corresponds to a very short half-life of ^{131}I (approximately 7.5 h) in rat prostate carcinomas, which has also been described by Nakamoto et al. for human mammary carcinomas, with a calculated biological half life of 3.6 h. In contrast, differentiated thyroid carcinoma showed a biological half-life of less than 10 days and normal thyroid of approximately 60 days (Berman et al. 1968).

However, in-vitro clonogenic assays revealed selective killing of NIS-expressing cells in some studies (Mandell et al. 1999; Boland et al. 2000; Spitzweg et al. 2000;

Carlin et al. 2000). Also, bystander effects have been suggested in three-dimensional spheroid cultures (Carlin et al. 2000). In-vivo experiments in stably transfected human prostate carcinoma cells showed a long biological half-life of 45 h (Spitzweg et al. 2000). This resulted in a significant tumor reduction $(84 \pm 12\%)$ after a single intraperitoneal application of a very high ^{131}I dose of 111 MBq (Spitzweg et al. 1999, 2000, 2001). The authors concluded that transfer of the NIS gene causes effective radioiodine doses in the tumor and might therefore represent a potentially curative therapy for prostate cancer. In order to improve therapy outcome, Smit et al. (2002) investigated the effects of low-iodide diets and thyroid ablation on iodide kinetics. The half-life in NIS-expressing human folliculary thyroid carcinomas without thyroid ablation and under a regular diet was very short at 3.8 h. In thyroid-ablated mice kept on a low-iodide diet, the half-life of radioiodide was increased to 26.3 h, which may be due to diminished renal clearance of radioiodine and lack of iodide trapping by the thyroid. Subcutaneous injection of 74 MBq in thyroid-ablated nude mice, kept on a low-iodide diet, postponed tumor development. However, 9 weeks after therapy, tumors had developed in four of the seven animals. The estimated tumor dose in these animals was 32.2 Gy (Smit et al. 2002).

However, these studies used very high doses: in a mouse, 74 MBq and 111 MBq correspond to administered doses of $11,100 \text{MBq/m}^2$ and $16,650 \text{MBq/m}^2$, respectively. This is far more than the doses used in patients. In rat prostate carcinomas treatment with amounts of ^{131}I corresponding to those given to patients $(1,200 \text{MBq}^{131}\text{I/m}^2$ and $2,400 \text{MBq}^{131}\text{I/m}^2)$ resulted in only a 3-Gy absorbed dose in the genetically modified tumors (Haberkorn et al. 2003). Since approximately 80 Gy have been described as necessary to achieve elimination of metastases in patients with thyroid cancer, this is not likely to induce a significant therapeutic effect in the tumors. Furthermore, the experiments were performed under ideal conditions with 100% NIS-expressing cells in the tumors. Given the low infection efficiency of currently viral vectors in vivo, the absorbed dose in a clinical study would be considerably lower.

There are also other differences in these studies: tracer administration, time of treatment, animal and tumor models. Therefore, differences in the biodistribution of iodide and the biochemical properties of the tumor cells may lead to differences in iodide retention.

In order to prolong the iodine retention time in tumors, some authors tried to simultaneously transfer the NIS and the thyroperoxidase gene (Boland et al. 2000, Huang et al. 2001). Boland et al. (2000) observed iodide organification in cells coinfected with both the NIS and the TPO gene in the presence of exogenous hydrogen peroxide. However, the levels of iodide organification obtained were too low to significantly increase the iodide retention time. In a variety of different cell lines, including human anaplastic thyroid carcinoma and rat hepatoma cells, we were not able to measure TPO enzyme activity or enhanced accumulation of iodide irrespective of very high amounts of hTPO protein after retroviral transfer of the human TPO gene (Haberkorn et al. 2001a). Moreover, only minimal enzymatic activity of the recombinant hTPO was determined in individual cell lines as shown by low levels of guaiacol oxidation. This suggests that the recombinant gene is either expressed as a functionally inactive protein or that a functional protein becomes inactive in a nonoptimal cellular milieu. In most in vitro systems, the hTPO introduced by cDNA-directed gene expression was detected by means of immunohistology, immunoblotting or autoantibodies of patients with thyroid autoimmune disease. However, the production of catalytically active hTPO was not achieved, irrespective of the expression system and cell culture system employed for the experimental approach (Hidaka et al. 1996; Kaufman et al. 1996; Kimura et al. 1989; Guo et al. 1998). The function and activity of the hTPO are probably influenced by the multimerization of the protein as well as by additional factors, including the incorporation of heme, the glycosylation, the localization of the enzyme, and the thyroglobulin content of the cells. In contrast, Huang et al. (2001) observed an increased radioiodide uptake (by a factor of 2.5) and retention (by a factor of 3) and enhanced tumor cell apoptosis after transfection of non-small cell lung cancer cells with both human NIS and TPO genes. However, a 72% efflux occurred in vitro during the first 30 min, indicating a very low hTPO activity in the genetically modified cells. Therefore, the transduction of the hTPO gene per se is not sufficient to induce the iodide accumulation in human anaplastic carcinoma cells and a low enzymatic activity in the recombinant cell lines is supposed to account for it. Studies are currently performed to define additional factors required for iodide uptake in undifferentiated thyroid tumor cells.

A further option to increase therapy outcome is the use of biologically more effective isotopes. Dadachova et al. (2002) compared ^{188}Re-perrhenate with ^{131}I for treatment of NIS-expressing mammary tumors. In a xenografted breast cancer model in nude mice, ^{188}Re-perrhenate exhibited NIS-dependent uptake into the mammary tumor. Dosimetry showed that ^{188}Re-perrhenate delivered a 4.5-times higher dose than ^{131}I and, therefore, may provide enhanced therapeutic efficacy. Furthermore, the high LET-emitter astatine-211 has been suggested as an isotope with high radiobiological effectiveness (Petrich et al. 2002). First experiments showed that the tracer uptake in NIS-expressing cell lines increased up to 350-fold for ^{123}I, 340-fold for ^{99m}TcO$_4^-$ and 60-fold for ^{211}At. Although all radioisotopes showed a rapid efflux, higher absorbed doses in the tumor were found for ^{211}At compared with ^{131}I (Petrich et al. 2002).

In conclusion, a definitive proof of therapeutically useful absorbed doses in vivo after transfer of the NIS gene is still lacking. Further studies have to examine pharmacological modulation of iodide efflux or the use of the hNIS gene as an in-vivo reporter gene.

Another approach of a genetically modified isotope treatment is the transfer of the norepinephrine gene. ^{131}I-meta-iodobenzylguanidine (MIBG), a metabolically stable false analogue of norepinephrine, has been widely used for imaging and targeted radiotherapy in patients suffering from neural crest-derived tumors such as neuroblastoma or pheochromocytoma. In the adrenal medulla and in pheochromocytoma, MIBG is stored in the chromaffin neurosecretory granules. The transport of MIBG by the human norepinephrine transporter (hNET) seems to be the critical step in the treatment of MIBG-concentrating tumors. The mechanism of MIBG uptake, which is qualitatively similar to that of norepinephrine, has been studied in a variety of cellular systems and two different uptake systems have been postulated. While most tissues accumulate MIBG by a nonspecific, nonsaturable diffusion process, cells of the neuroadrenergic tissues and in malignancies derived thereof exhibit an active uptake of the tracer which is mediated by the noradrenalin transporter. The clinical use of the MIBG radiotherapy is so far restricted to neural crest-derived malignancies and, due to insufficient ^{131}I-MIBG uptake therapy in these tumor patients, is not curative.

The effect of hNET gene transfection was investigated in a variety of cells, including COS-1 cells, HeLa cells, glioblastoma cells or rat hepatoma cells, and a threefold to 36-fold increase of ^{131}I-MIBG or noradrenaline accumulation was achieved (Glowniak et al. 1993; Pacholczyk et al. 1991; Boyd et al. 1999; Altmann et al. 2003). In-vivo experiments performed with nude mice bearing both the hNET-expressing and wild-type tumor showed a tenfold higher accumulation of ^{131}I-MIBG in the transfected tumors compared with the wild-type tumors. Furthermore, in rat hepatoma cells, when compared with previous studies concerning the efflux of ^{131}I from hNIS-expressing cells, a longer retention of MIBG in the hNET-transfected cells was observed (Altmann et al. 2003). Nevertheless, 4 h after incubation with MIBG an efflux of 43% of the radioactivity was determined for the recombinant cells, whereas wild-type cells had lost 95% of the radioactivity. In view of an MIBG radiotherapy in non-neuroectodermal tumors, an intracellular trapping of the tracer is required to achieve therapeutically sufficient doses of radioactivity in the genetically modified tumor cells. In that respect, a positive correlation has been observed between the content of chromaffin neurosecretory granules and the uptake of radiolabeled MIBG (Bomanji et al. 1987).

Human glioblastoma cells transfected with the bovine NET gene were killed by doses of 0.5–1 MBq/ml ^{131}I-MIBG in monolayer cell culture as well as in spheroids (Boyd et al. 1999). Accordingly, the authors expected the intratumoral activity in a 70-kg patient to be 0.021%. This corresponds to the range of MIBG uptake usually achieved in neuroblastoma. However, data obtained from in-vitro experiments can not be applied to the in-vivo situation. In contrast to stable in-vitro conditions, the radioactive dose delivered to the tumor in vivo differs due to decreasing radioactivity in the serum and due to heterogeneity within the tumor tissue. In order to calculate the radiation dose in a particular tumor more precisely, an in-vivo dosimetry is superior. Using 14.8 MBq ^{131}I-MIBG for the application in tumor-bearing mice, corresponding to 2,200 MBq/m^2 in humans, a radiation dose of 605 mGy in the hNET-expressing tumor and 75 mGy in the wild-type tumor was calculated (Altman et al. 2003). With regard to the treatment of patients suffering from a non-neuroectodermal tumor transfected by the hNET gene, this absorbed dose is too low to evoke any tumor response. In addition, as with most gene transfer studies, the in-vivo experiments were performed with animals that had been transplanted with 100% stable hNET-expressing cells. Therefore, due to the low in-vivo infection efficiency of virus particles, infection of tumor cells in vivo will result in even lower radiation doses.

Future development should comprise pharmacologic modulation of MIBG retention or interaction with competing catecholamines. Employment of the recombinant hNET gene product as an in-vivo reporter is not promising because the images showed high background and relatively faint appearance of the genetically modified tumor (Altman et al. 2003). Finally, it has been speculated as to whether the transfer of the NET gene into pheochromocytoma or neuroblastoma cells may enhance the efficiency of MIBG therapy (Boyd et al. 1999).

4 Antisense Oligonucleotides

The estimation of gene function using the tools of the genome program has been referred to as "functional genomics," which can be seen as describing the processes leading from a gene's physical structure and its regulation to the gene's role in the whole organism. Many studies in functional genomics are performed by analysis of differential gene expression using high throughput methods, such as DNA chip technology. These methods are used to evaluate changes in the transcription of many or all genes of an organism at the same time, in order to investigate genetic pathways for normal development and disease. However, the assessment and modification of the mRNA content of single genes is also of interest in functional studies.

Antisense RNA and DNA techniques were originally developed to modulate the expression of specific genes. These techniques originated from studies in bacteria, demonstrating that these organisms are able to regulate gene replication and expression by the production of small complementary RNA molecules in an opposite (antisense) direction. Base pairing between the oligonucleotide and the corresponding target mRNA leads to highly specific binding and specific interaction with protein synthesis. Thereafter, several laboratories showed that synthetic oligonucleotides complementary to mRNA sequences could downregulate the translation of various oncogenes in cells (Zamecnik and Stephenson 1978; Mukhopadhyay et al. 1991).

Silencing of genes can also be obtained by a mechanism which is based on double-stranded RNA (dsRNA). Double-stranded RNA is cleaved by a ribonuclease named Dicer, to yield short RNAs of 21–25 nucleotide length (siRNA). After interaction of these siRNAs with a complex of cellular proteins to form an RNA-induced silencing complex (RISC), the RISC binds to the complementary RNA and inhibits its translation into a protein. This is known as RNA interference (RNAi) and can be used for treatment either by application of synthetic oligonucleotides or after introduction of DNA-bearing vectors that produce RNA hairpins in vivo, which are cleaved in the cell to the corresponding siRNAs (Hannon 2002).

Besides their use as therapeutics for specific interaction with RNA processing, oligonucleotides have been proposed for diagnostic imaging and the treatment of tumors. Assuming a total human gene number between 24,000 and 30,000, calculations which take into account alternative polyadenylation and alternative splicing result in an mRNA number of between 46,000 and 85,000 (Claverie 2003). It is expected that an oligonucleotide with more than 12 nucleobases (12-mer) represents a unique sequence in the whole genome (Woolf et al. 1992). Since these short oligonucleotides can easily be produced, antisense imaging using radiolabeled oligonucleotides offers a high number of new tracers with high specificity. Prerequisites for the use of radiolabeled antisense oligonucleotides are ease of synthesis, stability in vivo, uptake into the cell, accumulation of the oligonucleotide inside the cell, interaction with the target structure, and minimal nonspecific interaction with other macromolecules. For the stability of radiolabeled antisense molecules, nuclease resistance of the oligonucleotide, stability of the oligo-linker complex and a stable binding of the radionuclide to the complex are required. In this respect, modifications of the phosphodiester backbone, such as phosphorothioates, methylphosphonates, peptide nucleic acids or gapmers (mixed backbone oligonucleotides), result in at least a partial loss of cleavage by RNAses.

Evidence has been presented of receptor-coupled endocytosis as the low capacity mechanism by which oligonucleotides enter cells. Subcellular fractionation experiments showed a sequestration of the oligonuleotides in the nuclei and the mitochondria of cervix carcinoma (HeLa) cells. This phenomenon of fractionation, problems with in-vivo stability of the oligonucleotides as well as the stability of the hybrid oligo-RNA structures may prevent successful imaging of gene expression. Furthermore, binding to other polyanions, such as heparin, based on charge interaction, results in nonspecific signals.

However, successful antisense imaging has been reported in several studies: accumulation of ^{111}In-labeled c-myc antisense probes with a phosphorothioate backbone occurred in mice bearing c-myc overexpressing mammary tumors (Dewanjee et al. 1994). Imaging was also possible with a transforming growth factor α antisense oligonucleotide, an antisense phosphorothioate oligodeoxynucleotide for the mRNA of glial fibrillary acidic protein and a ^{125}I-labeled antisense peptide nucleic acid targeted to the initiation codon of the luciferase mRNA in rat glioma cells permanently transfected with the luciferase gene (Cammilleri et al. 1996; Kobori et al. 1999; Shi et al. 2000; Urbain et al. 1995). Furthermore, positron emission tomography (PET) was used for the assessment of the biodistribution and kinetics of ^{18}F-labeled oligonucleotides (Tavitian et al. 1994). In addition, ^{90}Y labeled phosphorothioate antisense oligonucleotides may be applied as targeted radionuclide therapeutic agents for malignant tumors (Watanabe et al. 1999).

However, data obtained from messenger RNA (mRNA) profiling do not faithfully represent the proteome because the mRNA content seems to be a poor indicator of the corresponding protein levels. Direct comparison of mRNA and protein levels in mammalian cells either for several genes in one tissue or for one gene product in many cell types revealed only poor correlations with up to 30-fold variations. This might lead to misinterpretation of mRNA profiling results. Furthermore, mRNA is labile, leading to spontaneous chemical degradation as well as to degradation by enzymes which may be dependent on the specific sequence and result in nonuniform degradation of RNA. This phenomenon introduces quantitative biases that are dependent on the time after the onset of tissue stress or death. In contrast, proteins are generally more stable, and exhibit slower turnover rates in most tissues. A substantial fraction of interesting intracellular events is located at the protein level for example operating primarily through phosphorylation/dephosphorylation and the migration of proteins. Also, proteolytic modifications of membrane-bound precursors appear to regulate the release of a large series of extracellular signals, such as angiotensin or tumor necrosis factor.

Since protein levels often do not reflect mRNA levels, antisense imaging may be not a generally applicable approach for a clinically useful description of biological properties of tissues. Expression profiling data would be more useful, if mRNA samples could be enriched for transcripts that are being translated. This can be achieved by fractionation of cytoplasmic extracts in sucrose gradients, which leads to the separation of free mRNPs (ribonucleoprotein particles) from mRNAs in ribosomal pre-initiation complexes and from mRNAs loaded with ribosomes (polysomes). Since only the polysomes represent actively translated transcripts, this fraction should be directly correlated with de-novo synthesized proteins. Polysome imaging with nuclear medicine procedures has not been tried to date or even may be not possible. Therefore, antisense imaging for the determination of transcription by hybridization of the labeled antisense probe to the target mRNA makes sense in cases where RNA and protein content are highly correlated. Successful imaging was possible in cases where the expression of the protein was proven or the gene of interest was introduced by an expression vector (Dewanjee et al. 1994; Cammilleri et al. 1996; Kobori et al. 1999; Shi et al. 2000; Urbain et al. 1995). In the absence of such a correlation between mRNA and protein content, the diagnostic use of antisense imaging seems questionable. Therapeutic applications may use triplex oligonucleotides with therapeutic isotopes, such as Auger electron emitters, which can be brought near to specific DNA sequences to induce DNA strand breaks at selected loci. Imaging of labeled siRNAs makes sense if these are used for therapeutic purposes in order to assess the delivery of these new drugs to their target tissue.

References

Alauddin MM, Shahinian A, Kundu RK, Gordon EM, Conti PS (1999) Evaluation of 9-[(3-^{18}F-fluoro-1-hydroxy-2-propoxy)methyl]guanine ([^{18}F]-FHPG) in vitro and in vivo as a probe for PET imaging of gene incorporation and expression in tumors. Nucl Med Biol 26:371–376

Altmann A, Kissel M, Zitzmann S et al (2003) Increased MIBG uptake after transfer of the human norepinephrine transporter gene in rat hepatoma. J Nucl Med 44:973–980

Altmann A, Schulz RB, Glensch G, Eskerski H, Zitzmann S, Eisenhut M, Haberkorn U (2005) Effects of Pax8 and TTF-1 Thyroid transcription factor gene transfer in hepatoma cells: imaging of functional protein-protein interaction and iodide uptake. J Nucl Med 46:831–839

Berman M, Hoff E, Barandes M (1968) Iodine kinetics in man: a model. J Clin Endocrinol Metab 28:1–14

Bogdanov A, Petherick P, Marecos E, Weissleder R (1997) In vivo localization of diglycylcysteine-bearing synthetic peptides by nuclear imaging of oxotechnetate transchelation. Nucl Med Biol 24:739–742

Bogdanov A, Simonova M, Weissleder R (1998) Design of metal-binding green fluorescent protein variants. Biochim Biophys Acta 1397:56–64

Bomanji J, Levison DA, Flatman WD et al (1987) Uptake of iodine-123 MIBG by pheochromocytomas, paragangliomas, and neuroblastomas: a histopathological comparison. J Nucl Med 28:973–978

Boland A, Ricard M, Opolon P, Bidart JM, Yeh P, Filetti S, Schlumberger M, Perricaudet M (2000) Adenovirus-mediated transfer of the thyroid sodium/Iodide symporter gene into tumors for a targeted radiotherapy. Cancer Res 60:3484–3492

Boyd M, Cunningham SH, Brown MM, Mairs RJ, Wheldon TE (1999) Noradrenaline transporter gene transfer for radiation cell kill by ^{131}I meta-iodobenzylguanidine. Gene Ther 6:1147–1152

Cammilleri S, Sangrajrang S, Perdereau B, Brixy F, Calvo F, Bazin H, Magdelenat H (1996) Biodistribution of iodine-125 tyramine transforming growth factor β antisense oligonucleotide in athymic mice with a human mammary tumor xenograft following intratumoral injection. Eur J Nucl Med 23:448–452

Carlin S et al (2000) Experimental targeted radioiodide therapy following transfection of the sodium iodide symporter gene: effect on clonogenicity in both two-and three-dimensional models. Cancer Gene Ther 7:1529–1536

Cho JY, Xing S, Liu X, Buckwalter TLF, Hwa L, Sferra TJ, Chiu IM, Jhiang SM (2000) Expression and activity of human Na + /I-symporter in human glioma cells by adenovirus-mediated gene delivery. Gene Ther 7:740–749

Claverie JM (2001) What if there are only 30,000 human genes? Science 291:1255–1257

Dadachova E et al (2002) Rhenium-188 as an alternative to Iodine-131 for treatment of breast tumors expressing the sodium/iodide symporter (NIS). Nucl Med Biol 29:13–18

Dewanjee MK, Ghafouripour AK, Kapadvanjwala M, Dewanjee S, Serafini AN, Lopez DM, Sfakianakis GN (1994) Noninvasive imaging of c-myc oncogene messenger RNA with indium-111-antisense probes in a mammary tumor-bearing mouse model. J Nucl Med 35:1054–1063

de Vries EF, van Waarde A, Harmsen MC, Mulder NH, Vaalburg W, Hospers GA (2000) [11C]FMAU and [18F]FHPG as PET tracers for herpes simplex virus thymidine kinase enzyme activity and human cytomegalovirus infections. Nucl Med Biol 27:113–119

Gambhir SS, Barrio JR, Phelps ME, Iyer M, Namavari M, Satyamurthy N, Wu L, Green LA, Bauer E, MacLaren DC, Nguyen K, Berk AJ, Cherry SR, Herschman HR (1999) Imaging adenoviral-directed reporter gene expression in living animals with positron emission tomography. Proc Natl Acad Sci U S A 96:2333–2338

Gambhir SS, Bauer E, Black ME et al (2000) A mutant herpes simplex virus type 1 thymidine kinase reporter gene shows improved sensitivity for imaging reporter gene expression with positron emission tomography. Proc Natl Acad Sci U S A 97:2785–2790

Gati WP, Misra HK, Knaus EE, Wiebe LI (1984) Structural modifications at the 2' and 3' positions of some pyrimidine nucleosides as determinants of their interaction with the mouse erythrocyte nucleoside transporter Biochem Pharmacol 33:3325–3331

(6) Germann C, Shields AF, Grierson JR, Morr I, Haberkorn U (1998) 5-Fluoro-1-(2'-deoxy-2'-fluoro-ß-D-ribofuranosyl)uracil trapping in Morris hepatoma cells expressing the herpes simplex virus thymidine kinase gene. J Nucl Med 39:1418–1423

Glowniak JV, Kilty JE, Amara SG, Hoffman BJ, Turner FE (1993) Evaluation of metaiodobenzylguanidine uptake by the norepinephrine, dopamine and serotonin transporters J Nucl Med 34:1140-1146

Guo J, McLachlan SM, Hutchinson S, Rapoport B (1998) The greater glycan content of recombinant human thyroid peroxidase of mammalian than of insect cell origin facilitates purification to homogeneity of enzymatically protein remaining soluble at high concentration. Endocrinology 139:999–1005

Haberkorn U (1999) Monitoring of gene transfer for cancer therapy with radioactive isotopes. Ann Nucl Med 13:369–377

Haberkorn U, Altmann A (2003) Noninvasive imaging of protein-protein interaction in living organisms. Trends Biotechnol 21:241–243

Haberkorn U, Oberdorfer F, Gebert J et al (1996) Monitoring of gene therapy with cytosine deaminase: in vitro studies using ^{3}H-5-fluorocytosine. J Nucl Med 37:87–94

Haberkorn U, Altmann A, Morr I et al (1997) Gene therapy with herpes simplex virus thymidine kinase in hepatoma cells: uptake of specific substrates. J Nucl Med 38:287–294

Haberkorn U, Khazaie K, Morr I, Altmann A, Müller M, Kaick G. van (1998) Ganciclovir uptake in human mammary carcinoma cells expressing herpes simplex virus thymidine kinase. Nucl Med Biol 25:367–373

Haberkorn U, Altmann A, Jiang S, Morr I, Mahmut M, Eisenhut M (2001a) Iodide uptake in human anaplastic thyroid carcinoma cells after transfer of the human thyroid peroxidase gene. Eur J Nucl Med 28:633–638

Haberkorn U, Henze M, Altmann A, Jiang S, Morr I, Mahmut M, Peschke P, Debus J, W. Kübler, Eisenhut M (2001b) Transfer of the human sodium iodide symporter gene enhances iodide uptake in hepatoma cells. J Nucl Med 42:317–325

Haberkorn U, Altmann A, Eisenhut M (2002) Functional genomics and proteomics — the role of nuclear medicine. Eur J Nuc Med 29:115–132

Haberkorn U, Kinscherf R, Kissel M et al (2003) Enhanced iodide transport after transfer of the human sodium iodide symporter gene is associated with lack of retention and low absorbed dose. Gene Ther 10:774–780

Hannon GJ (2002) RNA interference. Nature 418:244–251

Haubner R, Avril N, Hantzopoulos PA, Gansbacher B, Schwaiger M (2000) In vivo imaging of herpes simplex virus type 1 thymidine kinase gene expression: early kinetics of radiolabelled FIAU. Eur J Nucl Med 27:283–291

Hidaka Y, Hayashi Y, Fisfalen ME, Suzuki S, Takeda T, Refetoff S, DeGroot LJ (1996) Expression of thyroid peroxidase in EBV-transformed B cell lines using adenovirus. Thyroid 6:23–28

Huang M et al (2001) Ectopic expression of the thyroperoxidase gene augments radioiodide uptake and retention mediated by the sodium iodide symporter in non-small cell lung cancer. Cancer Gene Ther 8:612–618

Hustinx R, Shiue CY, Alavi A, McDonald D, Shiue GG, Zhuang H, Lanuti M, Lambright E, Karp JS, Eck S (2001) Imaging in vivo herpes simplex virus thymidine kinase gene transfer to tumour-bearing rodents using positron emission tomography and (^{18}F)FHPG. Eur J Nucl Med 28:5–12

Iwashina T, Tovell DR, Xu L, Tyrrell DL, Knaus EE, Wiebe LI (1988) Synthesis and antiviral activity of IVFRU, a potential probe for the non-invasive diagnosis of herpes simplex encephalitis. Drug Des Deliv 3:309–321

Iyer M et al (2001) Two-step transcriptional amplification as a method for imaging reporter gene expression using weak promoters. Proc Natl Acad Sci U S A 98:14595–14600

Kaufman KD, Filetti S, Seto P, Rapoport B (1990) Recombinant human thyroid peroxidase generated in eukaryotic cells: a source of specific antigen for the immunological assay of antimicrosomal antibodies in the sera of patients with autoimmune thyroid disease. J Clin Endocrinol Metab 70:724–728

Kimura S, Kotani T, Ohtaki S, Aoyama T (1989) cDNA-directed expression of human thyroid peroxidase. FEBS Lett 250:377–380

Kobori N, Imahori Y, Mineura K, Ueda S, Fujii R (1999) Visualization of mRNA expression in CNS using ^{11}C-labeled phosphorothioate oligodeoxynucleotide. Neuroreport 10:2971–2974

La Perle KMD et al (2002) In vivo expression and function of the sodium iodide symporter following gene transfer in the MATLyLu rat model of metastatic prostate cancer. Prostate 50:170–178

Luker GD et al (2002) Noninvasive imaging of protein-protein interactions in living animals. Proc Natl Acad Sci U S A 99:6961–6966

MacLaren DC, Gambhir SS, Satyamurthy N et al (1999) Repetitive non-invasive imaging of the dopamine D2 receptor as a reporter gene in living animals. Gene Ther 6:785–791

Mahony WB, Domin BA, McConnel RT, Zimmerman TP (1988) Acyclovir transport into human erythrocytes. J Biol Chem 263:9285–9291

Mandell RB, Mandell LZ, Link CJ (1999) Radioisotope concentrator gene therapy using the sodium/iodide symporter gene. Cancer Res 59:661–668

Mukhopadhyay T, Tainsky M, Cavender AC, Roth JA (1991) Specific inhibition of K-ras expression and tumorigenicity of lung cancer cells by antisense RNA. Cancer Res 51:1744–1748

Nakamoto Y et al (2000) Establishment and characterization of a breast cancer cell line expressing Na+/I-symporters for radioiodide concentrator gene therapy. J Nucl Med 41:1898–1904

Pacholczyk T, Blakely RD, Amara SG (1991) Expression cloning of a cocaine- and antidepressant-sensitive human noradrenaline transporter. Nature 350:350–354

Paulmurugan R, Umezawa Y, Gambhir SS (2002) Noninvasive imaging of protein-protein interactions in living subjects by using reporter protein complementation and reconstitution strategies. Proc Natl Acad Sci U S A 99:15608–15613

Petrich T et al (2002) Establishment of radioactive astatine and iodine uptake in cancer cell lines expressing the human sodium iodide symporter. Eur J Nucl Med 29:842–854

(Raben D, Buchsbaum DJ, Khazaeli MB et al (1996) Enhancement of radiolabeled antibody binding and tumor localization through adenoviral transduction of the human carcinoembryonic antigen gene. Gene Ther 3:567–580

Ray P et al (2002) Noninvasive quantitative imaging of protein-protein interactions in living subjects. Proc Natl Acad Sci U S A 99:3105–3110

Saito Y, Price R, Rottenberg DA, Fox JJ, Su TL, Watanabe KA, Philipps FA (1982) Quantitative autoradiographic mapping of herpes simplex virus encephalitis with radiolabeled antiviral drug. Science 217:1151–1153

Schellingerhout D, Bogdanov A Jr, Marecos E, Spear M, Breakefield X, Weissleder R (1998) Mapping the in vivo distribution of herpes simplex virions. Hum Gene Ther 9:1543–1549

Shi N, Boado RJ, Pardridge WM (2000) Antisense imaging of gene expression in the brain in vivo. Proc Natl Acad Sci U S A 97:14709–14714

Shimura H et al (1997) Iodide uptake and experimental ^{131}J therapy in transplanted undifferentiated thyroid cancer cells expressing the Na + /I-symporter gene. Endocrinology 138:4493–4496

Sieger S, Jiang S, Schönsiegel F et al (2003) Tumour specific activation of the Sodium/Iodide Symporter Gene under Control of the Glucose Transporter Gene 1 Promoter (GTI-1.3). Eur J Nucl Med 30:748–756

Simonova M, Weissleder R, Sergeyev N, Vilissova N, Bogdanov A (1999) Targeting of green fluorescent protein expression to the cell surface. Biochem Biophys Res Commun 262: 638–642

Smit JW et al (2000) Reestablishment of in vitro and in vivo iodide uptake by transfection of the human sodium iodide symporter (hNIS) in a hNIS defective human thyroid carcinoma cell line. Thyroid 10:939–943

Smit JWA et al (2002) Iodide kinetics and experimental ^{131}I therapy in a xenotransplanted human sodium-iodide symporter-transfected human follicular thyroid carcinoma cell line. J Clin Endocrinol Metab 87:1247–1253

Spitzweg C, Zhang S, Bergert ER et al (1999) Prostate-specific antigen (PSA) promoter-driven androgen-inducible expression of sodium iodide symporter in prostate cancer cell lines. Cancer Res 59:2136–2141

Spitzweg C et al (2000) Treatment of prostate cancer by radioiodine therapy after tissue-specific expression of the sodium iodide symporter. Cancer Res 60:6526–6530

Spitzweg C et al (2001) In vivo sodium iodide symporter gene therapy of prostate cancer. Gene Ther 8:1524–1531

Tavitian B, Terrazzino S, Kühnast B, Marzabal S, Stettler O, Dolle F, Deverre JR, Jobert A, Hinnen F, Bendriem B, Crouzel C, Di Giamberardino L (1998) In vivo imaging of oligonucleotides with positron emission tomography. Nat Med 4:467–471

Tjuvajev JG, Stockhammer G, Desai R, Uehara H, Watanabe K, Gansbacher B, Blasberg RG (1995) Imaging the expression of transfected genes in vivo. Cancer Res 55:6126–6132

Tjuvajev JG, Avril N, Oku T et al (1998) Imaging herpes virus thymidine kinase gene transfer and expression by positron emission tomography. Cancer Res 58:4333–4341

Urbain JL, Shore SK, Vekemans MC, Cosenza SC, DeRiel K, Patel GV, Charkes ND, Malmud LS, Reddy EP (1995) Scintigraphic imaging of oncogenes with antisense probes: does it make sense? Eur J Nucl Med 22:499–504

(79) Watanabe N, Sawai H, Endo K, Shinozuka K, Ozaki H, Tanada S, Murata H, Sasaki Y (1999) Labeling of phosphorothioate antisense oligonucleotides with yttrium-90. Nucl Med Biol 26:239–243

Weissleder R, Simonova M, Bogdanova A et al (1997) MR imaging and scintigraphy of gene expression through melanin induction. Radiology 204:425–429

Wiebe LI, Morin KW, Knaus EE (1997) Radiopharmaceuticals to monitor gene transfer. Q J Nucl Med. 41:79–89

Wiebe LI, Knaus EE, Morin KW (1999) Radiolabelled pyrimidine nucleosides to monitor the expression of HSV-1 thymidine kinase in gene therapy. Nucleosides Nucleotides 18: 1065–1066

Woolf TM, Melton DA, Jennings CGB (1992) Specificity of antisense oligonucleotides in vivo. Proc Natl Acad Sci U S A 89:7305–7309

Wu JC et al (2001) Noninvasive optical imaging of firefly luciferase reporter gene expression in skeletal muscles of living mice. Mol Ther 4:297–306

Zamecnik PC, Stephenson ML (1978) Inhibition of Rous sarcoma virus replication and cell transformation by a specific oligodeoxynucleotide. Proc Natl Acad Sci U S A 75:280–285

Zinn KR, Douglas JT, Smyth CA, Liu HG, Wu Q, Krasnykh VN, Mountz JD, Curiel DT, Mountz JM (1998) Imaging and tissue biodistribution of ^{99m}Tc-labeled adenovirus knob (serotype 5). Gene Ther 5:798–808

Zinn KR, Buchsbaum DJ, Chaudhuri, TR, Mountz JM, Grizzle WE, Rogers-BE (2000) Noninvasive monitoring of gene transfer using a reporter receptor imaged with a high-affinity peptide radiolabeled with ^{99m}Tc or [188]Re. J Nucl Med 41:887–895

Environment-sensitive and Enzyme-sensitive MR Contrast Agents

Manuel Querol and Alexei Bogdanov, Jr.(✉)

Abstract The majority of approved MR contrast agents belong to the class of paramagnetic chelates. These small molecules are uniquely suited to respond to changes in the microenvironment in vivo. These contrast agents can also function as substrates for several classes of enzymes. In both cases, the chelates can be designed in a way that the relaxivity — i.e., the ability of chelated paramagnetic metal cations to shorten the relaxation times of water — is directly affected by changes in the microenvironment. This chapter summarizes a variety of MR contrast agent designs that enable "sensing" of metal cations, pH and enzymatic activity.

1 Introduction

Magnetic resonance imaging (MRI) is routinely used as a tool of clinical radiology. However, discrimination between pathological and normal tissue often requires the use of contrast agents (CAs) that induce local decreases of longitudinal (T_1) and transverse (T_2) relaxation times of the water protons. Such a reduction in relaxation times produces a localized contrast enhancement that allows discrimination of similar types of tissue (Caravan et al. 1999).

Alexei Bogdanov

UMASS Medical School, S2-808 Department of Radiology, 55 Lake Avenue North, Worcester, MA 01655, USA

alexei.bogdanov@umassmed.edu

W. Semmler and M. Schwaiger (eds.), *Molecular Imaging II.*
Handbook of Experimental Pharmacology 185/II.
© Springer-Verlag Berlin Heidelberg 2008

CAs can be divided into two categories depending whether they affect T_1 or T_2. T_1 agents are predominantly based on gadolinium (Gd), whereas T_2 agents include a variety of iron oxide nanoparticles. In 1999, approximately 30% of all clinical MRI protocols used either form of CA (Caravan et al. 1999), currently this ratio has increased 40–50% with Gd-based CAs being by far the most commonly used. Gadolinium is highly paramagnetic due to seven unpaired f-electrons and has a long electronic relaxation time, which makes it the perfect candidate for the development of T_1-CAs. The main problem associated with the use of Gd salts is toxicity. This problem has been solved by chelating Gd^{3+} to various organic ligands with high thermodynamic stability constants, eliminating its toxicity. Figure 1 shows Gd chelating compounds designed for contrast-assisted MRI that were approved for human use.

The first convincing demonstration of tissue-specific contrast by using chelated Gd in vivo was obtained in 1982 (Gries et al. 1982). The research, development and applications of Gd coordination chemistry in medicine was boosted with the first comprehensive survey of paramagnetic metal complexes for NMR imaging by Lauffer (1987) as well as later comprehensive reviews of the field (Lauffer 1990a, 1990b, 1991; Parker and Williams 1996; Aime et al. 1998, 1999a; Aime et al. 1999b, 2002; Caravan et al. 1999, 2001; Louie and Meade 2000; Toth et al. 2002; Caravan 2003; Meade Thomas et al. 2003; Zhang et al. 2003).

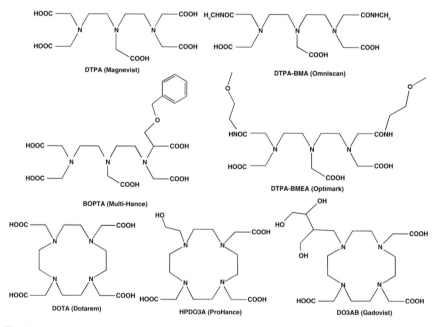

Fig. 1 Chelating compounds and the corresponding Gd contrast agents approved for human use

Relaxivity (molar relaxivity, $r_{i=1,2}$) is the central parameter that reflects the ability of a given CA to generate imaging signal contrast. The relaxivity is defined as relaxation rate of water protons in a 1 mmol/l solution of CA and its value is expressed in mmol l^{-1} s^{-1}. Relaxivity is defined as $1/T_{1,2obs} = 1/T_{1,2d} + r_{1,2}[CA]$, where $T_{1,2obs}$ is the observed relaxation time of a sample in a MR experiment, $T_{1,2d}$ is the diamagnetic contribution to either T_1 or T_2, [CA] is the concentration of contrast agent. The total magnetic relaxation rate enhancement of free water protons (R_1^{obs}) is obtained from three main contributions: one diamagnetic contribution and two paramagnetic contributions. In general, R_1^{obs} is expressed as $R_1^{obs} = R_{1d} + R_{1p}^{IS} + R_{1p}^{OS}$. Diamagnetic contribution (R_{1d}) usually is very similar to the relaxation of pure water. R_{1p}^{IS} is the paramagnetic contribution of the inner coordination sphere and it arises from the exchange of water molecules from the inner coordination sphere with the bulk of water. R_{1p}^{OS} accounts for the paramagnetic effects associated to water molecules that diffuse in the outer coordination sphere of the paramagnetic center. Most of the efforts towards molar relaxivity improvement of Gd have focused on the understanding and tuning of various parameters associated with inner sphere relaxation. R_{1p}^{IS} can be understood as the addition of three factors: reorientation time of the CA (τ_R), i.e., the tumbling time of the CA in the bulk; exchange time (τ_m), i.e., the rate in which a molecule of water at the paramagnetic center exchanges with the bulk; the electronic correlation time (τ_s), which is a parameter that depends on the paramagnetic center and its coordination (Merbach and Toth 2001). Figure 2 shows a representation of all these parameters.

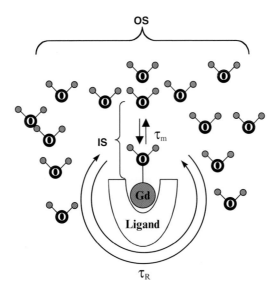

Fig. 2 Schematic representation of parameters influencing relaxivity. *OS* outer sphere, *IS* inner sphere, τ_R reorientation time (tumbling), τ_m exchange time

In the design of new CAs it is usually assumed that relaxivity increase could be theoretically achieved by decreasing τ_R and/or increasing τ_m; i.e., by slowing down the tumbling of the CA in the media and/or increasing the rate of coordinated water exchange with non-coordinated water in the bulk. As water exchange rate depends on the coordination number and geometry of the paramagnetic center, several mechanisms of exchange can be envisioned depending on the paramagnetic coordination number and the steric encumbrance around the coordinated water molecule/s. Two main mechanisms have been proposed: associative and dissociative. The dissociative mechanism is described for a gadolinium center coordinated to only one molecule of water and a dissociative mechanism is mainly anticipated for a gadolinium center coordinated to two water molecules. Between these two extremes, a variety of hybrid mechanisms can be proposed. In general, CAs with a coordination number of 7, i.e., CAs with two molecules of water would have higher relaxivity than its counterpart with only one water molecule coordinated. Generally, the latter statement is true but from a practical point of view, CAs with coordination number 7 tend to be unstable and release gadolinium, which is undesirable (Brucher and Sherry 2001). Nevertheless, recently CAs with coordination number 7 were developed with stability high enough to be used in vivo (Fig. 3) (Aime et al. 1997, 2000, 2004).

The second strategy of CA relaxivity increase is to decrease internal rotation with respect to the solvent. In this scenario several approaches have been undertaken. A first general approach consists of increasing the actual size of the CA. This has been accomplished through the synthesis of polymeric (Kornguth et al. 1990; Marchal et al. 1990; Wang et al. 1990; Van Hecke et al. 1991; Curtet et al. 1998) or dendrimeric (Dong et al. 1998; Clarke et al. 2000) scaffolds that not only are already large and therefore have characteristically slow internal motion but also are capable

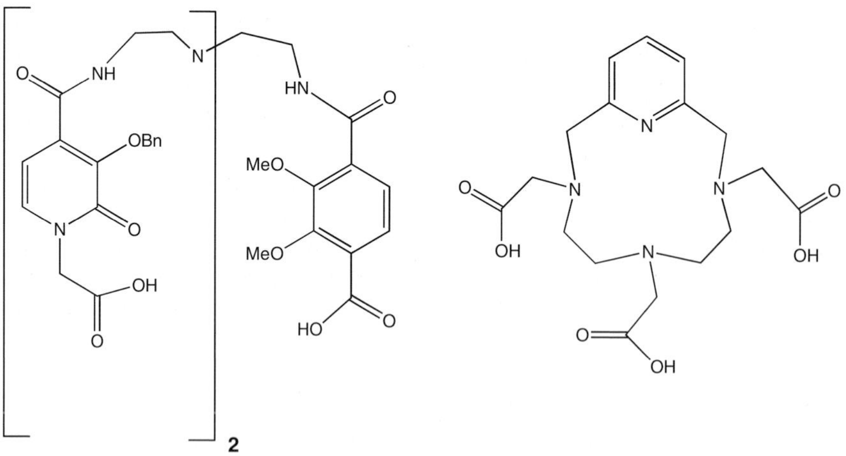

Fig. 3 Chelating units able to form stable (nontoxic) gadolinium complexes with coordination number = 7

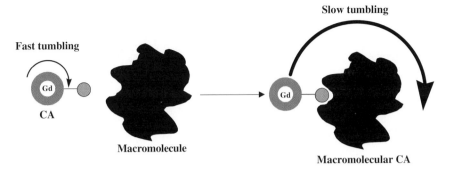

Fig. 4 Change in tumbling rate as a consequence of binding to a macromolecule: a "small" CA before conjugation becomes a "large" CA after conjugation

of hosting large payloads of paramagnetic ions. The second general approach used to decrease the rotational time is based on the concept shown in Fig. 4.

The general principle is in conjugating or noncovalent binding of CA to large molecules [proteins (Sipkins et al. 1998)]. Similar effects have been obtained by synthesizing CA with recognition sintons that can bind to specific receptors (i.e., cell surface receptors) (Artemov et al. 2004), producing as an overall effect the increase of imaging signal mainly due to the effect discussed in this paragraph.

Other strategies based on the formation of supramolecular assemblies, i.e., micelles (Andre et al. 1999), inclusion of CA into liposomes (Fossheim et al. 1998), protein assembly bearing tightly-associated CAs (Frias et al. 2004), supramolecular adduct formation via cyclodextrins (Aime et al. 1991, 1999c) have also been proposed in the literature over the last few years for increasing relaxivity via tuning of rotational times.

In all the examples mentioned so far, the MRI signal enhancement is constant. The relaxivity is either defined by a priori chemical design (relaxivity is considered an intrinsic parameter associated with CA itself) or is a product of a chemical reaction that completely changes the nature of the final CA (formation of a large bioconjugate). Below we present what could be seen as a second generation of CAs whose relaxivity is enhanced in situ by the action of an external stimulus. The external stimuli are functioning as catalysts triggering a cascade of evens that will end up with a change in relaxivity while keeping (within certain parameters) the basic topology of the CA unchanged. From a formal point of view the CAs to be discussed here can be seen as MRI sensors of physiological events having an "off" state associated with low relaxivity in the absence of the stimulus and an "on" state associated with high relaxivity in the presence of the stimulus. The above contrast agents are frequently referred to as "smart" (Fig. 5). At this point, two main stimuli types could be envisioned: stimuli arising from subtle environmental changes, as well as from specific enzymatic catalysis.

First generation CAs

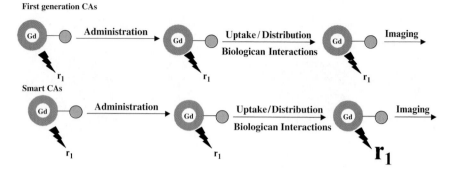

Fig. 5 "Traditional" fix r_1 along the experiment (*top*) versus "smart" variable r_1 along the experiment (*bottom*)

2 Environment-dependent Activatable Contrast Agents

2.1 pH-activatable CAs

It is known that pH in tumor tissue, due to the elevated glycolytic activity, is somewhat lower than in normal tissue. The local tissue pH values range from approximately 7.4 in healthy tissues to about 6.8–6.9 in cancer lesions. This difference, although small, may produce measurable differences in relaxivity by using properly functionalized CAs. A general approach is based on using the acid/base ionization capabilities of certain organic molecules adequately attached to the CA framework in such a way that, depending on their protonation state, they will be able to act as paramagnetic center chelating arms or not. The addition/removal of a chelating arm will induce a change in water coordination number (q) and therefore a pH-induced change in relaxivity (Fig. 6).

This approach was first envisioned by D. Parker and S. Aime (Bruce et al. 2000; Lowe et al. 2001). The principle is in that CA had a Gd-DOTA modified framework bearing a substituted phenyl group attached via a sulphonamide linkage as acid/base-sensing group. The protonation/deprotonation of the sulphonamide unit could be finely tuned by adding various moieties to a phenyl group in the para position to the sulphonamide bond (Fig. 7). This first prototype showed the potential of monitoring pH changes by means of longitudinal relaxation time measurements. The basic structure was further modified to avoid toxicity issues associated to Gd release and also to avoid the possibility of external anion binding to the paramagnetic center. The latter would result in a decrease in relaxivity associated with the increase in the number of inner-sphere water molecules. In general, this approach yielded compounds showing a continuous relaxivity change over the whole pH scale. When the compounds where essayed in solutions mimicking physiological conditions, various relaxivity values were measured at pH = 6.8 and pH = 7.4 and suggested the feasibility of the approach.

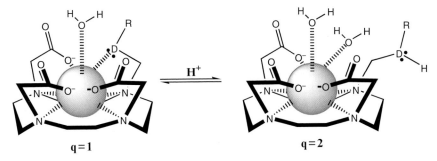

Fig. 6 Scheme of change in coordination number due to protonation/deprotonation

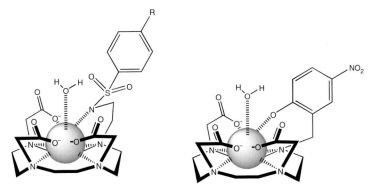

Fig. 7 Examples of pH-activatable CAs: structures proposed in Bruce et al. (2000) and Lowe et al. (2001) (*left*), and in Woods et al. (2004) (*right*)

A similar approach was used by Woods et al. (2004) (Fig. 7). The pH responsive arm of the complex contained a nitrophenyl group, where protonation/deprotonation of phenol served as the driving force for relaxivity change. A Gd(III) complex of a DOTA tetramide was prepared having pH responsiveness along the pH scale (Zhang et al. 1999). The relaxivity of the above pH-sensitive contrast agent increased if pH was increased from 4 to 6, followed by a decrease in the range of pH 6–8.5 and stayed constant between 8.5 to 10.5. This rather unusual pH dependence of relaxivity could be understood in terms of the presence of uncoordinated phosphonate groups of the ligand. The proton of these ionizable groups catalyzes the exchange of protons between the bound water molecule and the bulk by providing an efficient hydrogen bond network in the range of pH 6–9. This network could be disrupted at lower pH by further protonation.

In another approach, tuning of water distribution in the second coordination sphere around the paramagnetic center has been used to prepare yet another pH-dependent CA. The pH sensitivity has been achieved by attaching a hydroxypyridyl moiety to DOTA tetramide chelate (Fig. 8). Depending upon protonation of CA constituents, various relaxivities could be obtained (Woods et al. 2003).

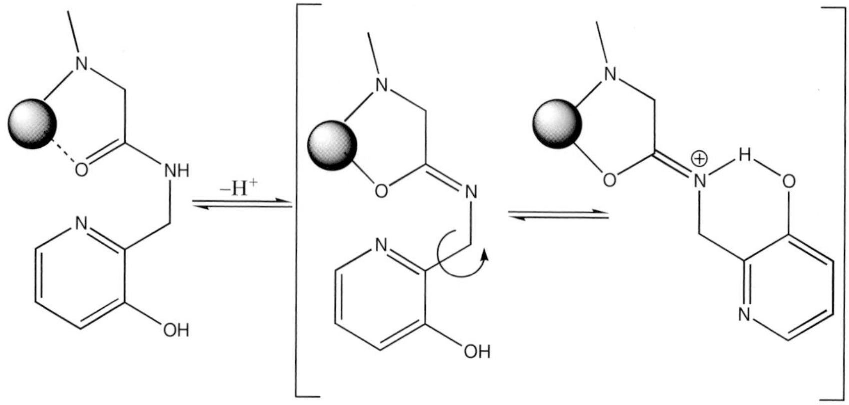

Fig. 8 Hydroxypyridyl moiety equilibria along the pH scale

A fundamentally different approach was used for obtaining pH-responsive poly-meric CA agents. (Aime et al. 1999): 30 Gd-containing chelates were attached to a polymer containing 114 ornitine residues. At pH below 4 the relaxivity was $23\,\mathrm{mM^{-1}s^{-1}}$. This value increased to $32\,\mathrm{mM^{-1}s^{-1}}$ by raising the pH to 8. The difference in relaxivity was rationalized in terms of the effect played by ornitine protonation on rotational time of the CA. It was hypothesized that at the higher pro-tonation level (low pH) the degree of intermolecular association would be low and, therefore, the system would keep a high degree of mobility, while at higher pH val-ues intermolecular association would occur, thereby lowering the degree of freedom of the CA, resulting in an increase in relaxivity.

Acidity-dependent modulation of macromolecular aggregates formation by CAs bearing long alkyl chains mimicking phospholipid structures enabled pH sensitivity (Hovland et al. 2001). Upon pH change the lipophilicity of the individual mole-cules was undergoing a change and so did their ability to form colloidal aggregates. Prominent relaxivity changes (from $7.9\,\mathrm{mM^{-1}s^{-1}}$ at pH below 6 to $19.1\,\mathrm{mM^{-1}s^{-1}}$ at pH above 8) were observed as a result.

The agent based on a microenvironment-responsive polyionic complex formed by a mixture of two polymers (Mikawa et al. 2000) has also been reported. The complex exhibits a 50% increase in relaxivity upon decreasing pH from 7.0 to 5.0. The mechanism of this effect is unknown; however, the complex is detectable in the presence of tumors in mice but is not detectable in their absence.

A pH-responsive CA with activation/deactivation due to changes in proton ex-change rate instead of the water exchange itself was described by Hall et al. (1998). The CA has a strictly planar geometry; this geometry was disrupted by the forma-tion of dinuclear complexes via υ-dioxo bridges at high pH values. By lowering the pH the oxygen in the bridge becomes protonated, breaking the above assembly. This CA showed a steady and reversible relaxivity variation from pH 6 to 7 (Fig. 9).

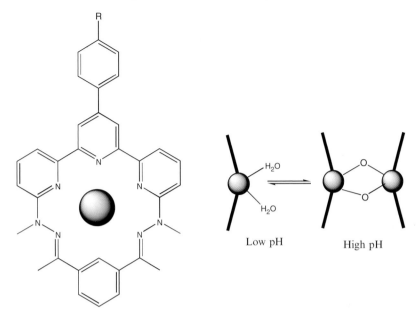

Fig. 9 CA mononuclear structure (*left*). Equilibrium between mononuclear and dinuclear species (*right*)

In another approach, the paramagnetic center of CA was encapsulated in a C_{60} fullerene (Toth et al. 2005). In this case the relaxivity dependence has been explained by variability in degrees of self-association along the pH scale.

By encapsulating Gd within liposomes, a nano-sized pH sensitive agent could be obtained (Lokling et al. 2001). At high pH the relaxivity was low probably due to the lack of surrounding water molecules inside the liposome. By decreasing the pH, the liposome structure changed producing a leakage of CA to the media resulting in a sixfold relaxivity increase. Further studies using this approach showed the instability of the above liposomes at physiological pH. Nevertheless, the leakage of CA at physiological pH has been modulated by adding certain cations (calcium or magnesium) to improve the robustness of the liposomes at the pH of interest.

2.2 Small Ion-responsive CA (Ion-selective Agents)

Many biological signaling events involve divalent cations, i.e., Ca (II), Zn (II) or Fe (II). Because of ultimate biological relevance of cation fluxes and fluctuations, different groups successfully attempted to monitor the presence of cations by using NMR. Calcium (II) is an intracellular secondary messenger involved in many signal transduction mechanisms. Calcium-sensing NMR agent described in (Li et al. 1999, 2002) is based on a well-known calcium fluorescence sensor (Grynkiewicz et al. 1985).

The structure of Ca-sensing molecule contains two classes of functional units, i.e., a specific calcium-chelating unit and two Gd-DOTA derivatives attached to the former one (Fig. 10). Due to the high binding constant of the calcium-chelating moiety in the presence of Ca (II) iminocarboxylates coordinate calcium cation, while in the absence of Ca (II) the same carboxylates rearrange and further stabilize Gd cation chelated by DOTA subunits. Thus, calcium-mediated rearrangements result in q values of 1 or 0, and therefore, depending on Ca(II) concentration, various relaxivity values are obtained.

A similar approach has been suggested by Hanaoka et al. (2002) for developing Zn (II)-sensing agent for MRI (Fig. 11). To impart cation selectivity, two carboxyls of the Gd-DTPA moiety have been functionalized at both ends with Zn (II) chelating units. The Zn (II) chelating unit presents an iminocarboxylate arm that can be either used to chelate Zn (II) or to assist in Gd chelation by the DTPA basic framework. As before, rearrangement of carboxylates results in q-value variability and, therefore, "tunes" relaxivity.

The ability of iron (III) cations to coordinate three bidentate ligands with the formation of an octahedral complex was used to design iron-sensing CAs (Aime et al. 1993; Comblin et al. 1999) via two different mechanisms: (1) the attachment of the paramagnetic chelate to salicylate or phenantroline unit has resulted in the assembly of three individual CA units into a larger supramolecular entity with a slower tumbling rate (Fig. 12); (2) the use of a molecule formed by three paramagnetic centers

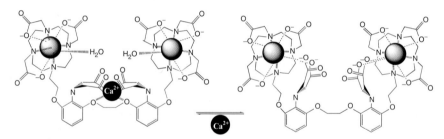

Fig. 10 Calcium-sensitive CA

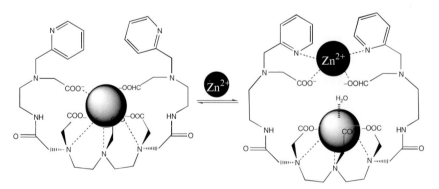

Fig. 11 Zinc-sensitive CA

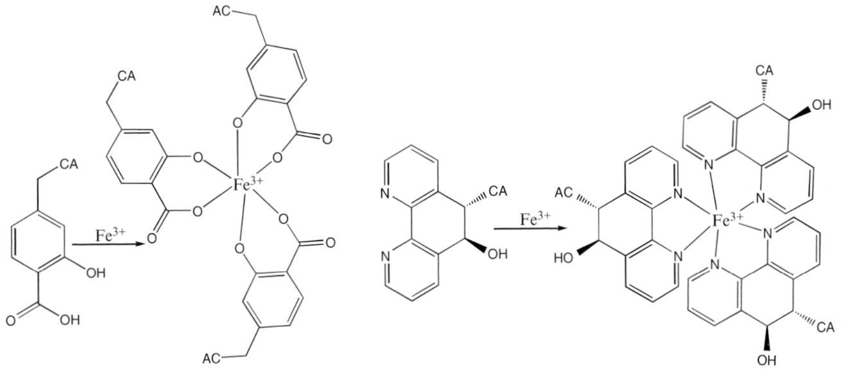

Fig. 12 Iron-sensitive CA

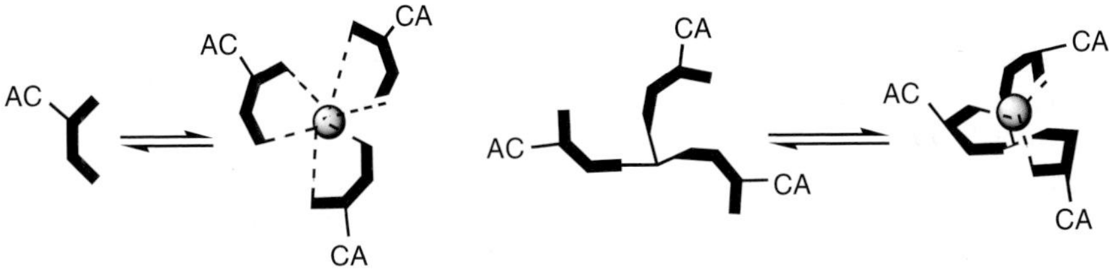

Fig. 13 Alternative approaches to modification of size/rigidity around the paramagnetic center

linked together by a tris-hydroxamate moiety (Fig. 13 *left*). Upon iron chelation by tris-hydroxamate the whole system becomes highly rigid, thereby restricting the free rotation at the gadolinium center and, hence, increasing the relaxivity without any significant size increase (Jacques and Desreux 2002).

Recently, a similar concept was used for preparing supramolecular systems containing two (Costa et al. 2005) or six (Livramento et al. 2005) gadolinium centers. The first system is based on a terpyridine bearing a DTPA-like chelating unit. Chelation to various metals through terpyridine nitrogen achieves the inclusion of two different gadolinium centers on the same aggregate (Fig. 14 *left*). The above approach has been extended to the formation of structures with six gadolinium atoms. Here, two gadolinium chelating units have been attached to a bipyridine (Fig. 14 *right*). Coordination of bipyridine with various metals resulted in six different gadolinium centers contained in "a small molecular space".

2.3 Other Sensing Agents

Temperature and oxygen concentration in blood have also been pursued as sensing agents in the past. First, constant temperature monitoring during tumor hyperthermia therapy was pursued in the past. Although the usefulness of MRI for

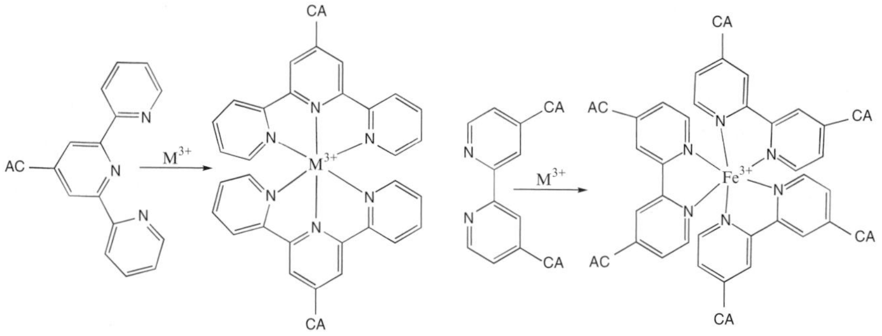

Fig. 14 The use of terpyridines and bipyridines coordination for obtaining multinuclear CAs

monitoring the above therapy is purely hypothetical, a Yb (III) chelate bearing a methyl group whose ^{1}H chemical shift was temperature-dependent (Aime et al. 1996). The report showed a linear dependence of MR signal on temperature within the range studied. Later it was discovered that observed dependence was not exclusively temperature-dependent, but also tissue-dependent. A different approach was later suggested by Fossheim et al. (2000). In this approach, the temperature-dependence of gel-to-liquid crystalline-phase transition in lipid bilayers was used. Liposome-based CA was prepared in such a way that the permeability of the liposome membrane changed in a temperature-controlled fashion, producing a change in water concentration around the encapsulated paramagnetic centers. The above change in water accessibility resulted in relaxivity changes.

The discovery of the paramagnetic properties of deoxyhemoglobin and the widespread use of blood oxygenation effects in functional imaging resulted in attempts to modify the ratio between hemoglobin T and R forms, since these two forms have different oxygen affinities and hence show different paramagnetic effects (Aime et al. 1995). The equilibrium between oxy- and deoxy- forms of hemoglobin is allosterically controlled by a natural effector (2,3-diphosphoglycerate) that binds via electrostatic interactions. The substitution of this effector by a polyphosphonated paramagnetic chelate produced a remarkable fivefold change in relaxivity (Aime et al. 1995).

The redox properties of oxygen where further exploited in (Burai et al. 2000, 2002) by using molecular oxygen to reduce Eu (III) center of a CA to its Gd (III) isoelectronic form Eu (II). This process augmented not only the number of unpaired electrons in the CA but also accounted for a faster water exchange process. The combination of these two effects resulted in a net increase in relaxivity. Aime and co-workers used a similar O_2-mediated redox approach (Aime et al. 2000). The system was based on Mn-porphyrin and the redox equilibrium between Mn (II) and Mn (III). Depending upon the redox state of Mn, different degrees of porphyrin aggregation were obtained, resulting in measurable relaxivity differences associated with variations in tumbling rates.

3 Enzyme-sensitive MR Contrast Agents

In the previous section we included examples of CAs that become activated with no covalent bond formation or cleavage involved. In the current section the ability of certain enzymes to form or to cleave bonds was used as driving force in CA activation. The above mode of activation is probably the most attractive due to the relevance of enzymatic activity as disease biomarkers. Despite its potential, the approach is still at the early stage of development. Nonetheless, several applications of enzyme-sensing CAs have already been well documented. The seminal work appeared in 1997 when β-galactosidase-sensitive paramagnetic substrates were first reported (Moats et al. 1997). A Gd-DOTA derivative was suggested in which the access of water to the paramagnetic gadolinium was hindered by the presence of a galactopyranose moiety attached to the chelating unit via an ether linkage. In the original state, the number of water molecules directly attached to the paramagnetic center (q) was 0.7. After β-galactosidase-mediated cleavage of the ether bond between the chelating unit and the galactopyranose moiety, q reached a value of 1.2. Therefore, enzymatic catalysis resulted in a higher degree of exposure of gadolinium to the surrounding water (Fig. 15). The increase of q value from 0.7 to 1.2 resulted in a relaxivity increase of 40%. Introduction of a methyl group in the arm of a group that was involved in enzymatically cleavable bond formation dramatically improved the rigidity of the system showing a relaxivity increase of ~200%. The apparent change in relaxivity and resultant MR signal intensity allowed successful imaging of *lacZ* gene expression in *X. laevis* embryos. Although CA was introduced into the embryos by microinjection, which circumvented the issue of cell uptake, the potential of this approach appears to be clearly established (Louie et al. 2000).

Recently, the same group reported a similar compound targeted to β-glucuronidase (Duimstra et al. 2005). β-Glucuronic acid has been linked to one of the CA agent arms via an ether bond using a self-immolating spacer as a linker. In this case, enzymatic catalysis resulted in a CA with a lower q value than the original substrate. The mechanism of relaxivity decrease could be summarized as follows: the cleavage of an ether bond in β-glucuronic acid activated a self-immolating cascade reaction from the spacer that freed the chelating arm that was used to interact

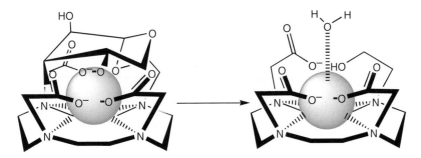

Fig. 15 β-galactosidase-responsive CA proposed in Moats et al. (1997)

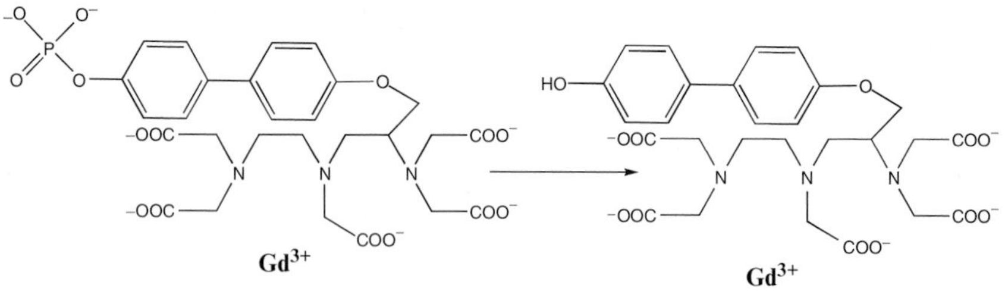

Fig. 16 Alkaline phosphatase-mediated CA activation

with β-glucuronic acid, and this elimination provided the chelating unit with another coordination arm, resulting in an increase in coordination number equivalent
to a decrease in q value.

Further, imaging of other hydrolases via very different approaches for achieving
relaxivity increase has been suggested. While previously hydrolysis of a bond in a
CA was shown to yield various q values, the enzyme was used to change CA binding
to human serum albumin (HSA). In the above scenario, the ultimate end result of
the enzymatic activity is the formation of a supramolecular bioconjugate with slow
rotational times and, hence, with higher relaxivity. This approach exploits the ability
of a hydrophobic group to bind to HSA. The first example is based on the attachment
of a modified 1,1'-dihydroxybiphenyl unit to Gd-DTPA derivative (Lauffer et al.
1997), as shown in Fig. 16. One of the hydroxyl groups of the biphenyl unit was
used to bind a chelating group via an ether bond, while the other hydroxyl group is
blocked by the formation of a hydrophilic phosphonate ester. Alkaline phosphatase-
mediated hydrolysis of the phosphonate ester produces a more hydrophobic form of
the biphenyl moiety, increasing the affinity of the contrast agent to HSA. The overall
affect is a reduction in tumbling time with a concomitant relaxivity increase.

The second example in this category benefits from a very similar approach. In the
latter case, a biphenyl group has been substituted by a short peptide containing HSA
binding sequence attached to trilysine as a terminus (Nivorozhkin et al. 2001). Due
to the charged nature of the peptide attached to the CA, the affinity towards HSA is
low; after enzymatic cleavage [by thrombin activatable fibrinolysis inhibitor (TAFI)]
of the lysine sequence, the remaining peptide chain becomes a suitable target for
HSA binding (Fig. 17). Depending on the exact substitution of the remaining peptide
sequence, the relaxivity increase varied from 2.2-fold (diphenylalanine derivative)
to 2.7-fold (5-diiodotyrosine derivative).

Activatable CAs, which utilize stearase activity in macrophages, have also been
reported. Enzymatic catalysis in this case resulted in changes that completely change
the solubility properties of the CA, transforming a completely insoluble material,
and therefore inactive, into a soluble CA. The design consists in the attachment of
long alkyl chains to both ends of Gd-DTPA via ester linkage (Fig. 18). Due to the
presence of these long aliphatic chains the initial form of the CA is insoluble. Once
the CA has been internalized, the presence of intracellular stearases hydrolyze the
ester linkages, producing the active form of the contrast agents (Aime et al. 2002).

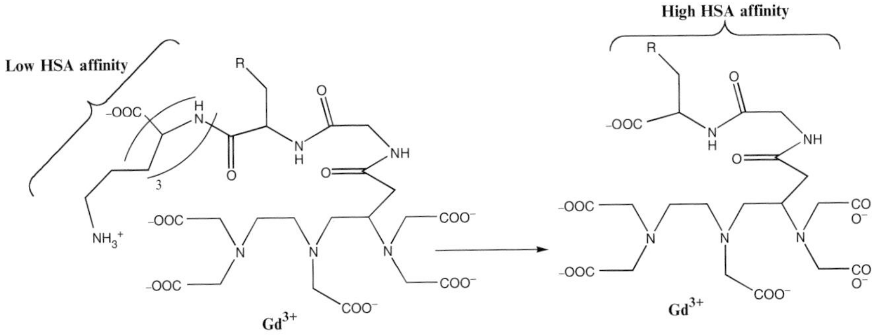

Fig. 17 TAFI-mediated CA activation

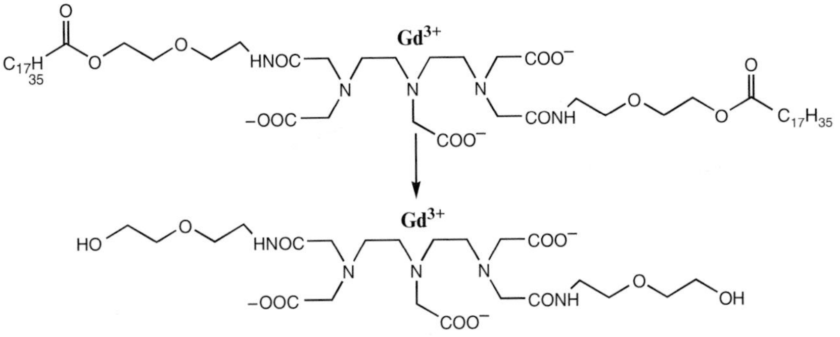

Fig. 18 Stearase-mediate CA activation

Although not many details have been published about this approach, its theoretical scope can be easily envisioned in the imaging of inflammatory processes where the presence of macrophages is ubiquitous.

The strategies shown so far in this section share a common pattern based on the ability of certain enzymes to break specific chemical bonds. However, the above strategy is applicable exclusively for hydrolases, i.e., enzymes that exhibit hydrolytic activity. Recently, a novel CA activation mechanism by means of the oppositely acting enzymes (polymerases and some oxidoreductases) has been suggested. These enzymes catalyze chemical bond formation, either directly or indirectly (Bogdanov et al. 2002). The original concept suggested the possibility of enzyme-mediated in situ oligomerization of specifically functionalized paramagnetic substrates. The hypothesis was that CAs could be activated on site via enzyme-mediated oxidation with subsequent generation of highly reactive species. Thereby generated reactive products would recombine with the formation of oligomers, i.e., larger molecules with longer rotational correlation times. Initially, a monofunctional Gd-DOTA derivative bearing hydroxytyramide (catechol) moiety was tested as a substrate of peroxidase (Fig. 19). Catechols are known to be very efficient in

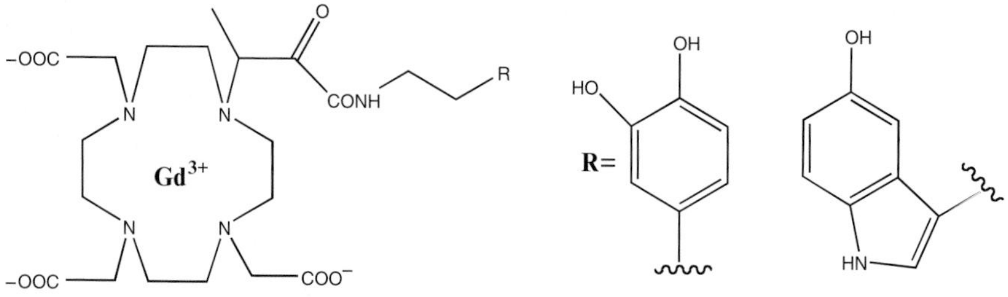

Fig. 19 DOTA-based paramagnetic substrates for peroxidase sensing

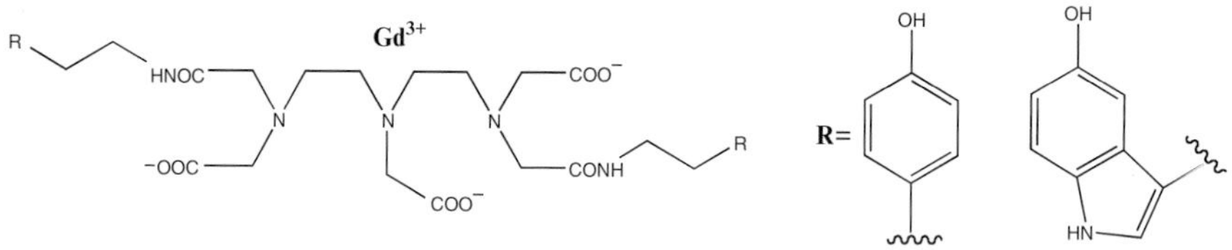

Fig. 20 DTPA-based paramagnetic substrates for peroxidase sensing

reducing oxidized peroxidases. The role of enzymes in such reactions was in the formation of radicals that trigger the oligomerization reaction cascade that results in overall higher molar relaxivity.

In initial feasibility experiments, horseradish peroxidase (HRP) enzyme detection limits were tested and found to be in the nanomolar range. By using a highly specific first antibody, followed by a secondary antibody conjugate with HRP, a targeted imaging concept has been tested using inducible E-selectin expression on the surface of endothelial cells (Bogdanov et al. 2002).

The initial feasibility experiments were followed by substituting the catechol moiety by a serotonin moiety (Chen et al. 2004). Serotonin is a naturally occurring neuromediator that functions in the above case, as a reducing substrate for inflammation-related enzyme myeloperoxidase. Myeloperoxidase is present in vulnerable atherosclerotic plaque (Brennan et al. 2003). The feasibility of sensing MPO in vivo has been tested (Chen et al. 2004) and, therefore, the possibility of imaging atherosclerotic vulnerable plaque recently began to emerge. The above enzyme-mediated oligomerization concept has been further expanded to include CAs bearing two reducing and oligomerizable moieties (Querol et al. 2005). For testing purposes, Gd-DTPA bis-amide derivatives bearing either tyramide or 5-hydroxytryptamide-(serotonin) groups linked to two carboxyls have been prepared (Fig. 20).

The inclusion of two oligomerizable moieties was expected to produce two main beneficial effects, i.e., the increase of the oligomerization degree as well as the induction of potential covalent interaction of oxidized CAs with proteins present in the MPO-rich area (Fig. 21). The preliminary results of the studies that used HRP as a model oxidoreductase have shown higher levels of relaxivity enhancement that in the case of mono-substituted CAs (Querol et al. 2005).

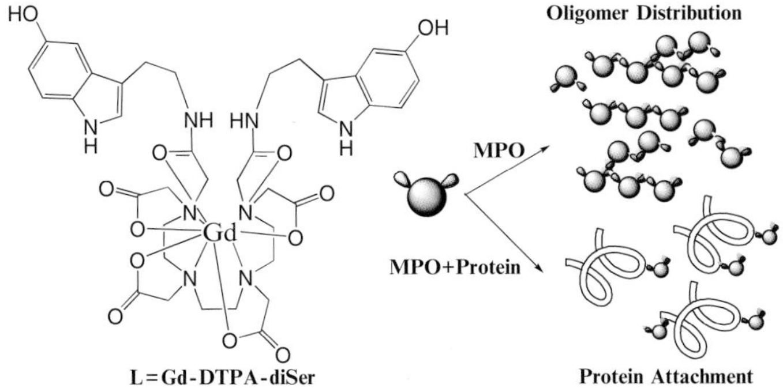

Fig. 21 Proposed mechanism for MPO sensing using DTPA-based paramagnetic substrates

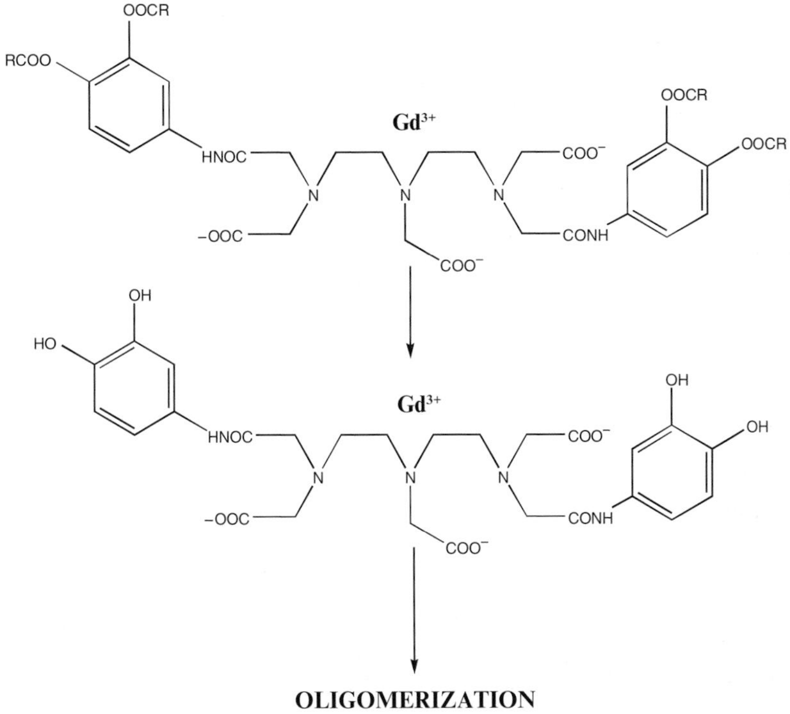

OLIGOMERIZATION

Fig. 22 Stearase/tyrosinase-mediated CA activation

The compounds have been tested in animal models using MPO-containing implants or injected with lipopolysaccharide to induce experimental myositis. Promising MR imaging results were obtained that suggested noninvasive detection of inflammation.

An approach based on oligomerization of oxidized substrates bearing catechol groups for sensing tyrosinase activity has been mentioned by Aime et al. (2002), Fig. 22.

4 Conclusion

The research summarized above suggests that paramagnetic molecules can be potentially employed for probing microenvironments when using MRI in vivo. The reporting ability of MR contrast agents is certainly not limited to paramagnetic probes as superparamagnetic nanoparticles undergo aggregation-disaggregation transitions in response to various stimuli and could function as "probes" of the biological milieu as well. However, paramagnetic chelates are more versatile and controllable in that the structure of small molecules can be fine-tuned through the design to undergo either intramolecular transitions or to be engaged in intermolecular interactions resulting in relaxivity changes in response to structural rearrangements induced by pH, temperature, cations of biologically relevant metals and enzymatic activity. Paramagnetic molecules thus have a potential to become reporter-type MR contrast agents for the needs of research and clinical imaging.

References

Aime S, Ascenzi P et al (1995) Molecular recognition of R- and T-states of human adult hemoglobin by a paramagnetic Gd (III) complex by means of the measurement of solvent water proton relaxation rate. J Am Chem Soc 117(36):9365–9366

Aime S, Botta M et al (1991) Inclusion complexes between b-cyclodextrin and b-benzyloxy-a-propionic derivatives of paramagnetic DOTA- and DTPA-gadolinium (III) complexes. Magn Reson Chem 29(9): 923–927

Aime S, Botta M et al (1993) Paramagnetic gadolinium (III)-iron (III) heterobimetallic complexes of DTPA-bis-salicylamide. Spectrochimica Acta, Part A: Molecular and Biomolecular Spectroscopy 49A(9):1315–1322

Aime S, Botta M et al (1996) A new ytterbium chelate as contrast agent in chemical shift imaging and temperature sensitive probe for MR spectroscopy. Magn Reson Med 35(5):648–651

Aime S, Botta M et al (1997) Synthesis and NMR studies of three pyridine-containing triaza macrocyclic triacetate ligands and their complexes with lanthanide ions. Inorg Chem 36(14): 2992–3000

Aime S, Botta M et al (1999a) 1H and 17O-NMR relaxometric investigations of paramagnetic contrast agents for MRI. Clues for higher relaxivities. Coord Chem Rev 185-186:321–333

Aime S, Botta M et al (1999b) Prototropic and water-exchange processes in aqueous solutions of Gd (III) chelates. Accounts Chem Res 32(11):941–949

Aime S, Botta M et al (1999c) Contrast agents for magnetic resonance imaging: a novel route to enhanced relaxivities based on the interaction of a GdIII chelate with poly-b-cyclodextrins. Chem Eur J 5(4):1253–1260

Aime S, Botta M et al (1999d) Novel paramagnetic macromolecular complexes derived from the linkage of a macrocyclic Gd (III) complex to polyamino acids through a squaric acid moiety. Bioconj Chem 10(2):192–199

Aime S, Botta M et al (2000a) [GdPCP2A(H(2)O)(2)](-): a paramagnetic contrast agent designed for improved applications in magnetic resonance imaging. J Med Chem 43(21):4017–4024

Aime S, Botta M et al (2000b) A p(O2)-responsive MRI contrast agent based on the redox switch of manganese (II/III)-porphyrin complexes. Ang Chem, Intl Ed 39(4):747–750

Aime S, Cabella C et al (2002) Insights into the use of paramagnetic Gd (III) complexes in MR-molecular imaging investigations. J Magn Res Imag 16(4):394–406

Aime S, Cavallotti C et al (2004) Mannich reaction as a new route to pyridine-based polyaminocarboxylic ligands. Org Lett 6(8):1201–1204

Aime S, Fasano M et al (1998) Lanthanide (III) chelates for NMR biomedical applications. Chem Soc Rev 27(1):19–29

Andre JP, Toth E et al (1999) High relaxivity for monomeric Gd(DOTA)-based MRI contrast agents, thanks to micellar self organization. Chem Eur J 5(10):2977–2983

Artemov D, Bhujwalla ZM et al (2004) Magnetic resonance imaging of cell surface receptors using targeted contrast agents. Curr Pharm Biotechnol 5(6):485–494

Bogdanov A Jr, Matuszewski L et al (2002) Oligomerization of paramagnetic substrates result in signal amplification and can be used for MR imaging of molecular targets. Mol Imaging 1(1):16–23

Brennan ML, Penn MS et al (2003) Prognostic value of myeloperoxidase in patients with chest pain. New England J Med 349(17):1595–1604

Bruce JI, Dickins RS et al (2000) The selectivity of reversible oxy-anion binding in aqueous solution at a chiral europium and terbium center: signaling of carbonate chelation by changes in the form and circular polarization of luminescence emission. J Am Chem Soc 122(40): 9674–9684

Brucher E, Sherry AD (2001) Stability and toxicity of contrast agents. In: Merbach AE, Toth E (eds) The chemistry of contrast agents in medical magnetic resonance imaging. Wiley, Chichester, pp 243–281

Burai L, Toth E et al (2000) Solution and solid-state characterization of Eu (II) chelates: a possible route towards redox responsive MRI contrast agents. Chemistry 6(20):3761–3770

Burai L, Scopelliti R et al (2002) EuII-cryptate with optimal water exchange and electronic relaxation: a synthon for potential pO2 responsive macromolecular MRI contrast agents. Chem Commun (20): 2366–2367

Caravan P, Ellison JJ et al (1999) Gadolinium (III) Chelates as MRI contrast agents: structure, dynamics, and applications. Chem Rev 99(9):2293–2352

Caravan P, Zhang Z et al (2001) Paradigms for increasing the relaxivity of MRI contrast agents. Abstracts of Papers, 222nd ACS National Meeting, Chicago, August 26-30, 2001, INOR-213

Caravan P (2003) Targeted molecular imaging with MRI. Abstracts of Papers, 226th ACS National Meeting, New York, September 7–11, 2003, INOR-541

Chen JW, Pham W et al (2004) Human myeloperoxidase: a potential target for molecular MR imaging in atherosclerosis. Magn Reson Med 52(5):1021–1028

Clarke SE, Weinmann HJ et al (2000) Comparison of two blood pool contrast agents for 0.5-T MR angiography: experimental study in rabbits. Radiology 214(3):787–794

Comblin V, Gilsoul D et al (1999) Designing new MRI contrast agents: a coordination chemistry challenge. Coordination Chem Rev 185–186:451–470

Costa J, Ruloff R et al (2005) Rigid MIIL2Gd2III (M = Fe, Ru) complexes of a terpyridine-based heteroditopic chelate: a class of candidates for MRI contrast agents. J Am Chem Soc 127(14):5147–5157

Curtet C, Maton F et al (1998) Polylysine-Gd-DTPAn and polylysine-Gd-DOTAn coupled to anti-CEA F(ab')2 fragments as potential immunocontrast agents. Relaxometry, biodistribution, and magnetic resonance imaging in nude mice grafted with human colorectal carcinoma. Invest Radiol 33(10):752–761

Dong Q, Hurst DR et al (1998) Magnetic resonance angiography with gadomer-17. An animal study original investigation. Invest Radiol 33(9):699–708

Duimstra JA, Femia FJ et al (2005) A gadolinium chelate for detection of beta-glucuronidase: a self-immolative approach. J Am Chem Soc 127(37):12847–12855

Fossheim SL, Fahlvik AK et al (1998) Paramagnetic liposomes as MRI contrast agents: influence of liposomal physicochemical properties on the in vitro relaxivity. Mag Reson Imag 17(1): 83–89

Fossheim SL, Il'yasov KA et al. (2000) Thermosensitive paramagnetic liposomes for temperature control during MR imaging-guided hyperthermia: in vitro feasibility studies. Acad Radiol 7(12):1107–1115

Frias JC, Williams KJ et al (2004) Recombinant HDL-like nanoparticles: a specific contrast agent for MRI of atherosclerotic plaques. J Am Chem Soc 126(50):16316–16317

Gries H, Rosember D et al (1982). Paramagnetische Komplexsalze deren Herstellung and Verwendung bei der NMR-Diagnostik.EP 0 071 564 A1

Grynkiewicz G, Poenie M et al (1985) A new generation of Ca2+ indicators with greatly improved fluorescence properties. J Biol Chem 260(6):3440–3450

Hall J, Haener R et al (1998) Relaxometric and luminescence behavior of triaquahexaazamacrocyclic complexes, the gadolinium complex displaying a high relaxivity with a pronounced pH dependence. New J Chem 22(6):627–631

Hanaoka K, Kikuchi K et al (2002) Design and synthesis of a novel magnetic resonance imaging contrast agent for selective sensing of zinc ion. Chem Biol 9(9):1027–1032

Hovland R, Glogard C et al (2001) Gadolinium DO3A derivatives mimicking phospholipids; preparation and in vitro evaluation as pH responsive MRI contrast agents. J Chem Soc, Perkin Trans 2 (6):929–933

Jacques V, Desreux JF (2002) In: Krause W (ed) Contrast agents I. Springer, Heidelberg Berlin New York

Kornguth S, Anderson M et al (1990) Glioblastoma multiforme: MR imaging at 1.5 and 9.4 T after injection of polylysine-DTPA-Gd in rats. AJNR Am J Neuroradiol 11(2):313–318

Lauffer RB (1987) Paramagnetic metal complexes as water proton relaxation agents for NMR imaging: theory and design. Chem Rev 87(5):901–927

Lauffer RB (1990a) Magnetic resonance contrast media: principles and progress. Magn Reson Q 6(2):65–84

Lauffer RB (1990b) Mechanisms of magnetic resonance contrast enhancement by relaxivity and magnetic susceptibility agents. Invest Radiol 25 Suppl 1:S32–S33

Lauffer RB (1991) Targeted relaxation enhancement agents for MRI. Magn Reson Med 22(2): 339–342

Lauffer RB, McMurry TJ et al (1997). Bioactivated diagnostic imaging contrast agents. Application: WO, (Epix Medical, USA)

Li W-h, Fraser SE et al (1999) A calcium-sensitive magnetic resonance imaging contrast agent. J Am Chem Soc 121(6):1413–1414

Li W-h, Parigi G et al (2002) Mechanistic studies of a calcium-dependent MRI contrast agent. Inorg Chem 41(15):4018–4024

Livramento JB, Toth E et al (2005) High relaxivity confined to a small molecular space: a metallostar-based, potential MRI contrast agent. Angew Chem Int Ed Engl 44(10):1480–1484

Lokling KE, Fossheim SL et al (2001) pH-sensitive paramagnetic liposomes as MRI contrast agents: in vitro feasibility studies. Mag Reson Imag 19(5):731–738

Louie AY, Huber MM et al. (2000) In vivo visualization of gene expression using magnetic resonance imaging. Nat Biotech 18(3):321–325

Louie AY, Meade TJ (2000) Recent advances in MRI: novel contrast agents shed light on in vivo biochemistry. Trends Biochem Sci, pp 7–11

Lowe MP, Parker D et al (2001) pH-dependent modulation of relaxivity and luminescence in macrocyclic gadolinium and europium complexes based on reversible intramolecular sulfonamide ligation. J Am Chem Soc 123(31):7601–7609

Marchal G, Bosmans H et al (1990) MR angiography with gadopentetate dimeglumine-polylysine: evaluation in rabbits. AJR Am J Roentgenol 155(2):407–411

Meade TJ, Taylor AK, Bull SR (2003) New magnetic resonance contrast agents as biochemical reporters. Curr Opin Neurobiol 13(5):597–602

Merbach AE, Toth E (2001) The chemistry of contrast agents in medical magnetic resonance imaging. Wiley, Chichester

Mikawa M, Miwa N et al (2000) Gd(3+)-loaded polyion complex for pH depiction with magnetic resonance imaging. J Biomed Mater Res 49(3):390–305

Moats RA, Fraser SE et al (1997) A "smart" magnetic resonance imaging agent that reports on specific enzymic activity. Angew Chem, Int Ed 36(7):726–728

Nivorozhkin A L, Kolodziej AF et al (2001) Enzyme-activated Gd3+ magnetic resonance imaging contrast agents with a prominent receptor-induced magnetization enhancement. Angew Chem, Int Ed 40(15):2903–2906

Parker D, Williams JAG (1996) Getting exited about lanthanide complexation chemistry. J Chem Soc, Dalton Transactions (18):3613–3628

Querol M, Chen JW et al (2005) DTPA-bisamide-based MR sensor agents for peroxidase imaging. Org Lett 7(9):1719–1722

Sipkins DA, Cheresh DA et al (1998) Detection of tumor angiogenesis in vivo by alphaVbeta3-targeted magnetic resonance imaging. Nat Med 4(5):623–626

Toth E, Helm L et al (2002) Relaxivity of MRI contrast agents. Top Curr Chem 221:61–101

Toth E, Bolskar RD et al (2005) Water-soluble gadofullerenes: toward high-relaxivity, pH-responsive MRI contrast agents. J Am Chem Soc 127(2):799–805

Van Hecke P, Marchal G et al. (1991) NMR imaging study of the pharmacodynamics of polylysine-gadolinium-DTPA in the rabbit and the rat. Magn Reson Imaging 9(3):313–321

Wang SC, Wikstrom MG et al (1990) Evaluation of Gd-DTPA-labeled dextran as an intravascular MR contrast agent: imaging characteristics in normal rat tissues. Radiology 175(2):483–488

Woods M, Zhang S et al (2003) pH-sensitive modulation of the second hydration sphere in lanthanide (III) tetraamide-DOTA complexes: a novel approach to smart MR contrast media. Chem Eur J 9(19):4634–4640

Woods M, Kiefer GE et al (2004) Synthesis, relaxometric and photophysical properties of a new pH-responsive MRI contrast agent: the effect of other ligating groups on dissociation of a p-nitrophenolic pendant arm. J Am Chem Soc 126(30):9248–9256

Zhang S, Wu K et al (1999) A novel pH-sensitive MRI contrast agent. Angew Chem, Int Ed 38(21):3192–3194

Zhang S, Merritt M et al (2003) PARACEST agents: modulating MRI contrast via water proton exchange. Accounts of Chem Res 36(10):783–790

Part IV
Molecular Targets and Biomarkers for Imaging

Peptides, Multimers and Polymers

I. Dijkraaf and H.J. Wester(✉)

Abstract Due to their favorable properties and pharmacokinetics, peptides are often regarded as "agents of choice" for imaging and radiotherapy. Chemical strategies have been developed that allow their site specific labeling with various radionuclides for PET and SPECT, without compromising their biological integrity. Together with the overexpression of a wide range of peptide receptors and binding

H.J. Wester
Department of Nuclear Medicine, Technische Universität München, Ismaninger Strasse 22, 81675 München, Germany
h.j.wester@lrz.tum.de

W. Semmler and M. Schwaiger (eds.), *Molecular Imaging II.*
Handbook of Experimental Pharmacology 185/II.
© Springer-Verlag Berlin Heidelberg 2008

sites on tumor cells or matrix components, this class of compounds offers multiple imaging applications. Furthermore, radiolabeled peptides have great potential as carrier molecules for site-specific delivery of other signalling units, such as fluorescent moieties, cyctotoxic compounds or metals for magnetic resonance imaging. In addition, great efforts have been made to exploit the favorable characteristics of peptides for the development of larger constructs, such as multimeric ligands, polymer-peptide conjugates and "peptide-coated" liposomes and nanoparticles. Some peptides have already entered clinical routine application; some are currently being evaluated in clinical studies. However, a variety of peptides is still "waiting" to enter the imaging arena. This chapter presents a brief overview of the highly active field of peptide radiopharmaceuticals and the future potential of multimeric and polymeric peptide constructs.

1 Introduction

Antibodies have become valuable and important probes for radioimmunoimaging and, especially, radioimmunotherapy. In addition, great efforts have been made to develop medium-sized proteins and even small peptides to generate high-affinity probes with improved pharmacokinetics. Consequently, an impressive collection of peptide constructs is currently being evaluated to overcome the drawback connected with the application of intact antibodies (Huhalov and Chester 2004; Sharkey and Goldenberg 2005). Table 1 summarizes major characteristics of peptides and

Table 1 The major characteristics of peptides and proteins and the particular role and potential of peptides for the development of radiopharmaceuticals

Peptides	Proteins
Small size (5–20 amino acids)	Large size (IgG: $\sim 1,500$ amino acids)
Easy preparation via solution- or solid phase peptide synthesis (SPPS)	Laborious recombinant production in bacteria or mammalian cell lines
Easy radiolabeling with diverse radiolabeling techniques	Restricted palette of radiolabeling strategies
Toleration of harsh conditions during chemical modification or radiolabeling	Reactions only possible in aqueous media under mild conditions
Easy purification of radiolabeled peptides (n.c.a. preparations)	Separation of radiolabeled protein from unlabeled precursor not possible (c.a. conditions unavoidable)
Possibility for easy and specific modification of any given amino acid in the sequence including the termini	Either nonspecific modification of a certain type of amino acid or time-consuming modification via site-directed mutagenesis
Tunable rate and route of excretion via chemical derivatization	Rate and route of excretion are determined by physicochemical properties of the protein
Rapid clearance from blood and nontarget organs ($t_{1/2}$ in blood <1 h)	Slow clearance from blood and nontarget organs
High tumor-to-background ratios	Low tumor-to-background ratios
High tumor penetration	Low tumor penetration
Low immunogenicity	Immunogenicity is not neglectable

proteins and highlights the particular role and potential of peptides for the development of radiopharmaceuticals. Peptides are large enough to tolerate direct radiolabeling or complexation of radiometals via conjugation of often bulky chelates, or can be used as vehicles for fluorescent groups or other site-specific targeting of a payload. If properly placed, even large modifications do not affect the receptor affinity. They are easily prepared by solid-phase peptide chemistry and thus allow a cost-effective large-scale production under GMP conditions (Wester et al. 2004; Krenning et al. 2004; Stefanidakis and Koivunen 2004). A variety of labeling techniques can be applied: on the resin (labeling on the solid support), direct (radioiodination), via prosthetic groups (site-specific and selective methods) or by attachment of chelates for radiolabeling with a battery of radiometals for PET, SPECT or therapeutic applications. In contrast to proteins, peptides withstand harsh conditions (low or high pH, high temperature, organic solvents, etc.) and can be prepared, if necessary, as no-carrier-added radiopharmaceuticals using standard HPLC equipment and conditions. They often exhibit excellent pharmacokinetics, fast blood clearance, low hepatobiliary excretion, and renal elimination. In contrast to proteins, they have excellent tissue penetration, minimal side effects and no antigenicity.

Owing to high affinity to their corresponding receptor, a usual high overexpression of the corresponding receptor and the fast elimination characteristics, peptides offer all basic requirements for reaching high target-to-background ratios in vivo.

Apart from solid-phase peptide synthesis and rational design, phage display has become an important tool to select and identify peptides with high affinity for new and relevant targets. Similar to endogenous peptide hormones, phage-displayed peptides consist of members of the 20 natural L-amino acids. Thus, a limited stability, due to rapid degradation by proteases in the circulation, is their major drawback. Consequently, except for a few examples (e.g., VIP), peptide radiopharmaceuticals are stabilized, e.g., by the introduction of D-amino acids, N-methylation, C-terminal amidation or reduction, N-terminal acylation or methylation, substitution of peptide bonds, the use of artificial (non-natural) amino acids, conjugation of sugar residues, cyclization or the formation of higher structures. Hence, radiolabeled peptides have been introduced as powerful radiopharmaceuticals into the diagnostic (Breeman et al. 2001; Haubner et al. 2005; Wester et al. 2004) and therapeutic field (de Jong et al. 2003; Signore et al. 2001), a development which generally corroborates the "peptide" concept.

2 Peptide Synthesis

2.1 Solid-phase Peptide Synthesis

Solid-phase peptide synthesis (SPPS) is currently the method of choice. Generally, this method is based on the sequential elongation of a solid-phase (resin)-bonded first amino acid by other amino acids. The functional groups of the side chains are commonly protected until the entire peptide is cleaved from the resin. Thus, the

1. Attachment of the first di-protected
   amino acid A to the resin

2. Selective deprotection,
   side chain remains protected

3. Coupling of a second di-protected
   amino acid B.

4. Repetition (n times) of step 2

5. Repetition (n times) of step 3

6. Cleavage of the peptide (C-B_n-A) from the resin
   and (simultaneous) deprotection of side chains
   (B represents different amino acids during the
   peptide elongation step)

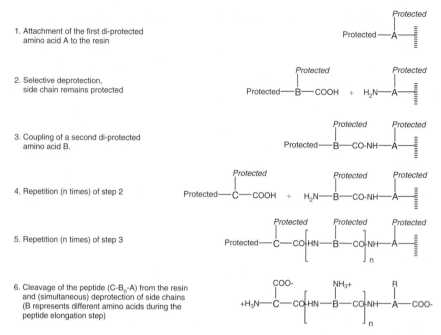

Fig. 1 Schematic representation of solid-phase peptide synthesis (SPPS) consisting of a resin-based elongation of the peptide by sequential couplings of amino acids followed by cleavage from the resin and (simultaneous) side chain deprotection

permanent side chain protection allows the selective deprotection of the functional group of the intermediate resin-bonded peptide chain necessary for coupling of the next amino acid. This process is repeated until the desired peptide is completely assembled and cleaved from the resin (Fig. 1).

The SPPS has several advantages over solution-phase peptide synthesis. Intermediate purification steps are fast (washing of the resins) and only minimum optimization of the reaction conditions is necessary (standardized procedures). Thus, automated peptide synthesizers are often used, although comparable results are also obtained manually by using disposable plastic syringes with suitable frits or flask shakers.

2.2 Phage Display

Phage-display technology is an approach to identify peptide molecules as potential pharmaceuticals (Smith 1985). A phage-display "library" is a mixture of various phages expressing different peptides on their surface. Although each phage clone displays only one special peptide, the entire library represents a huge variety of different peptides, which are expressed either as linear or constrained sequences.

To accomplish a selection of the phages which express peptides with high affinity to a receptor, an antibody or a tissue, the phage library is passed over the immobilized target molecules. The clones with high affinity are captured, while clones with low or no affinity are eluted though the column. After several cycles of selection, the primary structure of the foreign peptides (candidates) is characterized by sequencing the peptide-coding sequence in the viral DNA (Landon et al. 2004). Although this method allows for a fast selection of new peptides, one major drawback limits the usefulness of this methodology: since only L-amino acids are incorporated, phage-displayed peptides commonly exhibit only low in-vivo stability. Thus, high-affinity binders selected by phage display should be considered as first lead structures, and generally laborious and time-consuming optimizations (e.g., incorporation of D-amino acids, modification of lipophilicity, etc.) are necessary to obtain suitable in-vivo candidates.

A variation of this method, the in-vivo injection of a phage-display library and the analysis of the clones retained in a tissue of interest, has significantly contributed to the identification of new targets, which have been successfully used for directed vascular targeting in preclinical animal models (Hajitou et al. 2006).

3 Radiolabeling of Peptides

Most of the techniques developed for radiolabeling of peptides are also suitable for radiolabeling of larger proteins or monoclonal antibodies. According to George deHevesy's definition of a tracer, a good labeling method will not affect the biological properties, the affinity to the target, or the physicochemical properties (charge, hydrophilicity, size, etc.). Thus, a radiolabeled peptide synthesized by *isotopic* labeling (e.g., incorporation of ^{35}S-methionine) would result in an ideal tracer, but would not necessarily represent a valuable radiopharmaceutical. Thus, other features, such as stability of the label against in-vivo cleavage (e.g., deiodination, defluorination, transcomplexation), stability of the prosthetic group, ease and yield of labeling or amount of peptide necessary for labeling, are more important for peptide radiopharmaceuticals.

3.1 Radioiodination

Similar to proteins, direct introduction of radioiodine by electrophilic iodination of tyrosine residues using Iodogen or chloramine-T is the most straightforward approach to produce valuable experimental radiopeptides for first-line in-vitro and in-vivo evaluation. If there are no tyrosine residues present in the peptide sequence, phenylalanines can often be replaced by tyrosines without significant effects. Since directly iodinated peptides usually suffer from fast deiodination in vivo, prosthetic groups such as N-succinimidyl 3-iodobenzoates or 5-iodo-3-pyridinecarboxylate

(SIPC) have been developed. They allow the production of radioiodinated peptides with high stability against deiodination via amide formation with free lysine residues. In most cases (i.e., with small peptides), this improvement is accompanied by a significant increase in lipophilicity, which in turn generates the need for further optimizations, e.g., the introduction of a pharmacokinetic modifier (polyethylene glycol or carbohydrates).

3.2 Radiofluorination

Due to the limitations of nucleophilic ^{18}F-fluorination, prosthetic group labeling is the only reasonable route to peptides with high specific activity. Direct electrophilic fluorination methods are unsuitable, since the products exhibit low specific activity. Thus, these preparations are of limited value for imaging of saturable biological targets with low capacity, e.g., receptors.

The commonly used methodology for efficient peptide ^{18}F-labeling includes the preparation of ^{18}F-labeled synthons (prosthetic groups), which are subsequently activated or, in a few cases, conjugated to the peptides or proteins without activation. Acylation procedures have been found to be the most valuable methods with respect to overall yields, remote-controlled synthesis, and in-vivo stability and, thus, have been successfully applied to the labeling of some interesting peptides. However, the multistep procedures employed are time-consuming and necessitate some practice. Very recently a novel and promising two-step methodology was developed for the chemoselective ^{18}F-labeling of peptides (Fig. 2). By using the oxime ligation, this ^{18}F-labeling approach was successfully applied for the high-yield routine ^{18}F-labeling and clinical imaging.

3.3 Radiolabeling with ^{68}Ga

Inspired by the excellent image quality of $[^{68}\mathrm{Ga}]$DOTATOC PET studies and the commercial availability of small-sized ^{68}Ge/^{68}Ga-generators ($t_{1/2}$ ^{68}Ge $= 268$d), this isotope has gained considerable attention in recent years. Furthermore, with the two other Ga-isotopes of interest (^{66}Ga : $t_{1/2} = 9.5$h; ^{67}Ga : $t_{1/2} = 78.3$h) the field of potential applications is broad. DOTA (1,4,7,10-tetraazacyclododecane-1,4,7,10-tetraacetic acid) is commonly used as chelator for gallium and has found widespread application for peptide labeling (Fig. 3). Detailed studies on the optimization of the labeling conditions for DOTA-peptides (pH, buffer, conventional or microwave heating) have been published (Velikyan et al. 2004). Another chelator successfully evaluated in animal models is 1,4,7-tricarboxymethyl-1,4,7-triazacyclononane (NOTA). A trithiolate tripodal bifunctional ligand for the radiolabeling of peptides with gallium has recently been developed but still has to show suitability in vivo (Luyt and Katzenellenbogen 2002).

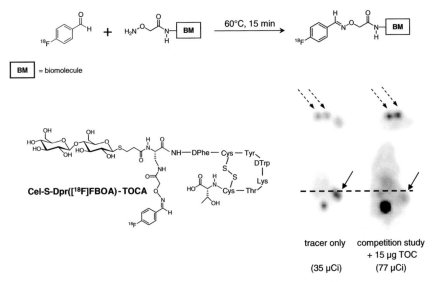

Fig. 2 *Upper panel*: Chemoselective oxime formation between n.c.a. 4-[¹⁸F]fluoro-benzaldehyde and an aminooxyacetyl-functionalized biomolecule. *Lower panel*: Structure of Cel-*S*-Dpr([¹⁸F]FBOA)TOCA and axial (*upper images*) and coronar (*lower images*) PET images of AR42J tumor-bearing nude mice 45–65 min p.i. of Cel-*S*-Dpr([¹⁸F]FBOA)TOCA. For control, only the ¹⁸F-labeled peptide was injected. For competition studies, 15 μg of cold Tyr³-octreotide (TOC) were coinjected. The amount of activity injected is given *in parentheses*. *Solid arrows* indicate the tumor, *dashed arrows* indicate the kidneys. The *dashed line* in the coronar images represents the plane of the axial image above

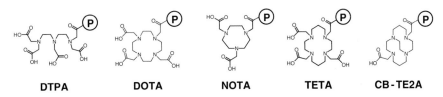

Fig. 3 Structures of chelators commonly used for peptide radiometallation. The *P* on the upper right side of the respective chelators indicates the site of attachment to the peptide via an amide bond

3.4 Radiolabeling with Cu

The advantage of ^{64}Cu ($T_{1/2} = 12.7$ h) is that it has b$^-$ (0.579 MeV, 39%) and b$^+$ (0.653 MeV, 17%) emission and can be made by a reactor or medical cyclotron ($S_A = 222$–1850 GBq/nmol). In addition, a number of other isotopes suitable for imaging and targeted radiotherapy are available (^{60}Cu, ^{62}Cu, ^{67}Cu). For complexation, macrocyclic ligands such as TETA (1,4,8,11-tetraazacyclotetradecane-N,N',N'',N'''-tetraacetic acid) and CB-TE2A (4,11-bis(carboxymethyl)-1,4,8,11-tetraazabicyclo[6.6.2]hexadecane) have been evaluated (Smith 2004) (Fig. 3). CB-TE2A was found to be an attractive alternative to TETA and a superior chelator for ^{64}Cu compared with TETA. Compared with ^{64}Cu-TETA-Y3-TATE, ^{64}Cu-CB-TE2A-Y3-TATE showed improved liver and blood clearance, resulting in higher tumor-to-tissue ratios. Further modifications to CB-TE2A to reduce the net positive charge of the Cu(II) complex may additionally improve in-vivo behavior of those conjugates (Sprague et al. 2004).

3.5 Radiolabeling with ^{99m}Tc

Although direct labeling has also been investigated for the synthesis of ^{99m}Tc-labeled peptides, examples are rare and have not found entrance into clinical studies so far. For direct labeling, the same agent responsible for the in-situ reduction of ^{99m}TcO$_4^-$ from the generator is used for reducing disulfide bridges into free thiols subsequently used to bind ^{99m}Tc. Direct labeling usually results in peptides with unclear coordination chemistry and poor in-vivo stability.

Indirect methods exploit bi-functional chelating agents (BFCAs), which are attached to the peptide (during or after SPPS). One part of the molecule coordinates the technetium, whereas the second function covalently binds the chelator to the peptide, often by introduction of a suitable spacer. The most widely applied BFCAs are based on a combination of nitrogen (amide, amine, imine) and sulfur (thiol, thioether) donors to give the class of N$_x$S$_{4-x}$ ligands. These ligands coordinated $[^{99m}$Tc=O$]^{3+}$ very efficiently and at low concentrations. A prominent member is MAG$_3$ (mercapto acetyl-glycyl-glycyl-glycine) (Fig. 4). One alternative to the

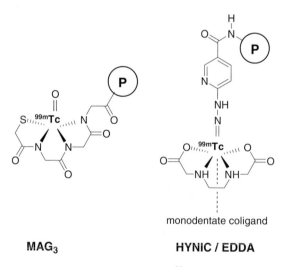

monodentate coligand

MAG$_3$ **HYNIC / EDDA**

Fig. 4 Structures of chelates most commonly used for ^{99m}Tc-labeling of peptides. The *P* on the upper right side of the respective chelates indicates the site of attachment to the peptide via an amide bond

N_xS_{4-x} ligands is the three-plus-one approach, using a monodentate (thiol) and a tridentate (SXY; X=O,N,S, Y=N,S) ligand to coordinate $[^{99m}Tc=O]^{3+}$. Another route for labeling with ^{99m}Tc, the HYNIC (hydrazine nicotinic acid) approach, is widely used but its coordination chemistry not well understood. The structure depicted in Fig. 4 is rationalized on the basis of the need for auxiliary ligands to stabilize the complex, such as ethylene diamine tetraacetic acid (EDDA) or tricine. Further improvement of stability has been reached by additional mondentate coligands, such as phosphines. A more recent route employs tridentate BFCAs to introduce the $[^{99m}Tc(CO_3)]^+$ core into peptide pharmaceuticals. $[^{99m}Tc(CO_3)]^+$ can easily be synthesized via a kit procedure (IsoLink, Mallinckrodt). Histidine is a highly efficient ligand, allowing easy labeling of His-tagged molecules. A variety of ligands have been developed, and the first $[^{99m}Tc(CO_3)]^+$ peptides have already been applied in first human studies. For a detailed review of the ^{99m}Tc-labeling chemistry, *see* Alberto (2003, 2007) and references therein.

4 Peptides for Imaging

4.1 Somatostatin

The physiological action of somatostatin (SS-14 and SS-28) is mediated by the five G-protein-coupled receptor (GPCR) subtypes sst1–sst5. Each of the subtypes is coupled to different intracellular signaling systems. The antimitotic activity of somatostatin derivatives has been related to sst1 and sst2, sst3 has been found to induce apoptosis, and sst5 inhibits cell proliferation. As GPCR, ssts, after internalization, are directed to the endosomes and either recycled to the cell membrane or degraded to lysosomes. Ssts have been found to form homo- and heterodimers (Krantic et al. 2004).

Because sstr was found to be highly expressed in a variety of tumors (Reubi 2003), the somatostatin receptor system and the corresponding ligands have been extensively studied and evaluated.

The cyclic octapeptide octreotide was the first peptide to be evaluated as an imaging agent for in-vivo tumor targeting. Although initial studies were successful using the radioiodinated derivative $[^{123}I]Tyr^3$-octreotide (Krenning et al. 1989), subsequent studies demonstrated the major drawback of this tracer, i.e., unsuitable pharmacokinetics and clearance (Bakker et al. 1996). In contrast, radiometallated peptides offer the advantage of fast and "kit"-like radiolabeling and were also found to possess superior imaging properties, i.e., reduced lipophilicity. Consequently, a ^{111}In-labeled derivative (^{111}In-DTPA-octreotide, Octreoscan) was the first agent for peptide-receptor imaging on the market. Due to the higher sst2 affinity, octreotide was replaced in most of the following studies by the Tyr^3 analogue (TOC). Today, further analogues, such as $[^{68}Ga]DOTA$-Tyr^3-octreotide [DOTA-TOC] (Hofmann et al. 2001; Henze et al. 2001; Maecke et al. 2005), as well as

[90Y]DOTATOC (de Jong et al. 1997; Stolz et al. 1997; Kwekkeboom et al. 2005; Bodei et al. 2004) and [177Lu]DOTATOC (and their Thr[8] analogues DOTATATE (Kwekkeboom et al. 2001; de Jong et al. 2001), have gained significant clinical relevance for PET imaging and peptide receptor radiotherapy. In addition, ^{18}F-labeled compounds with excellent properties for in-vivo imaging and quantification were developed and evaluated in animal models and patients (Wester et al. 2003; Schottelius et al. 2004, 2005). In analogy to data obtained with RGD peptides, conjugation with carbohydrates was found to be the method of choice for making the originally too lipophilic peptides valuable tracers (Meisetschlager et al. 2006) (Figs. 2 and 5).

Compared with most of the existing sst radiotracers, which exhibit high affinity only for the somatostatin receptor subtype 2 (sst$_2$), [68Ga]DOTANOC is a first

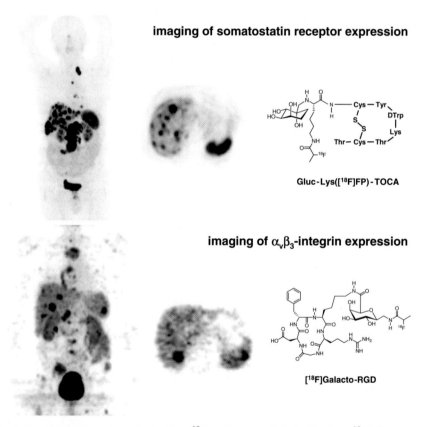

Fig. 5 *Upper panel*: Structure of Gluc-Lys([18F]FP)TOCA and (*left*) Gluc-Lys([18F]FP)TOCA-PET of a patient with an intestinal carcinoid with extended hepatic metastasis as well as mediastinal and paraaortal lymph node metastases; accumulation in the spleen is physiological; *middle*: corresponding axial view trough liver and spleen. *Lower panel*: Structure of [18F]Galacto-RGD and (*left*) [18F]Galacto-RGD-PET (maximum intensity projection) of a patient with a carcinoid of the lung and multiple osseous, hepatic and lienal metastases; *middle*: corresponding axial view trough liver and spleen

compound for PET imaging with high affinity for sst2 and sst5 (Wild et al. 2003) (IC_{50} nM: sst2, 1.9 ± 0.4; sst5, 7.2 ± 1.6). Compared with DOTATOC, more lesions were visible with this new tracer. The difference was attributed to different receptor-binding profiles of the ligands and the corresponding receptor-expression profiles of the metastases (Wild et al. 2005b).

Although being the most extensively studied receptor system in vivo, it seems as though the somatostatin receptor system is still not fully understood. Recently, the ^{111}In-labeled DOTA-conjugated somatostatin receptor-selective peptide antagonists [NH_2-CO-c(DCys-Phe-Tyr-DAgl^8(Me,2-naphthoyl)-Lys-Thr-Phe-Cys)-OH (sst3-ODN-8) and DOTA-[4-NO_2-Phe-c(DCys-Tyr-DTrp-Lys-Thr-Cys)-DTyr-NH_2] (sst2-ANT)] have been evaluated in mice bearing sst3- and sst2-expressing tumors (Ginj et al. 2006). High accumulation of ^{111}In-DOTA-sst3-ODN-8 was observed in sst3-expressing tumors, reaching up to 60% of the injected radioactivity per gram of tissue at 1 h post injection (p.i.). It remained at a high level for >72 h. In contrast, the potent agonist ^{111}In-DOTA–[1-Nal^3]-octreotide, with high affinity to sst3-binding and agonistic behavior, i.e., internalization properties, showed a much lower and shorter-lasting uptake in this tumor model. Similarly, compared with the sst2-selective agonist ^{111}In-DTPA-TATE, ^{111}In-DOTA-sst2-ANT showed a considerably higher tumor uptake. In addition, the authors showed by Scatchard analyses that the antagonists labeled many more sites on the cell surface than agonists. These data are in contradiction to the current opinion that agonists, due to their internalization, are better tracers than antagonists. Further studies will show whether antagonists for other receptor systems will show the same imaging properties and whether these experiments will lead to a general paradigm shift for targeting of peptide receptors.

In addition to the use of receptor imaging in oncology, peptides have also been studied as probes for reporter gene imaging (Buchsbaum 2004; Buchsbaum et al. 2004). In this genetic approach it is attempted to specifically increase the number of receptors on tumor cells that normally express a receptor, or to specifically induce expression on tumor cells that do not ordinarily express the receptor by the use of genetic transduction. The potential advantages of this approach are: (1) constitutive expression of a tumor-associated receptor is not required; (2) tumor cells are altered to express a target receptor at levels which may significantly improve tumor-to-normal tissue targeting of radiolabeled peptides.

Recently, an adenovirus (Ad) encoding the gene for sst2 under control of the cytomegalovirus promoter (AdCMVhSSTr2) was developed (Rogers et al. 1999). Subsequently, the in-vitro binding of ^{125}I-somatostatin and ^{111}In-DTPA-D-Phe^1-octreotide to cell membrane preparations of SK-OV-3.ip1 human ovarian cancer cells and A-427 human non-small-cell lung cancer cells infected with AdCMVhSSTr2 was demonstrated (Rogers et al. 1999). In another study, the ability to induce receptor expression in vivo was studied. Therefore, AdCMVhSSTr2 was injected intraperitoneally (i.p.) to induce sst2 expression on SK-OV-3ip1 tumors 5 days after tumor cell inoculation in the peritoneum in nude mice. Two days later, tumor uptake of ^{111}In-DTPA-D-Phe^1-octreotide appeared to be 60.4 %ID/g at 4 h after i.p. injection. The tumor uptake was significantly lower (1.6 %ID/g) when a control Ad (AdCMVGPRr) was injected. Furthermore, mice with subcutaneous

A-427 tumors injected intratumorally (i.t.) with AdCMVhSSTr2, showed uptake of the intraveneously (i.v) injected ^{99m}Tc- and ^{188}Re-labeled somatostatin analogue P829 (Zinn et al. 2000) detected by gamma-camera imaging. No uptake was observed when the tumors were infected with a control Ad. These studies showed that tumor uptake of radiolabeled sst2 ligands could be achieved after infection of the tumor in vivo with AdCMVhSSTr2.

4.2 Neurotensin

Neurotensin (NT) is a neuropeptide consisting of 13 amino acids that was first isolated from bovine hypothalamus (Carraway and Leeman 1973). This peptide is expressed in both the central nervous system and the periphery. The physiological and biochemical actions of NT are mediated through binding to NT receptors (NTRs). Three neurotensin receptor subtypes have been cloned so far. The NTR1 subtype is overexpressed in several human cancers, such as meningiomas, Ewing's sarcomas, and in more than 75% of ductal pancreatic carcinomas (Reubi 2003). The potential application of neurotensin analogues in cancer diagnosis and therapy is limited due to its rapid degradation in vivo. Therefore, NT analogues with modified lysine and arginine derivatives to enhance stability were synthesized and coupled either to DTPA or DOTA (De Visser et al. 2003). It was found that only 2% of an NT analogue without stabilizing amino acid derivatives [NT(8–13)] was intact after 4 h incubation in human serum. In contrast, after incubation under the same conditions more than 93% of the stabilized peptides were intact. Furthermore, these stabilized peptides showed receptor-mediated internalization in NTR1-overexpressing HT29 tumor cells. The DOTA-conjugated stabilized peptide showed receptor-mediated tumor uptake in mice with HT29 tumors. This compound is, therefore, a candidate for peptide-receptor radionuclide therapy of these tumors. Recently, three new NT analogues (NT-XII, NT-XIII, and NT-XVIII) with stabilization on the cleavage bonds 8–9 and 11–12 were developed (Garcia-Garayoa et al. 2006). Although all showed long plasma stability, NT-XII was the most stable in tumor cells. In addition, this radiotracer had the highest affinity for NTRs, highest internalization rate, and longest retention time in tumor cells. In vivo, NT-XII had the highest tumor uptake (6.26 ± 1.53 %ID/g, 1.5 h p.i.) and the highest tumor-to-nontumor ratios. Clinical studies with this compound are ongoing.

In another study, a series of NT(8–13) derivatives with a branched structure were synthesized (Hultsch et al. 2006). The peptides containing NT(8–13) attached via the C-terminus showed poor receptor binding (>50 nM). However, the branched derivatives containing NT(8–13) attached via the N-terminus showed binding affinities in the low nanomolar or even submolar range as found with unmodified NT(8–13). Introduction of a PEG spacer between the core matrix and NT(8–13) moieties resulted in a tetrameric peptide with a high NTR binding affinity (0.4 ± 0.2 nM). Work on the radiolabeling of these compounds with ^{18}F and radiopharmacological investigations are currently in progress.

4.3 RGD-peptides

The $\alpha_v\beta_3$ integrin receptor is a transmembrane protein consisting of two nonco-valently bound subunits, α and β. The $\alpha_v\beta_3$ integrin is expressed on activated en-dothelial cells during tumor-induced angiogenesis, whereas it is absent on quiescent endothelial cells and normal tissues. Furthermore, this integrin is expressed on the cell membrane of various tumor cell types, such as ovarian cancer, neuroblastoma, breast cancer, and melanoma.

Radiolabeled ligands for this integrin could be used as tracers to noninvasively visualize $\alpha_v\beta_3$ expression in tumors. Noninvasive visualization of $\alpha_v\beta_3$ expression might supply information about the angiogenic process and the responsiveness of a tumor for antiangiogenic drugs. Furthermore, noninvasive determination of $\alpha_v\beta_3$ expression potentially can be used to monitor the effect of antiangiogenic drugs in patients.

The first radiolabeled $\alpha_v\beta_3$ antagonist for the investigation of angiogenesis and metastasis in vivo was $[^{125}I]$-3-iodo-D-Tyr^4-cyclo(-Arg-Gly-Asp-D-Tyr-Val-) (Haubner et al. 1999). This radioiodinated $\alpha_v\beta_3$ integrin antagonist had a high affinity for $\alpha_v\beta_3$; however, it was mainly excreted via the hepatobiliary route. Sub-sequently, a glycosylated version, cyclo(Arg-Gly-Asp-D-Tyr-Lys[SAA]), was syn-thesized in an attempt to produce a more hydrophilic compound that would clear predominantly via the kidneys (Haubner et al. 2001). In a mouse tumor model, the radioiodinated glycopeptide showed a longer circulatory half-life and a significantly reduced uptake in the liver compared with the nonglycosylated peptide. In addition, the glycosylated RGD peptide had a clearly enhanced uptake in the tumor. A stable hydrophilic ^{18}F-labeled galactosylated cyclic pentapeptide has recently been devel-oped, with a high affinity and selectivity for $\alpha_v\beta_3$, which accumulates specifically in $\alpha_v\beta_3$-positive tumors (Haubner et al. 2004). In a recent study it was shown that this PET-tracer can be used to visualize $\alpha_v\beta_3$ expression in tumors in patients (Haubner et al. 2005) (Fig. 5). In addition, comparison with immunohistochemical analysis of the tumor lesion indicated that PET using this tracer correctly identified the level of $\alpha_v\beta_3$ expression in tissue noninvasively (Beer et al. 2006).

To improve tumor-targeting efficacy and to obtain better in-vivo imaging proper-ties, several research groups aimed to enhance the affinity toward the $\alpha_v\beta_3$ integrin by using multimeric (dimers and tetramers) RGD peptides (Janssen et al. 2002a, b; Thumshirn et al. 2003; Poethko et al. 2004a, b; Chen et al. 2004b, e; Zhang et al. 2006; Wu et al. 2005). E[c(RGDfK)]$_2$ and derivatives thereof were the first dimeric RGD peptides to have been used as diagnostic and therapeutic radiotrac-ers (Janssen et al. 2002a, b). Subsequently, E[c(RGDyK)]$_2$ was used for prepara-tion of ^{64}Cu- and ^{18}F-based PET radiotracers. Recently, it was demonstrated that the ^{18}F-labeled dimeric RGD-peptide [c(RGDfE)HEG]$_2$-K-Dpr-[^{18}F]FBOA had a much higher binding affinity to the immobilized $\alpha_v\beta_3$ integrin compared with its monomeric analogue c(RGDfE)HEG-Dpr-[^{18}F]FBOA. The tetrameric RGD pep-tide {[c(RGDfE)HEG$_2$]K}$_2$-K-Dpr-[^{18}F]FBOA demonstrated strongly enhanced affinity for the $\alpha_v\beta_3$ integrin compared with its monomeric and dimeric counter-part (Poethko et al. 2004b). In addition, it was found that the $\alpha_v\beta_3$ integrin-binding affinity of the tetrameric RGD-peptide $E\{E[c(RGDfK)]_2\}$ ($IC_{50} = 15.1 \pm 1.1$ nM) was higher than that of its dimeric analogue $E[c(RGDfK)]_2$ ($IC_{50} = 32.2 \pm 2.1$ nM) (Wu et al. 2005) (Fig. 6).

These studies clearly demonstrated the multivalency effect, since the in-vivo affinity significantly increased in the series monomer < dimer < tetramer. Moreover, also with respect to tumor uptake and tumor-to-organ ratios, a similar increase monomer < dimer < tetramer was observed. These are promising results toward the development of integrin-targeted radionuclide therapy (Wester and Kessler 2005).

4.4 Bombesin

The bombesin receptors belong to the G-protein-coupled receptors and comprise four subtypes. Three subtypes have been found in humans: GRPr, neuromedin B receptor (NMB-R), and bombesin subtype-3 receptor (BB_3-R) (Kroog et al. 1995).

Bombesin (BN) is an amphibian 14-amino-acid neuropeptide with a high affinity for the BB_2 or gastrin-releasing peptide receptor (GRPr). The GRP receptor is overexpressed in a variety of tumors, including breast and prostate cancer (Reubi and Waser 2003). Consequently, various radiolabeled BN analogues have been investigated and proposed for use in the diagnosis and therapy of tumors (Smith et al. 2005). For example, in mice a ^{99m}Tc-labeled bombesin analogue, demobesin, showed rapid background clearance and high and prolonged localization in PC-3 human prostate cancer xenografts (Maina et al. 2005; Nock et al. 2003, 2005a). Recently, four demobesin analogues were developed: demobesins 3–6. In demobesin 3, Pyr[1] had been replaced by Pro[1]. Further substitution of Met[14] through Nle[14] resulted in demobesin 4. In nude mice with PC-3 xenografts, ^{99m}Tc]demobesin 3 and 4 showed high and rapid localization in the tumor and cleared mainly via the kidneys. [99m]Tc]demobesin 5 and 6, which are truncated peptides, showed lower tumor uptake and cleared mainly via the hepatobiliary route (Nock et al. 2005a).

To enable visualization of GRPr-positive tumors by PET, a few BN analogues have been developed. ^{64}Cu-DOTA-[Lys[3]]bombesin exhibited high GRPr-binding affinity and specifity and rapid internalization in PC-3 tumor cells. Specific localization of ^{64}Cu-DOTA-[Lys[3]]bombesin to GRPr-positive tumors and tissues was confirmed by biodistribution, microPET imaging, and autoradiography studies (Chen et al. 2004c). Another newly developed radiotracer for PET imaging of GRPr-positive tumors is ^{68}Ga-BZH3. This radiotracer had a high affinity for the GRPr and internalized rapidly in GRPr-positive AR42J cells. The diagnostic potential of ^{68}Ga-BZH3 was demonstrated in a mouse tumor model using PET (Schuhmacher et al. 2005). Recently, the radiotracer ^{177}Lu-AMBA showed the ability to bind GRPr and NMB-R with nanomolar affinity. In addition, this tracer had a low kidney retention and showed a very favorable risk-benefit profile. This tracer is currently in phase I clinical trails (Lantry et al. 2006; Waser et al. 2007). Furthermore, a ^{111}In-labeled DTPA-bombesin analogue appeared to be a promising radioligand for scintigraphy of GRP receptor-expressing tumors. Phase I studies in patients with

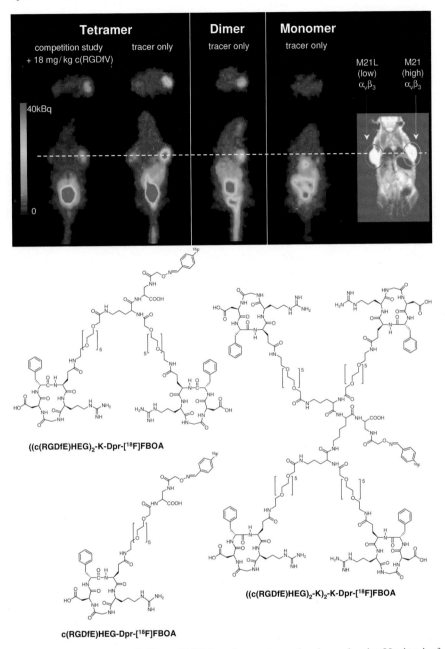

Fig. 6 Micro-PET images of M21- and M21-L-melanoma tumor-bearing nude mice 90 min p.i. of the [^{18}F]FBOA-labeled RGD-mono- (c(RGDfE)HEG-Dpr-[^{18}F]FBOA), -di- ((c(RGDfE)HEG)$_2$-K-Dpr-[^{18}F]FBOA) and -tetramer (((c(RGDfE)HEG)$_2$-K)$_2$-K-Dpr–[^{18}F]FBOA) (structures are depicted *below*). Specificity of tumor uptake of the tetramer is demonstrated in a competition study via coinjection of 18 mg/kg c(RGDfV). The MRI image on the *right* indicates the position of the respective tumor with high (M21) and low (M21L) $\alpha v \beta 3$ expression

invasive prostate carcinoma are currently being undertaken (Breeman et al. 2002). However, the loss of bombesin receptors upon dedifferentiation of prostate cancer cells from androgen-controlled to androgen-independent growth may hamper clinical utility (De Visser et al. 2005).

4.5 Cholecystokinin/gastrin

The cholecystokinin (CCK) receptor is expressed on a variety of tumors (Reubi et al. 1997). CCK receptors can be distinguished pharmacologically by their affinity for gastrin, a 33-amino-acid peptide hormone involved in gastric motility (Wank et al. 1994). The CCK_1, or formerly CCK-A, receptor has a low affinity for gastrin, whereas the CCK_2, or formerly CCK-B, receptor has a high affinity for gastrin. Medullary thyroid carcinomas, small-cell lung cancers, astrocytomas, or stromal ovarian cancers can frequently express CCK_2 receptors. The expression of CCK_1 receptors in humans is quite restricted. However, CCK_1 receptors are found in gastroenteropancreatic tumors, meningiomas, and neuroblastoma.

Several radiolabeled gastrin analogues have been developed and their potential for targeted diagnostic imaging and radionuclide therapy of CCK_2-receptor-expressing tumors has been investigated. The radioiodinated gastrin analogue $[^{131}I\text{-}Tyr^{12}]$gastrin-I showed high and specific uptake in mice with TT medullary thyroid cancer xenografts (Behr et al. 1998). Maximum tumor uptake was obtained 1 h after injection. This radiotracer cleared rapidly from the blood mainly via renal excretion and partly via biliary excretion. Initial therapeutic experiments with this radiotracer showed that tumor growth was retarded significantly compared with untreated controls. An initial clinical study showed that the radiotracer was well tolerated by a patient with metastatic MTC.

A series of nonsulfated CCK analogues which were conjugated with DTPA or DOTA were developed recently (Reubi et al. 1998). The most potent compounds were DTPA-$[Nle^{28,31}]$-CCK(26–33) (MP2286) and DTPA-$[D\text{-}Asp^{26}, Nle^{28,31}]$-CCK(26–33) (MP2288) with an IC_{50} value of 1.5 nM. Both compounds were conjugated at the N-terminus. Analogues with C-terminal DTPA had an IC_{50} value of > 100 nM. DOTA-conjugated MP2288 showed specific internalization in CCK_2-positive AR42J tumor cells. In rats, this ^{111}In-labeled radiotracer showed specific uptake in CCK_2-expressing tumor and stomach (de Jong et al. 1999). However, in medullary thyroid cancer (MTC) patients this CCK analogue had a relatively low uptake in the strong CCK receptor-positive stomach and small lesions could not be detected (Kwekkeboom et al. 2000).

The CCK analogue $[^{111}In\text{-}DTPA^0]$-minigastrin demonstrated high uptake in stomach and tumor lesions in metastatic MTC patients (Behr et al. 1999). The in-vivo properties of this compound were further improved by the coupling of DTPA to $[D\text{-}Glu^1]$-minigastrin (Béhé et al. 2003). The first clinical studies using $[^{111}In\text{-}DTPA\text{-}D\text{-}Glu^1]$-minigastrin showed that this CCK analogue is able to delineate metastatic MTC with high sensitivity (Béhé and Behr 2002; Gotthardt et al.

2006a). Recently, three new ^{99m}Tc-labeled minigastrin analogues modified with open-chain tetraamines at the N-terminus were evaluated for their suitability in the CCK_2/gastrin-R-targeted imaging of tumors (Nock et al. 2005b). In nude mice with AR42J tumors, these radiotracers, $[^{99m}$Tc]demogastrin 1–3, localized very rapidly in the tumor and in the stomach by a receptor-mediated process. The tumor-to-nontarget tissue ratios were high for all three analogues, but especially favorable for $[^{99m}$Tc]demogastrin 2. This compound provided excellent delineation of tumor deposits in a first patient with metastatic MTC.

4.6 SDF-1

The chemokine receptor CXCR4 is expressed in a wide range of normal tissues, such as lymphatic tissues, spleen, brain, and small intestine. This G-protein-coupled receptor was initially identified as a coreceptor for the entry of T-cell line tropic HIV-1 (Feng et al. 1996). Recent studies showed that CXCR4 is frequently upregulated on different tumor cell lines, including those of colorectal, breast, prostate, and lung cancer. This CXCR4 receptor and its ligand stromal cell-derived factor-1 (SDF-1 or CXCL12) are thought to play a crucial role in regulating the metastasis of many solid tumors. Gradients of the chemokine CXCL12 are proposed to attract CXCR4-expressing tumor cells to specific metastatic sites analogous to the directed homing of leukocytes. Organs that are commonly affected by metastasis, such as lung and liver, produce high amounts of the endogenous CXCR4 ligand, CXCL12 (Muller et al. 2001).

Radiolabeled CXCR4 ligands would be valuable tools for noninvasive investigation of the metastatic potential of tumors and determination of CXCR4 expression for individualized therapy. Recently, the ^{111}In-labeled 14-residue CXCR4 ligand ^{111}In-DTPA-Ac-TZ14011 was developed. This radioligand showed CXCR4-mediated tumor accumulation in a mouse pancreatic carcinoma model (Hanaoka et al. 2006). The utilization of cyclic pentapeptides libraries led to the finding that these cyclic peptides can have strong CXCR4 antagonistic activity (Fujii et al. 2003). Indeed, the radiolabeled cyclic pentapeptide CPCR4 showed the ability to bind to CXCR4 with high affinity and specificity (Koglin et al. 2006). This tracer showed CXCR4-mediated tumor uptake and rapid blood clearance in mice with $CMS5/CXCR4^+$ tumors. In addition, $CXCR4^+$ tumors could be clearly visualized using SPECT and PET imaging. Further ligands — i.e., radiofluorinated and radiometallated ligands — are currently under investigation.

4.7 Neuropeptide Y

Neuropeptide Y (NPY) is a 36-amino-acid peptide of the pancreatic polypeptide family. NPY is the most abundant neuropeptide in the central nervous system (Gehlert 1999; Wieland et al. 2000) and several physiological processes, such as increase in memory retention, inhibition of anxiety, and induction of food intake, have been attributed to NPY (Grundemar and Bloom 1997).

The NPY receptor belongs to the GPCR family and five distinct subtypes of this receptor (Y_1, Y_2, Y_4, Y_5, and y_6) have been cloned so far (Michel et al. 1998). Although these receptors are expressed in normal tissues, such as the central and peripheral nervous system, these receptors are interesting candidates for in-vivo tumor targeting as they are also overexpressed in various tumors. High expression of subtypes Y_1 and Y_2 was found in adrenal cortical tumors, ovarian sex cord-stromal tumors, breast cancer, and neuroblastoma (Reubi et al. 2001; Körner et al. 2004a, b). Several nonreceptor subtype-selective NPY radioligands and subtype-specific radioligands have been developed, such as the highly Y_5 receptor-selective radioligand $[^{125}I][hPP(1-17), Ala^{31}, Aib^{32}]$ NPY (Dumont et al. 2003). To overcome the high nonspecific binding of this ligand, the more specific Y_5 radioligand $[^{125}I][cPP(1-7), NPY(19-23), Ala^{31}, Aib^{32}, Gln^{34}]hPP$ has recently been developed (Dumont et al. 2004). Substitution of His^{26} by Ala in the Ac-$[Ahx^{5-24}, K^4$ $(^{99m}Tc(CO)_3$-2-picolylamine N,N-diacetic acid) (PADA)]-NPY, a selective and high-affinity ligand for the Y_2-receptor, resulted in the Y_1/Y_2 selective radioligand Ac-$[Ahx^{5-24}, K^4$ $(^{99m}Tc(CO)_3$-PADA, $A^{26})]$-NPY, which shows receptor-mediated internalization and suitable characteristics for future applications in tumor diagnosis and treatment (Langer et al. 2001).

4.8 GLP-1

The glucagon-like peptide 1 (GLP1) receptor is overexpressed in nearly all insulinomas and gastrinomas. In addition, this receptor is expressed in a large number of intestinal and bronchial carcinoids (Reubi and Waser 2003). GLP-1 is an intestinal hormone that stimulates postprandial insulin secretion from pancreatic β-cells. The radioiodinated GLP-1 and a GLP-1 receptor-selective analogue, exendin-3, showed successful tumor targeting in a rat insulinoma model (Gotthardt et al. 2002). Compared with GLP-1, radioiodinated exendin-3 demonstrated a more pronounced pancreatic uptake and tumor accumulation. Due to its higher metabolic stability, exendin-3 offered superior visualization compared with GLP-1. The first small animal SPECT studies using ^{111}In-labeled exendin-4 in rodents with pancreatic insulinomas showed promising results and will certainly initiate further in-vivo studies investigating GLP-1 receptors in primary human tumors known to express a very high GLP-1 receptor density, i.e., insulinomas (Wild et al. 2005a; Gotthardt et al. 2006b).

4.9 Substance P

Substance P is an 11-amino-acid neuropeptide that acts through the binding to three types of transmembrane G-protein-coupled receptors, denoted as NK1, NK2, and

NK3. Substance P plays an important role as a neurotransmitter in the peripheral and central nervous system. Receptors for substance P are mainly expressed in breast cancer, medullary thyroid cancer (MTC), small-cell lung cancer (SCLC), and in brain tumors such as astrocytoma and glioblastoma (Hennig et al. 1995). Severe side effects could occur after injection of substance P (Van Hagen et al. 1996) and intravenous application is not tolerated well by patients. However, local application into tumor tissue does not cause these problems. So far, radiolabeled substance P derivates have not been used for imaging, but have been exploited for intracavitary therapy of high-grade gliomas (Schumacher et al. 2002). Recently, the new targeting vector 1,4,7,10-tetraazacyclododecane-1-glutaric acid-4,7,10-triacetic acid substance P (DOTAGA-Arg^1-SP) was developed. This peptidic vector had a high affinity for NK1R ($IC_{50} = 0.88 \pm 0.34$ nM) and demonstrated specific internalization in LN319 glioblastoma cells. Clinically, the radiopharmaceutical was distributed according to tumor geometry. In addition, disease-stabilization and/or improved neurologic status was observed in 13 of 20 patients. Targeted radiotherapy using the radiolabeled diffusible peptidic vector DOTAGA-SP represents an innovative strategy for local control of malignant gliomas. This compound will be further examined for intratumoral and intracavitary injections in future clinical trials (Kneifel et al. 2006).

4.10 Melanocyte-stimulating Hormone

Wild-type alpha-melanocyte-stimulating hormone (α-MSH) is a tridecapeptide that is involved in the control of skin pigmentation (Cone et al. 1993). The biological activity of α-MSH is mediated through interactions with the melanocortin 1 (MC1) receptor (Hruby et al. 1993). The melanocortin receptors belong to the GPCR family, and five distinct subtypes (MC1-MC5) have been identified and cloned so far (Mountjoy et al. 1992; Gantz et al. 1993a, b; Barret et al. 1994; Desarnaud et al. 1994; Labbé et al. 1994; Fathi et al. 1995). α-MSH receptors are expressed in human and murine melanoma cell lines (Tatro and Reichlin 1987; Siegrist et al. 1989; Tatro et al. 1990). In addition, it has been shown that >80% of melanoma tumor samples from patients with metastatic lesions express α-MSH receptors (Siegrist et al. 1989). Initial studies with radiohalogenated α-MSH analogues for melanoma targeting showed very rapid tumor radioactivity washout due to lysosomal degradation of the radiohalogenated complex after internalization (Stein et al. 1995; Garg et al. 1995). Subsequently, a novel class of metal-cyclized α-MSH analogues has been developed. The cyclization of the peptide with ^{99m}Tc and ^{188}Re resulted in α-MSH analogues which were more resistant to chemical and proteolytic degradation (Giblin et al. 1998; Chen et al. 2000). These ^{99m}Tc/^{188}Re-cyclized peptides, Tc/Re-CCMSH, showed high tumor uptake, prolonged tumor retention, and high stability in mice with B16/F1 murine melanoma and in mice with TXM-13 human melanoma. The in-vivo results showed that the tumor uptake of ^{99m}Tc-CCMSH was significantly higher than that of ^{99m}Tc-labeled and radioiodinated linear NPD analogues. The tumor-to-blood ratio of ^{99m}Tc-CCMSH at 4 h p.i. was 6.3- and 21.5-fold higher than that of ^{99m}Tc-CGCG-NDP and [125]I-(Tyr[2])-NDP, respectively. In another study, [188]Re-CCMSH was optimized by substitution of Lys[11] through Arg[11] (Miao et al. 2002). [188]Re-(Arg[11])CCMSH had a significantly higher tumor uptake than [188]Re-CCMSH (20.44 ± 1.91 %ID/g and 15.03 ± 5.20 %ID/g at 1 h p.i., respectively). In addition, the kidney retention of [188]Re-(Arg[11])CCMSH was reduced by more than 50% compared with [188]Re-CCMSH. Recently, this compound was conjugated with DOTA to enable radiolabeling with a wider variety of radionuclides. DOTA-ReCCMSH(Arg[11]) had high melanoma uptake and lower kidney uptake than the corresponding DOTA-conjugated Lys[11] analogues (Cheng et al. 2002).

Another DOTA-conjugated short linear α-MSH analogue, [Nle[4], Asp[5], D-Phe[7]]-α-MSH$_{4-11}$ (NAPamide) was designed recently (Froidevaux et al. 2004). Compared with a previously reported DOTA-α-MSH analogue, DOTA-MSH$_{oct}$, ^{111}In-DOTA-NAPamide showed a higher tumor uptake in mice with B16F1 melanoma. Furthermore, it was observed that ^{111}In-DOTA-NAPamide had a lower kidney accumulation than ^{111}In-DOTA-MSH$_{oct}$. The clinical potential of DOTA-NAPamide was demonstrated in high-contrast images with ^{68}Ga-DOTA-NAPamide in mice with B16F1 melanoma. An interesting finding of this study was the role of the quantity of injected peptide on the tumor-to-background ratio. A fivefold increase in tumor uptake was observed by reducing the peptide dosage from 420 to 20 pmol, although kidney retention decreased by only 1.4-fold. This demonstrated the importance of the specific activity of the radiopeptide: the amount of administered peptide can only be kept low if the specific activity is high, resulting in a maximum tumor-to-background ratio.

5 From Small Peptides to Multimers and Polymers

Similar to examples in nature, such as antibody recognition, the DNA-DNA duplex formation by pairwise van der Waals interaction of nucleotides, or the presentation of numerous peptides by a virus, the binding of one molecule or particle with numerous binding sites onto the target (e.g., cell membrane, extracellular matrix) can serve to increase the binding interactions between "ligand" and "target". This concept can be used for the design of peptide radiopharmaceuticals by linking multiple copies of a peptide to a sort of common backbone, such as linear or dendritic peptides or polymers, liposomes or nanoparticles (Kessler et al. 1988, 1989; Kramer and Karpen 1998; Mammen et al. 1998; Kiessling et al. 2000; Handl et al. 2004). Two methods of interaction are expected: (1) the multimeric ligand interacts sequentially in a step-by-step fashion with the individual binding sites of a "high capacity" target (tumor cells with high receptor density, extracellular matrix components, etc.), resulting in a polyvalent interaction and, thus, increased avidity; (2) the low target density and, thus, the high medium distance between the binding sites makes a polyvalent interaction impossible. Although in the latter case the multimeric ligand can only interact in a monvalent fashion, an increase in the "apparent ligand concentration" at the target (cell membrane) may lead to increased "apparent affinity" and, thus, improved tracer binding.

It has been shown in several studies that the affinity of small molecules to their binding site is dramatically increased by formation of multimeric units (Kessler et al. 1988, 1989; Kramer and Karpen 1998; Mammen et al. 1998; Kiessling et al. 2000; Handl et al. 2004). Linear or branched polymers, dendrimers and star-like structures have been evaluated to enhance antigen-immunogenicity, binding affinity, cytotoxic potency or selectivity.

Whether a multimeric construct can bind in a simultaneous fashion depends on several characteristics of the construct: its overall size, the length of the linker between ligand and backbone, the flexibility and density of the linker, and the receptor density. When short linkers are used with low-molecular-weight multimers (dimers, tetramers, octamers), even high receptor densities or the formation of receptor clusters will hardly lead to polyvalent binding. Longer linkers may result in polyvalent binding after initial monovalent interaction, when receptor clustering occurs or is initiated by ligand binding (binding-induced clustering). Large flexible linkers seem to have the highest probability of polyvalent interaction of the entire construct, resulting in a decrease of K_{off} and, thus, long-lasting retention in the receptor-expressing tissue.

The concept of multimerization of peptides has already been tested on various systems, e.g., for the development of superactive activators of lysozyme release from human neutrophils (Kraus et al. 1984; Kraus and Menassa 1987). The EC_{50} in a lysozyme release assay was up to 15-fold lower for the tested tetrameric clusters. The data also indicate that the monomeric analogues were significantly less active on a molar basis than the tested tetramers assuming simple molar additivity as a controlling factor in the potencies of these clusters.

However, only one complete series of tracers has been developed which allows a valid comparison of the effects of multimerization and polymerization of peptide ligands on the pharmacokinetics and in-vivo behavior (Fig. 6). During the last decade, peptidomimetics, small cyclic and linear peptides, peptide dimers, tetramers, octamers, polymers, proteins and even larger structures, such as peptide-coated liposomes and even nanoparticles, have been designed for targeting the same protein, the $\alpha_v\beta_3$-integrin (Haubner and Wester 2004). Especially for integrin targeting, this "multimer-strategy" perfectly matches the molecular structure of the target, and especially with hypothesized structural changes after functional ligand binding. It is known that ligand binding to heterodimeric integrins initiates altered interactions of the α and β subunits (Gottschalk et al. 2002; Adair and Yeager 2002; Schneider and Engelman 2004). Studies on another integrin subtype, the $\alpha IIb\beta 3$-integrin, have shown that the heterodimeric integrin dissociates after ligand binding to form β-homotrimers and α-homodimers (Li et al. 2001, 2005). Thus, ligand binding initiates a structural reorganization, and a β-homotrimer is formed. We assume that such a mechanism is also valid for $\alpha_v\beta_3$. It is interesting to note that cell spreading and formation of focal adhesion has been shown to require a maximal distance of about 65 nm for single RGD units (Arnold et al. 2004). It can easily be calculated that the local concentration of a ligand tethered via a spacer to a second binding unit already interacting with a receptor is approximately 2.6 µM, assuming the above-mentioned distance of 65 nm. Thus, initial binding of ligand multimers can result in strong high local concentrations and, thus, to additional binding of the multivalent ligand, finally resulting in a very strong interaction (affinity) with the target structure.

To study the influence of ligand multimerization on the binding characteristics to integrins and to improve imaging, a variety of oligomeric structures were designed by tethering together multiple cyclo(-RGDfE-)-units via linkers (Jansen et al. 2002a; Thumshirn et al. 2003; Poethko et al. 2004a, b; Boturyn et al. 2004; Chen et al. 2004a, d).

Comparison of the IC_{50} of cyclo(-RGDfK-) and cyclo(-RGDfE-) containing monomers, dimers, tetramers and octamers for vitronectin binding to $\alpha_v\beta_3$ revealed significantly increasing affinity in the series monomer < dimer < tetramer < octamer (Janssen et al. 2002a, b; Poethko et al. 2004a, b). In contrast, the affinity of reference and control peptides carrying only one cyclo(-RGDfK-)- (or cyclo (-RGDfE-)-peptide, but otherwise cyclo(-RADfK-)- or cyclo(-RADfE-)-sequences, respectively, was lower or just similar to that of the corresponding monomers. Together, these experiments clearly demonstrate the "multimer effect" in vitro with similar molecular structures, and thus independent of differences in charge, size or shape. These data were subsequently confirmed in vivo in M21melanoma-tumor-bearing-mice (Poethko et al. 2004a, 2004b). Both tumor uptake and tumor-to-organ ratios increased in the series monomer < dimer < tetramer, leading to significantly improved imaging with the ^{18}F-labeled RGD-tetramer (Fig. 6).

Polymerization for improvement of tumor delivery was tested with RGD peptides coupled to a chitin backbone (Komazawa et al. 1993a, b, c). In these studies, the potency of monomeric RGD peptides and RGD peptides coupled to poly(carboxyethylmethacylamide) [poly(CEMA)] to inhibit spontaneous metastasis after subcutaneous inoculation of B16BL6 melanoma cells was investigated. Similar to the results obtained with polypeptides containing repetitive RGD sequences [poly(RGDS)], the polymeric integrin ligands inhibited experimental and spontaneous metastasis more efficiently than the corresponding monomer peptides. Furthermore, the effect of two monomeric peptides, YIGSR and RGD, and two polymeric compounds, poly(CEMA-RGDS) and 6Ocarboxymethyl-chitin-RGDS (CM-Chitin-RGDS), on the invasiveness and survival of mice after inoculations of peritoneal-seeding OCUM-2MD3 ($\alpha 2\beta 1^+$ und $\alpha 3\beta 1^+$) human scirrhous gastric carcinoma cells was investigated and compared. All peptides and especially the polymers significantly inhibited the invasiveness of OCUM-2MD3-cells and resulted in improved survival time (Matsuoka et al. 1998).

In a similar strategy, polyvalent high-affinity peptide binding was investigated for targeting the $\alpha_v\beta_3$-integrin expression during tumor angiogenesis. In this study uptake of a macromolecular methacrylamide polymer conjugated with RGD4C-peptides (Koivunen et al. 1995) and labeled via the $[^{99m}Tc(CO)_3]^+$ (IsoLink) approach was investigated in PC3 and DU145 prostate tumor xenografts and compared with the corresponding RGE4C polymers with no affinity to $\alpha_v\beta_3$ and monomeric

[99m]Tc-labeled RGD4C- and RGE4C-peptides (Mitra et al. 2004, 2005). In all afore-mentioned studies, a strong increase in binding affinity and target localization has been observed.

6 Multimeric Structures and Specificity of Uptake

Tumors are known to exhibit enhanced vascular permeability (Luo and Prestwich 2002; Maeda et al. 2003; Ferrari 2005), resulting in a facilitated permeability and influx of macromolecules into the interstitium. In addition to inadequate lymphatic drainage of solid tumors, macromolecular plasma components remain in the tumor for a long time, up to days (Landon et al. 2004; Maeda et al. 2000). Thus, and in accordance with this "enhanced permeability and retention effect" (EPR), bio-compatible macromolecules accumulated in much higher concentrations in tumor tissue (>sixfold) than in normal tissues and organs. EPR was found to be effective for molecules with a molecular size >45 kDa (Landon et al. 2004; Noguchi et al. 1998). Thus, EPR does not affect the uptake of small peptides, small multimers or even medium-size polymers. For larger peptide constructs, such as large poly-meric peptide tracers and even medium-sized proteins, antibody fragments or small nanoparticles, EPR contributes to tumor uptake.

However, since the uptake mediated by EPR is unspecific, accumulation of a large construct (e.g., a polymer) will not reflect a process addressed by the pep-tides conjugated to the vehicle, at least not early after injection. In addition, EPR is a slow process and significant uptake often takes several hours. Consequently, to overcome these uncertainties, imaging with the aim to receive target-specific infor-mation would have to be carried out very early or at late time-points after injection. Thus, compared with the large peptide-polymer conjugates, low-molecular-weight multimers exhibit striking pharmacokinetic advantages for imaging. The first human studies with ^{18}F-labeled tetrameric cyclo(-RGDfE-) revealed excellent and specific uptake, fast-clearance-kinetics, low background activity and high-contrast imaging 1 h p.i.; thus combining the advantages of multimerization with small size.

Although not ideal for peptide-receptor imaging, larger peptide-polymer con-jugates may generally be promising vehicles for strategies aiming to deliver a payload to tumors (Schiffelers et al. 2003; Kok et al. 2002; Burkhart et al. 2004). As already successfully demonstrated with $\alpha_v\beta_3$-targeted nanoparticles and lipo-somes for imaging of angiogenesis with MRI (Anderson et al. 2000; Winter et al. 2003; Dubey et al. 2004), targeting concepts with polyvalent vehicles may offer a suitable alternative for an integrin-targeted EPR-enhanced PRRT-radiotherapy. Here, EPR-mediated radiotherapy of the entire tumor would act in parallel with an RGD/integrin-mediated dose enhancement for the neovasculature and single tumor cells expressing $\alpha_v\beta_3$, and both the polyvalent binding and EPR would help to retain the activity over a long period inside the tumor.

In conclusion, the diversity of methods for the identification and synthesis of peptides, the wide field of approaches for the modification, stabilization, labeling, and construction of more complex derivatives, their use as targeting vectors either as single molecules, multimers or coupled to liposomes or nanoparticles, the high diversity of their corresponding binding sites, their ability to be internalized into cells and thus be accumulated make peptides perhaps the most flexible class of tracers and extremely valuable molecules with a broad spectrum of application — but only in the context of an appropriate chemical and pharmaceutical design.

References

Adair BD, Yeager M (2002) Three-dimensional model of the human platelet integrin $\alpha IIb\beta 3$ based on electron cryomicroscopy and x-ray crystallography. Proc Natl Acad Sci USA 99: 14059–14064

Alberto R, Abram U (2003) ^{99m}Tc: Labeling Chemistry and Labeled Compounds. A. Vertès, S. Nagy and Z. Klencsár (eds) Handbook of Nuclear Chemistry-Vol. 4, 211–256

Alberto R (2007) The particular role of radiopharmacy within bioorganicmetallic chemistry. J Organomet Chem 692:1179–1186

Anderson SA, Rader RK, Westlin WF et al (2000) Magnetic resonance contrast enhancement of neovasculature with alpha(v)beta(3)-targeted nanoparticles. Magn Reson Med 44:433–439

Arnold M, Cavalcanti-Adam E-A, Glass R et al (2004) Activation of integrin function by nanopatterned adhesive interfaces. Chem Phys Chem 5:383–388

Bakker WH, Breeman WA, van der Pluijm ME, de Jong M, Visser TJ, Krenning EP (1996) Iodine-131 labelled octreotide: not an option for somatostatin receptor therapy.Eur J Nucl Med 23(7):775–781

Barret P, MacDonald A, Helliwell R, Davidson G, Morgan P (1994) Cloning and expression of a new member of the melanocyte–stimulating hormone receptor family. J Mol Endocrinol 12:203–213

Beer AJ, Haubner R, Sarbia M, Goebel M, Luderschmidt S, Grosu AL, Schnell O, Niemeyer M, Kessler H, Wester HJ, Weber WA, Schwaiger M (2006) Positron emission tomography using $[^{18}F]$Galacto-rgd identifies the level of $\alpha_v\beta_3$ expression in man. Clin Cancer Res 12:3942–3949

Béhé M, Behr TM (2002) Cholecystokinin-B (CCK-B)/gastrin receptor targeting peptides for staging and therapy of medullary thyroid cancer and other CCK-B receptor expressing malignancies. Biopolymers 66: 399–418

Béhé M, Becker W, Gotthardt M, Angerstein C, Behr TM (2003) Improved kinetic stability of DTPA-Dglu as compared with monofunctional DTPA in chelating indium and yttrium: preclinical and initial clinical evaluation of radiometal labeled minigastrin derivatives. Eur J Nucl Med Mol Imaging 30:1140–1146

Behr TM, Jenner N, Radetzky S et al (1998) Targeting of cholecystokinin-B/gastrin receptors in vivo: preclinical and initial clinical evaluation of the diagnostic and therapeutic potential of radiolabeled gastrin. Eur J Nucl Med 25:424–430

Behr TM, Jenner N, Behe M et al (1999) Radiolabeled peptides for targeting cholecystokinin-B/gastrin receptor-expressing tumors. J Nucl Med 40:1029–1044

Bodei L, Cremonesi M, Grana C, Rocca P, Bartolomei M, Chinol M, Paganelli G (2004) Receptor radionuclide therapy with 90Y-[DOTA]0-Tyr3-octreotide (90Y-DOTATOC) in neuroendocrine tumours. Eur J Nucl Med Mol Imaging 31:1038–1046

Boturyn D, Coll J-L, Garanger E, Favrot M-C, Dumy P (2004) Template assembled cyclopeptides as multimeric systems for integrin targeting and endocytosis. J Amer Chem Soc 126:5730–5739

Breeman WA, de Jong M, Kwekkeboom DJ, Valkema R, Bakker WH, Kooij PP, Visser TJ, Krenning EP (2001) Somatostatin receptor-mediated imaging and therapy: basic science, current knowledge, limitations and future perspectives. Eur J Nucl Med 28:1421–1429

Breeman WAP, de Jong M, Erion JL, Bugaj JE, Srinivasan A, Bernard BF, Kwekkeboom DJ, Visser TJ, Krenning EP (2002) Preclinical comparison of ^{111}In-labeled DTPA- or DOTA-bombesin analogs for receptor-targeted scintigraphy and radionuclide therapy. J Nucl Med 43:1650–1656

Buchsbaum DJ (2004) Imaging and therapy of tumors induced to express somatostatin receptor by gene transfer using radiolabeled peptides and single chain antibody constructs. Sem Nucl Med 34:32–46

Buchsbaum DJ, Chaudhuri TR, Yamamoto M, Zinn KR (2004) Gene expression imaging with radiolabeled peptides. Ann Nucl Med 18:275–283

Burkhart DJ, Kalet BT, Coleman MP, Post GC, Koch TH (2004) Doxorubicin-formaldehyde conjugates targeting alphavbeta3 integrin. Mol Cancer Ther 3:1593–1604

Carraway R, Leeman SE (1973) The isolation of a new hypotensive peptide, neurotensin, from bovine hypothalami. J Biol Chem 248:6854–6861

Chen J, Cheng Z, Hoffman TJ, Jurisson SS, Quinn TP (2000) Melanoma–targeting Properties of [99m]Technetium-labeled cyclic α-melanocyte-stimulating hormone peptide analogues. Cancer Res 60:5649–5658

Chen X, Hou Y, Tohme M et al (2004a) Pegylated Arg–Gly–Asp peptide: 64Cu labeling and PET imaging of brain tumor alphavbeta3-integrin expression. J Nucl Med 45:1776–1783

Chen X, Liu S, Hou Y, Tohme M, Park R, Bading JR et al (2004b) MicroPET imaging of breast cancer αv-integrin expression with 64Cu-labeled dimeric RGD peptides. Mol Imaging Biol 6:350–359

Chen X, Park R, Hou Y, Tohme M, Shahinian AH, Bading JR, Conti PS (2004c) MicroPET and autoradiographic imaging of GRP receptor expression with ^{64}Cu-DOTA-[Lys[3]]bombesin in human prostate adenocarcinoma xenografts. J Nucl Med 45:1390–1397

Chen X, Park R, Shahinian AH, Bading JR, Conti PS (2004d) Pharmacokinetics and tumor retention of ^{125}I-labeled RGD peptide are improved by PEGylation. Nucl Med Biol 31:11–19

Chen X, Tohme M, Park R, Hou Y, Bading JR, Conti PS (2004e) Micro-PET imaging of αvβ3-integrin expression with 18F-labeled dimeric RGD peptide. Mol Imaging 3:96–104

Cheng Z, Chen J, Miao Y, Owen NK, Quinn TP, Jurisson SS (2002) Modification of the structure of a metallopeptide: synthesis and biological evaluation of ^{111}In-labeled DOTA-conjugated rhenium-cyclized α-MSH analogues. J Med Chem45:3048–3056

Cone RD, Mountjoy KG, Robbins LS et al (1993) Cloning and functional characterization of a family of receptors for the melanotropin peptides. Ann N Y Acad Sci 680:342–363

de Jong M, Bakker WH, Krenning EP, Breeman WA, van der Pluijm ME, Bernard BF, Visser TJ, Jermann E, Behe M, Powell P, Macke HR (1997) Yttrium-90 and indium-111 labelling, receptor binding and biodistribution of [DOTA0,d-Phe1,Tyr3]octreotide, a promising somatostatin analogue for radionuclide therapy. Eur J Nucl Med 24:368–371

de Jong M, Bakker WH, Bernard BF et al (1999) Preclinical and initial clinical evaluation of ^{111}In-labeled nonsulfated CCK8 analog: a peptide for CCK-B receptor-targeted scintigraphy and radionuclide therapy. J Nucl Med 40: 2081–2087

de Jong M, Breeman WA, Bernard BF, Bakker WH, Schaar M, van Gameren A, Bugaj JE, Erion J, Schmidt M, Srinivasan A, Krenning EP (2001) [177Lu-DOTA(0),Tyr3] octreotate for somatostatin receptor-targeted radionuclide therapy. Int J Cancer 92:628–633

de Jong M, Kwekkeboom D, Valkema R, Krenning EP (2003) Radiolabelled peptides for tumour therapy: current status and future directions. Plenary lecture at the EANM 2002. Eur J Nucl Med Mol Imaging 30:463–469

De Visser M, Janssen PJJM, Srinivasan A, Reubi JC, Waser B, Erion JL, Schmidt MA, Krenning EP, De Jong M (2003) Stabilised ^{111}In-labelled DTPA- and DOTA-conjugated neurotensin analogues for imaging and therapy of exocrine pancreatic cancer. Eur J Nucl Med Mol Imaging 30:1134–1139

De Visser M, Van Weerden WM, De Ridder CM, Reneman S, Wildeman N, Melis M, Krenning EP, De Jong M (2005) Androgen regulation of GRP receptor-expression in human prostate tumor xenografts. J Nucl Med 46:396P

Desarnaud F, Labbé O, Eggerickx D, Vassart G, Parmentier M (1994) Molecular cloning, functional expression and pharmacological characterization of a mouse melanocortin receptor gene. Biochem J 299:366–373

Dubey PK, Mishra V, Jain S, Mahor S, Vyas SP (2004). Liposomes modified with cyclic RGD peptide for tumor targeting. J Drug Target 12:257–264

Dumont Y, Thakur M, Beck-Sickinger A, Fournier A, Quirion R (2003) Development and characterization of a highly selective neuropeptide Y Y5 receptor agonist radioligand: [125I][hPP1-17, Ala31, Aib32]NPY. Br J Pharmacol 139:1360–1368

Dumont Y, Thakur M, Beck-Sickinger A, Fournier A, Quirion R (2004) Characterization of a new neuropeptide Y Y5 agonist radioligand: [^{125}I][cPP(1-7), NPY(19-23), Ala^{31}, Aib^{32}, Gln^{34}]hPP. Neuropeptides 38:163–174

Fathi Z, Iben LG, Parker EM (1995) Cloning, expression, and tissue distribution of a fifth melanocortin receptor subtype. Neurochem Res 20:107–113

Feng Y, Broder CC, Kennedy PE, Berger EA (1996) HIV-1 entry cofactor: functional cDNA cloning of a seven-transmembrane, G protein-coupled receptor. Science 272: 872–877

Ferrari M (2005) Cancer nanotechnology: opportunities and challenges. Nat Rev Cancer 5: 161–171

Froidevaux S, Calame-Christe M, Schuhmacher J, Tanner H, Saffrich R, Henze M, Eberle AN (2004) A gallium-labeled DOTA-α-melanocyte-stimulating hormone analog for PET imaging of melanoma metastases. J Nucl Med 45:116–123

Fujii N, Oishi S, Hiramatsu K, Araki T, Ueda S, Tamamura H, Otaka A, Kusano S, Terakubo S, Nakashima H, Broach JA, Trent JO, Wang ZX, Peiper SC (2003) Molecular-size reduction of a potent CXCR4-chemokine antagonist using orthogonal combination of conformation- and sequence-based libraries. Angew Chem Int Ed 42:3251–3253

Gantz I, Konda Y, Tashiro T, Shimoto Y, Miwa H, Munzert G, Watson SJ, Del Valle V, Yamada T (1993a) Molecular cloning of a novel melanocortin receptor. J Biol Chem 268:8246–8250

Gantz I, Miwa H, Konda Y, Shimoto Y, Tashiro T, Watson SJ, Del Valle V, Yamada T (1993b) Molecular cloning, expression, and gene localization of a fourth melanocortin receptor. J Biol Chem 268:15174–15179

Garcia-Garayoa E, Maes V, Bläuenstein P, Blanc A, Hohn A, Tourwé D, Schubiger PA (2006) Double-stabilized neurotensin analogues as potential radiopharmaceuticals for NTR-positive tumors. Nucl Med Biol 33:495–503

Garg PK, Alston KL, Zalutsky MR (1995) Catabolism of radioiodinated murine monoclonal antibody F(ab$'$)2 fragment labeled using N-succinimidyl 3-iodobenzoate and Iodogen methods. Bioconjug Chem 6:493–501

Gehlert DR (1999) Role of hypothalamic neuropeptide Y in feeding and obesity. Neuropeptides 33:329–338

Giblin MF, Wang N, Hoffman TJ, Jurisson SS, Quinn TP (1998) Design and characterization of α-melanotropin peptide analogs cyclized through rhenium and technetium metal coordination. Proc Natl Acad Sci U S A 95:12814–12818

Ginj M, Zhang H, Waser B, Cescato R, Wild D, Wang X, Erchegyi J, Rivier J, Macke HR, Reubi JC (2006) Radiolabeled somatostatin receptor antagonists are preferable to agonists for in vivo peptide receptor targeting of tumors. Proc Natl Acad Sci U S A 103:16436–16441

Gotthardt M, Fischer M, Holz JB, Jungclas H, Fritsch HW, Béhé M et al (2002) Use of the incretin hormone glucagon–like peptide–1 (GLP–1) for the detection of insulinomas: first experimental results. Eur J Nucl Med Mol Imaging 29: 597–606

Gotthardt M, Béhé MP, Beuter D, Battmann A, Bauhofer A, Schurrat T, Schipper M, Pollum H, Oyen WJG, Behr TM (2006) Improved tumour detection by gastrin receptor scintigraphy in patients with metastasised medullary thyroid carcinoma. Eur J Nucl Med Mol Imag 33: 1273–1279

Gotthardt M, Lalyko G, van Eerd-Vismale J, Keil B, Schurrat T, Hower M, Laverman P, Behr TM, Boerman OC, Goke B, Behe M (2006b) A new technique for in vivo imaging of specific GLP-1 binding sites: First results in small rodents. Regul Pept 137:162–167

Gottschalk K-E, Adams PD, Brunger AT, Kessler H (2002) Transmembrane signal transduction of the $\alpha_{IIb}\beta_3$ integrin. Protein Science11:1800–1812

Grundemar L, Bloom SR (1997) Neuropeptide Y and drug developments, vol 396. Academic Press, San Diego

Hajitou A, Pasqualini R, Arap W (2006) Vascular targeting: recent advances and therapeutic perspectives. Trends Cardiovasc Med 16:80–88

Hanaoka H, Mukai T, Tamamura H, Mori T, Ishino S, Ogawa K, Iida Y, Doi R, Fujii N, Saji H (2006) Development of a ^{111}In-labeled peptide derivative targeting a chemokine receptor, CXCR4, for imaging tumors. Nucl Med Biol 33:489–494

Handl HL, Vagner J, Han H, Mash E, Hruby VJ, Gillies RJ (2004) Hitting multiple targets with multimeric ligands. Expert Opin Ther Targets 8:565–586

Haubner R, Wester H-J (2004) Radiolabeled tracers for imaging of tumor angiogenesis and evaluation of anti-angiogenic therapies. Curr Pharm Des 10:1439–1455

Haubner R, Wester HJ, Reuning U, Senekowitsch-Schmidtke R, Diefenbach B, Kessler H et al (1999) Radiolabeled $\alpha_v\beta_3$ integrin antagonists: a new class of tracers for tumor targeting. J Nucl Med 40:1061–1071

Haubner R, Wester HJ, Burkhart F, Senekowitsch-Schmidtke R, Weber W, Goodman SL, Kessler H, Schwaiger M (2001) Glycosylated RGD-containing peptides: tracer for tumor targeting and angiogenesis imaging with improved biokinetics. J Nucl Med 42:326–336

Haubner R, Kuhnast B, Mang C, Weber WA, Kessler H, Wester HJ, Schwaiger M (2004) [18F]Galacto-RGD: synthesis, radiolabeling, metabolic stability, and radiation dose estimates. Bioconjugate Chem 15:61–69

Haubner R, Weber WA, Beer AJ et al (2005) Noninvasive visualization of the activated alphavbeta3 integrin in cancer patients by positron emission tomography and [18F]Galacto-RGD. PLoS Med. 2:244–254

Hennig IM, Laissue JA, Horisberger U, Reubi JC (1995) Substance P receptors in human primary neoplasms. Int J Cancer 61:786–792

Henze M, Schuhmacher J, Hipp P, Kowalski J, Becker DW, Doll J, Macke HR, Hofmann M, Debus J, Haberkorn U (2001) PET imaging of somatostatin receptors using [68GA]DOTA-D-Phe1-Tyr3-octreotide: first results in patients with meningiomas. J Nucl Med 42:1053–1056

Hofmann M, Maecke H, Borner R, Weckesser E, Schoffski P, Oei L, Schumacher J, Henze M, Heppeler A, Meyer J, Knapp H (2001) Biokinetics and imaging with the somatostatin receptor PET radioligand (68)Ga-DOTATOC: preliminary data. Eur J Nucl Med 28:1751–1757

Hruby VJ, Sharma SD, Toth K, Jaw JY, Al–Obeidi F, Sawyer TK, Hadley ME (1993) Design, synthesis, and conformation of superpotent and prolonged acting melanotropins. Ann N Y Acad Sci 680:51–63

Huhalov A, Chester KA (2004) Engineered single chain antibody fragments for radioimmunotherapy. Q J Nucl Med Mol Imaging 48:279–288

Hultsch C, Pawelke B, Bergmann, Wuest F (2006) Synthesis and evaluation of novel multimeric neurotensin(8-13) analogs. Bioorg Med Chem 14:5913–5920

Janssen ML, Oyen WJ, Dijkgraaf I, Massuger LF, Frielink C, Edwards DS et al (2002a) Tumor targeting with radiolabeled $\alpha v\beta3$ integrin binding peptides in a nude mouse model. Cancer Res 62:6146–6151

Janssen MLH, Oyen WJG, Massuger LFAG, Frielink C, Dijkgraaf I, Edwards DS et al (2002b) Comparison of a monomeric and dimeric radiolabeled RGD-peptide for tumor imaging. Cancer Biother Radiopharm 17:641–646

Kessler H, Haupt A, Schudok M (1988) structural optimization of peptides for cytoprotection of rat liver cells. In: Shiba T, Sakakibara S (eds) Peptide chemistry 1987 (Proc Jpn Symp Peptide Chem, Sept. 28 – Oct. 2, 1987, Kobe, Japan). Protein Research Foundation, Osaka, pp 627–630

Kessler H, Schudok M, Haupt A (1989) Dimerization of cyclic hexapeptides: strong increase of biological activity. In: Jung G, Bayer E (eds) Peptides 1988 (Proc 20th Eur Peptide Symp, Sept. 4–9, 1988, Tübingen). Walter de Gruyter, Berlin New York, pp 664–666

Kiessling LL, Gestwicki JE, Strong LE (2000) Synthetic multivalent ligands in the exploration of cell-surface interactions. Curr Opin Chem Biol 6:696–703

Kneifel S. Cordier D, Good S, Ionescu MCS, Ghaffari A, Hofer S, Kretzschmar M, Tolnay M, Apostolidis C, Waser B, Arnold M, Mueller–Brand J, Maecke HR, Reubi JC, Merlo A (2006) Local targeting of malignant gliomas by the diffusible peptidic vector 1,4,7,10-tetraazacyclododecane-1-glutaric acid-4,7,10-triacetic acid-substance P. Clin Cancer Res 12: 3843–3850

Körner M, Waser B, Reubi JC (2004a) Neuropeptide Y receptor expression in human primary ovarian neoplasms. Lab Invest 84:71–80

Körner M, Waser B, Reubi JC (2004b) High expression of NPY receptors in tumors of the human adrenal gland and extraadrenal paraganglia. Clin Cancer Res 10:8426–8433

Koglin N, Anton M, Hauser A, Saur D, Algul H, Schmid R, Gansbacher B, Schwaiger M, Wester HJ (2006) CXCR4 chemokine receptor SPECT/PET imaging with radiolabeled CPCR4: a promising approach for imaging metastatic processes. J Nucl Med 47(Suppl 1):505P

Kok RJ, Schraa AJ, Bos EJ et al (2002) Preparation and functional evaluation of RGD-modified proteins as alpha(v)beta(3) integrin directed therapeutics. Bioconjug Chem 13:128–135

Koivunen E, Wang B, Ruoslahti E (1995) Phage libraries displaying cyclic peptides with different ring sizes: ligand specificities of the RGD-directed integrins. Biotechnology (N Y) 13:265–270

Komazawa H, Saiki I, Aoki M et al (1993a) Synthetic Arg-Gly-Asp-Ser analogues of the cell recognition site of fibronectin that retain antimetastatic and anti-cell adhesive properties. Biol Pharm Bull 16:997–1003

Komazawa H, Saiki I, Igarashi Y et al (1993b) The conjugation of RGDS peptide with CM-chitin augments the peptide-mediated inhibition of tumor metastasis. Carbohydrate Polymers 21: 299–307

Komazawa H, Saiki I, Nishikawa N et al (1993c) Inhibition of tumor metastasis by Arg-Gly-Asp-Ser (RGDS) peptide conjugated with sulfated chitin derivative, SCM-chitin-RGDS. Clin Exp Metastasis 11:482–491

Kramer RH, Karpen JW (1998) Spanning binding sites on allosteric proteins with polymer-linked ligand dimers. Nature 395:710–713

Krantic S, Goddard I, Saveanu A, Giannetti N, Fombonne J, Cardoso A, Jaquet P, Enjalbert A (2004) Novel modalities of somatostatin actions. Eur J Endocrinol 151:643–655

Kraus JL, Menassa P (1987) Effect of new biologically active polypeptides on dihexadecyl phosphate vesicles. Pharmacol Res Commun 19:469–77

Kraus JL, DiPaola A, Belleau B (1984) Cyclic tetrameric clusters of chemotactic peptides as superactive activators of lysozyme release from human neutrophils. Biochem Biophys Res Commun 124:939–944

Krenning EP, Bakker WH, Breeman WA, Koper JW, Kooij PP, Ausema L, Lameris JS, Reubi JC, Lamberts SW (1989) Localisation of endocrine-related tumours with radioiodinated analogue of somatostatin. Lancet 1(8632):242–244

Krenning EP, Kwekkeboom DJ, Valkema R, Pauwels S, Kvols LK, De Jong M (2004) Peptide receptor radionuclide therapy. Ann N Y Acad Sci 1014:234–245

Kroog GS, Jensen RT, Battey JF (1995) Mammalian bombesin receptors. Med Res Rev 15: 389–417

Kwekkeboom DJ, Bakker WH, Kooij PPM et al (2000) Cholecystokinin receptor imaging using an octapeptide DTPA-CCK analogue in patients with medullary thyroid carcinoma. Eur J Nucl Med 27:1312–17

Kwekkeboom DJ, Bakker WH, Kooij PP, Konijnenberg MW, Srinivasan A, Erion JL,Schmidt MA, Bugaj JL, de Jong M, Krenning EP (2001) [177Lu-DOTAOTyr3]octreotate: comparison with [111In-DTPAo]octreotide in patients. Eur J Nucl Med 28:1319–1325

Kwekkeboom DJ, Mueller-Brand J, Paganelli G, Anthony LB, Pauwels S, Kvols LK, O'dorisio TM, Valkema R, Bodei L, Chinol M, Maecke HR, Krenning EP (2005) Overview of results of peptide receptor radionuclide therapy with 3 radiolabeled somatostatin analogs. J Nucl Med 46(Suppl 1):62S–66S

Labbé O, Desarnaud F, Eggerickx D, Vassart G, Parmentier M (1994) Molecular cloning of a mouse melanocortin 5 receptor gene widely expressed in peripheral tissues. Biochemistry 33:4543–4549

Landon LA, Zou J, Deutscher SL (2004) Is phage display technology on target for developing peptide - based cancer drugs? Curr Drug Discov Technol. 2004 Jan; 1(2):113–132

Langer M, La Bella R, Garcia-Garayoa E, Beck–Sickinger AG (2001) ^{99m}Tc-labeled neuropeptide Y as potential tumor imaging agents. Bioconjugate Chem12:1028–1034

Lantry LE, Cappelletti E, Maddalena ME, Fox JS, Feng W, Chen J, Thomas R, Eaton SM, Bogdan NJ, Arunachalam T, Reubi JC, Raju N, Metcalfe C, Lattuada L, Linder KE, Swenson RE, Tweedle MF, Nunn AD (2006) ^{177}Lu-AMBA: synthesis and characterization of a selective ^{177}Lu-labeled GRP-R agonist for systemic radiotherapy of prostate cancer. J Nucl Med 47:1144–1152

Li R, Babu CR, Lear JD, Wand AJ, Bennett JS, DeGrado WF (2001) Oligomerization of the integrin $\alpha IIb\beta 3$: roles of the transmembrane and cytoplasmic domains. Proc Natl Acad Sci U S A 98:12462–12467

Li W, Metcalf DG, Gorelik R et al (2005) A push-pull mechanism for regulating integrin function. Proc Natl Acad Sci U S A 102:1424–1429

Luo Y, Prestwich GD (2002) Cancer–targeted polymeric drugs. Curr Cancer Drug Targets 2: 209–226

Luyt LG, Katzenellenbogen JA (2002) A trithiolate tripodal bifunctional ligand for the radiolabeling of peptides with gallium(III). Bioconjug Chem 13:1140–1145

Maecke HR, Hofmann M, Haberkorn U (2005) (68)Ga-labeled peptides in tumor imaging. J Nucl Med 46(Suppl 1):172S–178S

Maeda H, Wu J, Sawa T, Matsumura Y, Hori K (2000) Tumor vascular permeability and the EPR-effect in macromolecular therapeutics: a review. J Control Release 65:271–284

Maeda H, Fang J, Inutsuka T, Kitamoto Y (2003) Vascular permeability enhancement in solid tumor: various factors, mechanisms involved and its implications. Int Immunopharmacol 3: 319–328

Maina T, Nock BA, Zhang H, Nikolopoulou A, Waser B, Reubi JC, Maecke HR (2005) Species differences of bombesin analog interactions with GRP-R define the choice of animal models in the development of GRP-R-targeting drugs. J Nucl Med 46:823–830

Mammen M, Choi SK, Whitesides M (1998) Polyvalent interactions in biological systems: implications for design and use of multivalent ligands and inhibitors. Angew Chem Int Ed 37: 2754–2794

Matsuoka T, Hirakawa K, Chung YS et al (1998) Adhesion polypeptides are useful for the prevention of peritoneal dissemination of gastric cancer. Clin Exp Metastasis 16:381–388

Meisetschlager G, Poethko T, Stahl A, Wolf I, Scheidhauer K, Schottelius M, Herz M, Wester HJ, Schwaiger M (2006) Gluc-Lys([18F]FP)-TOCA PET in patients with SSTR-positive tumors: biodistribution and diagnostic evaluation compared with [111In]DTPA-octreotide. J Nucl Med 47:566–573

Miao Y, Owen NK, Whitener D, Gallazi F, Hoffman TJ, Quinn TP (2002) In vivo evaluation of [188]Re-labeled alpha-melanocyte stimulating hormone peptide analogs for melanoma therapy. Int J Cancer 101:480–487

Michel MC, Beck-Sickinger A, Cox H, Doods HN, Herzog H, Larhammer D, Quirion R, Schwartz T, Westfall T (1998) XVI. International Union of Pharmacology recommendations for the nomenclature of neuropeptide Y, peptide YY, and pancreatic polypeptide receptors. Pharmacol Rev 50:143–150

Mitra A, Nan A, Ghandehari H, McNeill E, Mulholland J, Line BR (2004) Technetium-99m-Labeled N-(2-hydroxypropyl) methacrylamide copolymers: synthesis, characterization, and in vivo biodistribution. Pharm Res 21:1153–1159

Mitra A, Mulholland J, Nan A, McNeill E, Ghandehari H, Line BR (2005) Targeting tumor angiogenic vasculature using polymer-RGD conjugates. J Control Release 102:191–201

Mountjoy KG, Robbins LS, Mortrud MT (1992) Cone RD. The cloning of a family of genes that encode the melanocortin receptors. Science 257:1248–1251

Muller A, Homey B, Soto H, Ge N, Catron D, Buchanan ME, McClanahan T, Murphy E, Yuan W, Wagner SN, Barrera JL, Mohar A, Verastegui E, Zlotnik A (2001) Involvement of chemokine receptors in breast cancer metastasis. Nature 410:50–56

Nock B, Nikolopoulou A, Chiotellis E, Loudos G, Maintas D, Reubi JC, Maina T (2003) [99mTc]Demobesin 1, a novel potent bombesin analogue for GRP receptor-targeted tumour imaging. Eur J Nucl Med Mol Imaging 30:247–258

Nock BA, Nikolopoulou A, Galanis A, Cordopatis P, Waser B, Reubi JC, Maina T (2005a) Potent bombesin-like peptides for GRP-receptor targeting of tumors with 99mTc: a preclinical study. J Med Chem 48:100–110

Nock BA, Maina T, Béhé M, Nikolopoulou A, Gotthardt M, Schmitt JS, Behr TM, Mäcke HR (2005b) CCK-2/gastrin receptor-targeted tumor imaging with ^{99m}Tc-labeled minigastrin analogs. J Nucl Med 46:1727–1736

Noguchi Y, Wu J, Duncan R et al (1998) Early phase tumor accumulation of macromolecules: a great difference in clearance rate between tumor and normal tissues. Jpn J Cancer Res 89: 307–314

Poethko T, Schottelius M, Thumshirn G, Hersel U, Herz M, Henriksen G et al (2004a) Two-step methodology for high-yield routine radiohalogenation of peptides: 18F-labeled RGD and octreotide analogs. J Nucl Med 45:892–902

Poethko T, Schottelius M, Thumshirn G, Herz M, Haubner R, Henriksen G et al (2004b) Chemoselective pre-conjugate radiohalogenation of unprotected mono- and multimeric peptides via oxime formation. Radiochimica Acta 92:317–327

Reubi JC (2003) Peptide receptors as molecular targets for cancer diagnosis and therapy. Endocr Rev 24:389–427

Reubi JC, Waser B (2003) Concomitant expression of several peptide receptors in neuroendocrine tumours: molecular basis for in vivo multireceptor tumour targeting. Eur J Nucl Med Mol Imaging 30:781–793

Reubi JC, Schaer JC, Waser B (1997) Cholecystokinin(CCK)-A and CCK-B/gastrin receptors in human tumors. Cancer Res 57:1377–1386

Reubi JC, Waser B, Schaer JC et al (1998) Unsulfated DTPA- and DOTA-CCK analogs as specific high-affinity ligands for CCK-B receptor-expressing human and rat tissues in vitro and in vivo. Eur J Nucl Med 25:481–490

Reubi JC, Gugger M, Waser B, Schaer JC (2001) Y1-mediated effect of neuropeptide Y in cancer: breast carcinomas as targets. Cancer Res 61:4636–4641

Rogers BE, McLean SF, Kirkman RL, Della Manna D, Bright SJ, Olsen CC et al (1999) In vivo localization of [^{111}In]-DTPA-D-Phe^1-octreotide to human ovarian tumor xenografts induced to express the somatostatin receptor subtype 2 using an adenoviral vector. Clin Cancer Res 5:383–393

Schiffelers RM, Koning GA, ten Hagen TL et al (2003) Anti-tumor efficacy of tumor vasculature-targeted liposomal doxorubicin. J Control Release 91:115–122

Schneider D, Engelman DM (2004) Involvement of transmembrane domain interactions in signal transduction by α/β integrins. J Biol Chem 279:9840–9846

Schottelius M, Poethko T, Herz M, Reubi JC, Kessler H, Schwaiger M, Wester HJ (2004) First (18)F-labeled tracer suitable for routine clinical imaging of sst receptor-expressing tumors using positron emission tomography. Clin Cancer Res 10:3593–3606

Schottelius M, Reubi JC, Eltschinger V, Schwaiger M, Wester HJ (2005) N-terminal sugar conjugation and C-terminal Thr-for-Thr(ol) exchange in radioiodinated Tyr3-octreotide: effect on cellular ligand trafficking in vitro and tumor accumulation in vivo. J Med Chem 48:2778–2789

Schumacher T, Hofer S, Good S, Reubi JC, Maecke H, Mueller–Brand J et al (2002) Diffusible Brachytherapie mit 90Y–Substanz P bei High Grade Gliomen: Erste Beobachtungen. In: Brink I, Högerle S, Moser E (ed) Nuklearmedizin als Paradigma molekularer Bildgebung. Blackwell, Berlin, p 68

Schuhmacher J, Zhang H, Doll J, Mäcke HR, Matys R, Hauser H, Henze M, Haberkorn U, Eisenhut M (2005) GRP receptor-targeted PET of a rat pancreas carcinoma xenograft in nude mice with a ^{68}Ga-labeled bombesin(6-14) analog. J Nucl Med 46:691–699

Sharkey RM, Goldenberg DM (2005) Perspectives on cancer therapy with radiolabeled monoclonal antibodies. J Nucl Med. 46(suppl 1):115S–127S

Siegrist W, Solca F, Stutz S et al (1989) Characterization of receptors for alpha-melanocyte stimulating hormone on human melanoma cells. Cancer Res 49:6352–6358

Signore A, Annovazzi A, Chianelli M, Corsetti F, Van de Wiele C, Watherhouse RN (2001) Peptide
radiopharmaceuticals for diagnosis and therapy. Eur J Nucl Med 28:1555–1565

Smith GP (1985) Filamentous fusion phage: novel expression vectors that display cloned antigens
on the virion surface. Science 228:1315–1317

Smith CJ, Volkert WA, Hoffman TJ (2005) Radiolabeled peptide conjugates for targeting of the
bombesin receptor superfamily subtypes. Nucl Med Biol 32:733–740

Smith SV (2004) Molecular imaging with copper-64. J Inorg Biochem 98:1874–1901

Sprague JE, Peng Y, Sun X, Weisman GR, Wong EH, Achilefu S, Anderson CJ (2004) Preparation
and biological evaluation of copper-64-labeled tyr3-octreotate using a cross-bridged macrocyclic chelator. Clin Cancer Res 10:8674–8682

Stefanidakis M, Koivunen E (2004) Peptide-mediated delivery of therapeutic and imaging agents
into mammalian cells. Curr Pharm Des 10:3033–3044

Stein R, Goldenberg DM, Thorpe SR, Basu A, Mattes MJ (1995) Effects of radiolabeling monoclonal antibodies with a residualizing iodine radiolabel on the accretion of radioisotope in
tumors. Cancer Res 55:3132–3139

Stolz B, Smith-Jones P, Albert R, Tolcsvai L, Briner U, Ruser G, Macke H, Weckbecker G, Bruns C
(1997) Somatostatin analogues for somatostatin-receptor-mediated radiotherapy of cancer. Digestion 57 Suppl 1:17–21

Tatro JB, Reichlin S (1987) Specific receptors for alpha-melanocyte stimulating hormone are
widely distributed in tissues of rodents. Endocrinology 121:1900–1907

Tatro JB, Atkins M, Mier JW et al (1990) Melanotropin receptors demonstrated in situ in human
melanoma. J Clin Invest 85:1825–1832

Thumshirn G, Hersel U, Goodman SL, Kessler H (2003) Multimeric cyclic RGD peptides as potential tools for tumor targeting: solid-phase peptide synthesis and chemoselective oxime ligation.
Chemistry 9:2717–2725

Van Hagen PM, Breeman WAP, Reubi JC, Postema, PTE, van den Anker–Lugtenburg PJ, Kwekkeboom DJ et al (1996) Visualization of the thymus by substance P receptor scintigraphy in man.
Eur J Nucl Med 23:1508–1513

Velikyan I, Beyer GJ, Langstrom B (2004) Microwave-supported preparation of (68)Ga bioconjugates with high specific Radioactivity. Bioconjug Chem 15:554–560

Wank SA, Pisegna JR, de Weerth A (1994) Cholecystokinin receptor family. Molecular cloning,
structure, and functional expression in rat, guinea pig, and human. Ann N Y Acad Sci 713:
49–66

Waser B, Eltschinger V, Linder K, Nunn A, Reubi JC (2007) Selective in vitro targeting of GRP
and NMB receptors in human tumours with the new bombesin tracer ^{177}Lu-AMBA. Eur J Nucl
Med Mol Imaging 34:95–100

Wester HJ, Schottelius M, Scheidhauer K, Meisetschlager G, Herz M, Rau FC, Reubi JC,
Schwaiger M (2003) PET imaging of somatostatin receptors: design, synthesis and preclini-
cal evaluation of a novel 18F-labelled, carbohydrated analogue of octreotide. Eur J Nucl Med
Mol Imaging 30:117–122

Wester HJ, Schottelius M, Poethko T, Bruus-Jensen K, Schwaiger M (2004) Radiolabeled carbohydrated somatostatin analogs: a review of the current status. Cancer Biother Radiopharm
19(2):231–244

Wester HJ, Kessler H (2005) Molecular targeting with peptides or peptide-polymer conjugates: just
a question of size? J Nucl Med 46:1940–1945

Wieland HA, Hamilton BS, Krist B, Doods HN (2000) The role of NPY in metabolic homeostasis:
Implications for obesity therapy. Expert Opin Investig Drugs 9:1327–1346

Wild D, Schmitt JS, Ginj M, Macke HR, Bernard BF, Krenning E et al (2003) DOTA-NOC, a
high-affinity ligand of somatostatin receptor subtypes 2, 3 and 5 for labelling with various
radiometals. Eur J Nucl Med Mol Imaging 30:1338–1347

Wild D, Béhé M, Wicki A, Christofori G, Waser B, Gotthardt M et al (2005a) Preclinical evaluation of an In–111 labeled Exendin-4 derivative, a very promising ligand for glucagons-like peptide-1 (GLP-1) receptor targeting. Mol Imaging 4:328

Wild D, Macke HR, Waser B, Reubi JC, Ginj M, Rasch H, Muller-Brand J, Hofmann M (2005b) 68Ga-DOTANOC: a first compound for PET imaging with high affinity for somatostatin receptor subtypes 2 and 5. Eur J Nucl Med Mol Imaging 32:724

Winter PM, Morawski AM, Caruthers SD et al (2003) Molecular imaging of angiogenesis in early-stage atherosclerosis with alpha(v)beta3-integrin-targeted nanoparticles. Circulation 108: 2270–2274

Wu Y, Zhang X, Xiong Z, Cheng Z, Fisher DR, Liu S et al (2005) MicroPET imaging of glioma integrin $\alpha v \beta 3$ expression using 64Cu-labeled tetrameric RGD peptide. J Nucl Med 46: 1707–1718

Zhang X, Xiong Z, Wu Y, Cai W, Tseng JR, Gambhir SS, Chen X (2006) Quantitative PET imaging of tumor integrin $\alpha_v \beta_3$ expression with 18F-FRGD2. J Nucl Med 47:113–121

Zinn KR, Buchsbaum DJ, Chaudhuri T et al (2000) Noninvasive monitoring of gene transfer using a reporter receptor imaged with a high affinity peptide radiolabeled with ^{99m}Tc or [188]Re. J Nucl Med41:887–895

Small Molecule Receptors as Imaging Targets

Aviv Hagooly, Raffaella Rossin, and Michael J. Welch(✉)

Abstract The aberrant expression and function of certain receptors in tumours and other diseased tissues make them preferable targets for molecular imaging. PET and SPECT radionuclides can be used to label specific ligands with high affinity for the target receptors. The functional information obtained from imaging these receptors can be used to better understand the systems under investigation and for diagnostic and therapeutic applications. This review discusses some of the aspects of receptor imaging with small molecule tracers by PET and SPECT and reviews some of the tracers for the receptor imaging of tumours and brain, heart and lung disorders.

Michael J. Welch

Mallinckrodt Institute of Radiology, Washington University School of Medicine, 510 S. Kingshighway Blvd. Campus Box 8225, St. Louis, MO 63110

welchm@wustl.edu

W. Semmler and M. Schwaiger (eds.), *Molecular Imaging II.*
Handbook of Experimental Pharmacology 185/II.
© Springer-Verlag Berlin Heidelberg 2008

1 Introduction

Molecular imaging enables the viewing, measurement and characterization of biological processes at the cellular and sub-cellular (molecular) levels. Within the past few decades, the scientific community has witnessed the development of a plethora of imaging techniques. Some of these techniques provide mainly anatomical information, while others, such as PET and SPECT, allow functional studies at molecular levels.

Examples of commonly used SPECT radionuclides are the non-physiological elements ^{99m}Tc, ^{111}In, ^{123}I, and ^{67}Ga. These radionuclides have half-lives ranging from 6 h to almost 3 days and photon energies that allow the acquisition of high quality images (100–200 keV). On the other hand, the radionuclides used for PET include physiologically important elements such as ^{11}C, ^{15}O, and ^{13}N, with a half-life of up to 20 min. However, ^{18}F is the most used PET radionuclide as its half-life (110 min) allows both sophisticated chemistry and prolonged in vivo evaluation. Other non-standard positron-emitting radionuclides under evaluation for the production of PET radiotracers are listed in Table 1. More details about the production and application of radionuclides, radiochemistry, etc., can be found elsewhere (Valk et al. 2003; Welch and Redvanly 2003; Mazzi 2006).

In order for a radiotracer to be useful for imaging applications it must specifically accumulate at the target site and clear rapidly from the non-target tissues to decrease the background activity and reduce the dose to the patient. The accumulation at the target site can be achieved by using radiotracers with high affinity and selectivity for disease biomarkers, such as over-expressed receptors, antigens, transporters, mRNA, etc. In the following pages, some of the application of small molecule radiotracers for PET and SPECT receptor imaging in tumours, brain, heart, and lung will be discussed briefly.

2 Tumour Receptors

Cells perform and communicate via a multitude of protein-protein interactions which activate the complex pathways of cell signalling. Since cancer cells occasionally up-regulate specific receptors, high-affinity receptor ligands labelled with PET or SPECT radionuclides can be used to identify tumour lesions, to estimate the grade and aggressiveness of a tumour, and to assess the early response to anti-cancer agents in a non-invasive manner (Van Den Bossche and Van de Wiele 2004). To this aim, a series of extra- and intra-cellular receptors has been evaluated.

2.1 Folate Receptors

The folate receptor (FR) is a membrane-bound protein with a high affinity for the vitamin folic acid (Antony 1996). The FR-α isoform is an attractive target for

Table 1 Radionuclides for PET and SPECT (Welch and Redvanly 2003)

	$T_{1/2}$	Decay modes (%)	Main γ KeV (%)	β_{max} MeV (β_{ave})	Production
SPECT radionuclides					
^{99m}Tc	6.01 h	IT	140 (89.1)		^{99}Mo/^{99m}Tc generator
^{123}I	13.27 h	EC	159 (83.3)		^{124}Te(p,2n)^{123}I
^{67}Ga	78.27 h	EC	93 (39.2); 185 (21.2); 300 (16.8)		^{68}Zn(p,2n)^{67}Ga
^{111}In	67.31 h	EC	171 (90.7); 245 (94.1)		^{111}Cd(p,n)^{111}In ^{112}Cd(p,2n)^{111}In
^{201}Tl	72.91 h	EC	167 (10.0)		^{203}Tl(p,3n)^{201}Pb: ^{201}Tl
^{133}Xe	5.24 d	β^-	81 (38.0)	0.346 (0.100)	^{235}U fission
PET radionuclides					
^{11}C	20.39 min	β^+ (99.8) EC (0.2)	511 (199.5)	0.960 (0.386)	^{14}N(p,α)^{11}C
^{13}N	9.96 min	β^+ (99.8) EC (0.2)	511 (199.6)	1.198 (0.492)	^{16}O(p,α)^{13}N
^{15}O	122.24 s	β^+ (99.9) EC (0.1)	511 (199.8)	1.732 (0.735)	^{14}N(d,n)^{15}O ^{15}N(p,n)^{15}O
^{18}F	109.8 min	β^+ (97) EC (3)	511 (193.5)	0.633 (0.250)	^{18}O(p,n)^{18}F ^{20}Ne(d,α)^{18}F
^{124}I	4.18 d	β^+ (23) EC (77)	511 (46); 603 (62.9); 723 (10.3)	2.138 (0.820)	^{124}Te(p,n)^{124}I ^{124}Te(d,2n)^{124}I
^{75}Br	96.7 min	β^+ (73) EC (27)	287 (90); 511 (146)	2.008 (0.719)	^{76}Se(p,2n)^{75}Br ^{76}Se(d,3n)^{75}Br
^{76}Br	16.2 h	β^+ (55) EC (45)	511 (109); 559 (74.0); 657 (15.9); 1,854 (14.7)	3.941 (1.180)	^{76}Se(p,n)^{76}Br ^{76}Se(d,2n)^{76}Br
^{66}Ga	9.49 h	β^+ (56) EC (44)	511 (112); 1,039 (36.0); 2,752 (23.3)	4.153 (1.740)	^{63}Cu(α,n)^{66}Ga
^{68}Ga	67.71 min	β^+ (89) EC (11)	511 (178.3)	1.899 (0.829)	^{68}Ge/^{68}Ga generator
^{60}Cu	23.7 min	β^+ (93) EC (7)	511 (185); 826 (21.7); 1,332 (88.0); 1,792 (45.4)	3.772 (0.970)	^{60}Ni(p,n)^{60}Cu
^{61}Cu	3.33 h	β^+ (61) EC (39)	511 (123); 656 (10.8)	1.215 (0.500)	^{61}Ni(p,n)^{61}Cu
^{62}Cu	9.7 min	β^+ (97) EC (3)	511 (194.9)	2.926 (1.314)	^{62}Zn/^{62}Cu generator
^{64}Cu	12.7 h	β^+ (17) EC (44) β^- (39)	511 (34.8)	0.653 (0.278)	^{64}Ni(p,n)^{64}Cu
^{94m}Tc	52.0 min	β^+ (70) EC (30)	511 (140.4); 871 (94.2)	2.438 (1.072)	^{94}Mo(p,n)^{94m}Tc

Source: http://www.nndc.bnl.gov

diagnosis and therapy of cancer and other malignancies because it is physiologically expressed in limited regions of the body (kidney, placenta and apical surface of some normal epithelia), while it is over-expressed by a number of tumours, haematopoietic malignancies of myeloid origin, and activated macrophages. Furthermore, a strong correlation between FR expression and tumour grade was observed and high levels of FR in primary tumour masses were associated with poor prognosis in breast cancer patients (Ke et al. 2004; Hilgenbrink and Low 2005; Reddy et al. 2005). Folic acid is known to internalise macromolecules into cells via FR-mediated endocytosis (Leamon and Low 1991) and has been used to deliver a variety of anti-cancer drugs into tumour cells (Leamon and Reddy 2004).

For imaging purposes, folic acid has been labelled with Ga radioisotopes (Wang et al. 1996; Mathias et al. 2003), [111]In (Wang et al. 1997), [99m]Tc (Guo et al. 1999; Mathias et al. 2000; Leamon et al. 2002; Trump et al. 2002; Wedeking et al. 2002; Panwar et al. 2004; Liu et al. 2005; Müller et al. 2006; Okarvi and Jammaz 2006), [64]Cu (Ke et al. 1999), and [18]F (Bettio et al. 2006). All the radiolabelled folate conjugates retained affinity for the receptor in vitro and in vivo using FR-positive tumour models. In addition, a recent preliminary clinical study demonstrated that ^{111}In-DTPA-folate SPECT was able to identify both newly diagnosed and recurrent ovarian cancers with high sensitivity (Siegel et al. 2003), thus confirming the possible use of radiolabelled folate conjugates to diagnose malignancies. ^{99m}Tc-EC20, a new promising folate conjugate labelled with the more attractive SPECT radionuclide ^{99m}Tc, is currently undergoing clinical evaluation as an agent for detecting the locus of FR-positive cancers (Leamon et al. 2002; Reddy et al. 2004).

Due to folic acid's ability to internalise big payloads into tumour cells, the FR is also being evaluated as a target for imaging and drug delivery to tumours with folic acid conjugated liposomes and nanoparticles (Gabizon et al. 2004; Rossin et al. 2005; Dixit et al. 2006; Sun et al. 2006).

2.2 Sigma Receptors

Sigma receptors (σ-Rs) are membrane-bound proteins originally classified as subtypes of the opioid receptor (Martin et al. 1976). They are expressed in liver, kidney, endocrine glands, central nervous system, and other tissues (Ferris et al. 1991), and at least two subtypes of σ-Rs (σ_1 and σ_2), differing in molecular weight and stereospecificity, have been identified (Quirion et al. 1992). Their involvement in several neurological disorders, such as Alzheimer's disease, epilepsy, and schizophrenia, has been confirmed (Caveliers et al. 2001) and a number of radiotracers have been developed to non-invasively image these disorders (Hashimoto and Ishiwata 2006). Furthermore, the observed over-expression of σ-Rs in a variety of human tumours (Vilner et al. 1995) suggested the use of σ-specific imaging agents for tumour diagnosis (Caveliers et al. 2001). In particular, targeting of σ-Rs for breast cancer imaging was suggested in the mid 1990s, when binding experiments with the benzamide [^{125}I]4-IBP confirmed a high σ-R density in human breast cancer cells

(John et al. 1995). Since then, many σ_1/σ_2 ligands have been developed to target σ-R-rich tissues (Dence et al. 1997; Shiue et al. 1997; Huang et al. 1998; Kawamura et al. 2003; Waterhouse et al. 2003) and some have been proposed as promising tumour imaging agents (Waterhouse et al. 1997; John et al. 1999b; van Waarde et al. 2004, 2006; Berardi et al. 2005; Kawamura et al. 2005).

The discovery that σ_2-R expression is eight- to tenfold higher in proliferating tumour cells than in quiescent cells (Wheeler et al. 2000) suggested that this σ-R sub-type can serve as a biomarker for assessing the proliferative status of tumours non-invasively, and specific targeting of σ_2-R resulted in high contrast images (Mach et al. 2001). Therefore, high affinity and selective σ_2-R targeting ligands have been synthesized and evaluated as potential agents for breast tumour imaging with PET (Berardi et al. 2004; Colabufo et al. 2005) and SPECT (Choi et al. 2001; Hou et al. 2006). Recently, two new benzamide-based σ_2-R tracers labelled with ^{11}C (Tu et al. 2005) and ^{76}Br (Rowland et al. 2006) were evaluated in a breast cancer model and exhibited higher tumour uptake compared with that of $[^{18}F]FLT$, another candidate tracer for imaging tumour proliferation (Barthel et al. 2003).

To the best of our knowledge, the only clinical trial with σ-R-specific tracers in breast cancer patients was performed with a radio-iodinated benzamide ($[^{123}I]PIMBA$) expressing affinity for both σ-R sub-types (John et al. 1999a). In this pilot SPECT study, focal uptake of $[^{123}I]PIMBA$ was observed in patients with confirmed breast cancer and no uptake was found in fibrocystic disease or local inflammation (Caveliers et al. 2002). Although some false-negative results highlighted the need for a better understanding of receptor expression in breast cancer, the overall study confirms the feasibility of breast cancer imaging with σ-R targeting tracers.

2.3 Steroid Receptors

The steroid receptors are proteins located in both the cytoplasmic and nuclear fractions of the cell (Drummond 2006). Steroid hormones such as progestins, estrogens, and androgens are likely to influence carcinogenesis since they have profound effects on cellular proliferation, and up-regulation of steroid receptors may have clinical implications. Therefore, a variety of radiolabelled ligands have been produced in order to image the steroid receptors (Mankoff et al. 2000).

Estrogens regulate the growth, development and function of diverse tissues in both men and women. In women, target tissues are mostly in the reproductive apparatus (ovaries, uterus) as well as in select non-reproductive tissues expressing the estrogen receptors (ERs). The α and β ER and their isoforms (Kuiper et al. 1996) are members of the nuclear hormone receptor family of transcription factors (Landel et al. 1997), and bind both estrogen and the estrogen modulators (such as tamoxifen) used to treat ER-positive tumours (Forbes 1997). Two-thirds of patients with breast carcinoma have ER-positive primary tumours, and the presence of the receptor has been observed to be predictive of patient prognosis (Clark et al. 1987). In addition, tumour ER expression has been shown to correlate with response to hormonal therapy and is carefully considered when a patient's treatment is determined by a physician (Bennink et al. 2004). Therefore, development of non-invasive ER imaging protocols is highly attractive to determine the ER status of primary tumours and metastases and to assess efficacy of hormonal therapy relatively quickly.

The feasibility of functional ER status determination by in vivo imaging has been confirmed with 16α-[^{18}F]fluoroestradiol ([^{18}F]FES) and PET. Clinical studies have demonstrated a strong correlation between [^{18}F]FES uptake and tumour ER concentration (Dehdashti et al. 1995). [^{18}F]FES has shown high sensitivity in detecting ER-positive primary tumour lesions and metastatic foci in patients with known breast cancer (Mortimer et al. 1996). Furthermore, baseline tumour [^{18}F]FES uptake and a "flare" reaction, resulting in increased [^{18}F]FDG uptake after tamoxifen treatment, were determined to be important predictors of response to tamoxifen treatment of breast cancer (Mortimer et al. 2001).

[^{18}F]FES PET has also proven to be useful in monitoring the response to hormonal therapy in a population of heavily pre-treated metastatic breast and endometrial cancer patients (Linden et al. 2006; Yoshida et al. in press), and it was also used to non-invasively monitor gene therapy in vivo (Takamatsu et al. 2005) and in vitro (Furukawa et al. 2006) by using the human ER ligand binding domain as a reporter gene.

Despite these promising pre-clinical and human studies and the development of an automatic procedure to synthesize [^{18}F]FES on a cassette-type [^{18}F]FDG synthesizer (Mori et al. 2006), [^{18}F]FES PET still has not found widespread clinical application.

In order to reduce metabolism and improve tumour localization compared with [^{18}F]FES, a different series of estradiol derivatives (Hostetler et al. 1999; Jonson et al. 1999; Seimbille et al. 2002) and non-steroidal ER ligands (Seo et al. 2006) have been evaluated in pre-clinical and clinical trials. Derivatives of the ER antagonist fulvestrant labelled with ^{18}F were evaluated for imaging the response to hormonal therapy of ER-positive breast cancer, but suffered from decrease in binding affinity and low uptake (Seimbille et al. 2004).

The radio-iodinated estradiol derivative Z-[^{123}I]MIVE has been suggested as a candidate SPECT agent to detect ERs (Rijks et al. 1996). Preliminary clinical studies demonstrated a high sensitivity in detecting primary breast carcinoma lesions and a good correlation between Z-[^{123}I]MIVE uptake and ER histochemistry was also observed (Bennink et al. 2001). In addition, recent studies in patients confirmed the value of Z-[^{123}I]MIVE scintigraphy in assessing tumour response to tamoxifen therapy as early as 1 month after the beginning of treatment (Bennink et al. 2004). The addition of a cyano group to the 7α-position of the iodinated labelled estrogen did not improve its potential as a SPECT imaging agent (Ali et al. 2003b).

In order to increase the availability of ER-targeting tracers, a number of attempts have been made to synthesize ^{99m}Tc-labelled compounds (Skaddan et al. 2000; Mull et al. 2002; Arterburn et al. 2003; Luyt et al. 2003; Bigott et al. 2005; Takahashi et al. 2008). Many of these compounds exhibited excellent properties in vitro but performed poorly in vivo, producing low and non-specific uptake in ER-rich tissues.

Retrospective studies on the relation between ER sub-type expression in breast cancers and the clinical outcome have indicated the necessity to include an assessment of ER-β status in the patient evaluation (Palmieri et al. 2002; Murphy and Watson 2006). ER-β imaging was attempted with [18F]FEDPN in immature rodents and mice whose ER gene has been deleted. Despite specific binding to the receptor β sub-type in vivo, [18F]FEDPN exhibited a lower uptake in ER rich tissues compared with [18F]FES (Yoo et al. 2005).

The steroid hormone progesterone mediates its effects through the progesterone receptor (PgR), which belong to a large superfamily of ligand-activated nuclear receptors. Since its expression is induced by the ER, the PgR has been studied as a surrogate marker for ER activity and has been used as an additional predictive factor for hormonal therapy response in breast cancer (Cui et al. 2005). Several clinical studies have confirmed that elevated total PgR levels correlate with an increased probability of response to tamoxifen, longer time before treatment failure, and longer overall survival (Hopp et al. 2004). Furthermore, since tamoxifen therapy does not block PgR expression as it does with ER expression, PgR was suggested as a promising target for imaging of breast tumour during hormonal therapy (Johnston et al. 1995).

[123]I-Labelled nortestosterone derivatives displayed high binding affinity for the PgR in vitro (van den Bos et al. 1998) but no significant uptake was observed in animals with mammary tumours (Rijks et al. 1998), and only a few ^{18}F-labelled steroids were synthesized for PET imaging of PgR (Verhagen et al. 1991; Ali et al. 1994; De Groot et al. 1994). While [18F]FENP, a radiolabelled analogue of the potent progestin ORG2058, exhibited high uptake in PgR-rich tissues in rats (Pomper et al. 1988), low target/non-target ratios were obtained in patients with primary breast carcinomas and tracer uptakes were not correlated with PgR tumour expression (Dehdashti et al. 1991). In an effort to increase the in vivo stability and improve the tumour uptake, new halogenated derivatives of fluorofuranyl norprogesterone, a high affinity PgR-binding ligand, have been synthesised and are under evaluation (Verhagen et al. 1994).

Prostate cancer is the most diagnosed malignant growth in men and ranks as the second leading cause of male cancer deaths in the majority of western countries (Jemal et al. 2006). Although androgens are required for prostate development and normal prostate function, the androgen receptor (AR) is believed to be involved in prostate carcinogenesis (Denis and Griffiths 2000; Santos et al. 2004) and may act as a specific target for prostate cancer treatment (Heinlein and Chang 2004).

The main efforts for PET imaging of the AR in prostate cancers have focused on a variety of steroids. Dihydrotestosterone (Choe et al. 1995b; Labaree et al. 1999; Garg et al. 2001), testosterone (Choe and Katzenellenbogen 1995a), mibolerone (Liu et al. 1991), and other steroids (Liu et al. 1992; Bonasera et al. 1996) were labelled with ^{18}F and evaluated as radiotracers for the AR in animal models. [18F]Fluoro-dihydrotestosterone has proven to be an effective tracer for PET imaging of prostate tumours in humans, but further evaluation is needed in order to assess its value as a diagnostic agent during hormonal therapies (Larson et al. 2004; Zanzonico et al. 2004; Dehdashti et al. 2005). While dihydrotestosterone was also radio-iodinated for AR SPECT imaging (Labaree et al. 1997), attempts to radiolabel nortestosterone derivatives with ^{125}I resulted in low affinity for the AR in castrated rats (Ali et al. 2003a).

Androgen ablation therapy (chemical or surgical castration to suppress testosterone synthesis) is the main treatment for prostate cancer. However, following this procedure, most patients experience androgen-independent cancer progression or recurrence (Small et al. 2004). Since the development of resistance to non-steroidal AR antagonists cannot be completely understood by using radiolabelled steroidal agonists, experiments to image the AR with non-steroidal radiotracers and PET were recently conducted. Flutamide was the first non-steroidal anti-androgen drug approved for chemical castration of advanced prostate cancer patients (Katchen and Buxbaum 1975; McLeod 1993). Binding assays performed with ^{76}Br-labelled hydroxyflutamide, the active form of flutamide, showed higher AR affinity compared with that of the parent compound (Parent et al. 2006b). On the contrary, a ^{18}F-labelled derivative of the potent AR antagonist BMS-22 (3-F-NNDI) exhibited twofold lower receptor affinity compared with that of the parent compound (Parent et al. 2006a), and both of these compounds exhibited poor prostate uptake in rats, probably due to in vivo dehalogenation. Other derivatives of hydroxyflutamide labelled with the ^{11}C and ^{18}F were also synthesized, but need further evaluation as potential radiotracers for AR PET imaging (Jacobson et al. 2005, 2006).

3 Brain Neuroreceptors and Neurotransmitters

The first imaging studies of neurotransmission in the human brain were performed in the early 1980s (Wagner et al. 1983). Since then, the number of PET and SPECT studies on cerebral neurotransmission has grown rapidly. To date, nuclear medicine techniques are used for functional imaging studies of dementia, seizure, movement and psychiatric disorders, drug and alcohol addictions, and aging (Zisterer and Williams 1997; Camargo 2001; Wong and Brasic 2001; Burn and O'Brien 2003; Kessler 2003; Piccini and Whone 2004). The goal of neurotransmitter imaging is to elucidate the pathophysiology of mental and neurological disorders, delineate the mechanism of drug action at neurotransmitter sites (e.g., antidepressants, antipsychotics, etc.), evaluate the effects of potential neuroprotective drugs, and identify subjects with or at risk for specific neurodegenerative disorders (Talbot and Laruelle 2002). A multitude of specific imaging tracers have been developed to target brain physiology including the dopaminergic and the serotonergic systems, the benzodiazepine and the opioid receptors. Most of these tracers contain ^{123}I (Kung et al. 2003), ^{11}C and ^{18}F (Mazière and Halldin 2004), and are briefly reviewed in the following sections.

3.1 The Dopaminergic System

The neurotransmitter dopamine (DA) has been implicated in a number of neurodegenerative diseases, neuropsychiatric disorders, and in drugs abuse (Barrio et al.

1997; Nicolaas and Verhoeff 1999; Sanchez-Pernaute et al. 2002; Marek et al. 2003). For this reason, a variety of radiotracers for PET imaging of DA receptors have been developed (Elsinga et al. 2006).

Information on the DA metabolism and the integrity of dopaminergic neurons can be obtained by imaging the pre-synaptic dopaminergic activity in the brain with L-DOPA analogues such as $[^{18}F]$FDOPA (Garnett et al. 1983; Fischman 2005) and $[^{18}F]$FMT (Asselin et al. 2002; Murali et al. 2003; VanBrocklin et al. 2004).

Other families of imaging agents for pre-synaptic DA neurons target the DA transporter (DAT), and $[^{11}C]\beta$–CFT is the progenitor of a series of DAT imaging tracers containing the phenyl-tropane group of cocaine (Wong et al. 1993). Its iodinated analogue, $[^{123}I]\beta$-CIT (DopaScan), is the most widely used DAT imaging tracer for human brain (Boja et al. 1991). Another promising DAT tracer containing the phenyl-tropane moiety is the ^{99m}Tc radiopharmaceutical, TRODAT-1 (Kung 2001; Weng et al. 2004); its small size and optimal lipophilicity result in good penetration of the blood brain barrier. In addition, a kit for the synthesis of TRODAT-1, in conjunction with the low cost and wide availability of the ^{99}Mo$/^{99m}$Tc generator, is likely to allow more widespread and less expensive application of DAT imaging.

The vesicular monoamine transporter type 2 (VMAT2) is another molecular target used to image pre-synaptic dopaminergic activity. To this aim, ^{11}C- and ^{18}F-labelled derivatives of tetrabenazine, a monoamine-depleting drug with a strong affinity for VMAT2, have been extensively evaluated (DaSilva and Kilbourn 1992; De La Fuente-Fernández et al. 2003; Goswami et al. 2006).

Post-synaptic aspects of dopaminergic neurotransmission can be investigated in vivo with imaging tracers for the DA receptors. The DA receptors are classified in two families: the D_1-like (D_1, D_5) and the D_2-like (D_2, D_3, D_4) receptors (Sibley and Monsma 1992). The ^{11}C-labelled benzazepine SCH 23390 was the first high affinity ligand reported for PET imaging of the D_1 receptors (Halldin et al. 1986). Although $[^{11}C]$SCH 23390 was widely used for human studies, its neocortex-to-cerebellum uptake ratio in humans is low (<1.5) and this is not ideal for detailed in vivo examinations (Farde et al. 1987). Furthermore, $[^{11}C]$SCH 23390 interacts with serotonin receptors and is rapidly metabolised in vivo, resulting in a rapid wash-out from the brain with consequent poor test-retest reproducibility (Foged et al. 1996). For these reasons, several other radiotracers (benzazepine and non-benzazepine based) with improved stability and selectivity have been evaluated for mapping D_1 receptors in humans with both PET (Göran et al. 1991; Karlsson et al. 1993; Kassiou et al. 1995; DaSilva et al. 1996; Foged et al. 1996; Yang et al. 1996; Foged et al. 1998; Wu et al. 2005; Elsinga et al. 2006) and SPECT (Kung et al. 1988; Moerlein et al. 1990; Billings et al. 1992; Kassiou et al. 2001). To date, the most promising D_1 ligand is the ^{11}C-labelled benzazepine $(+)$-NNC 112, which has a 100-fold lower affinity for the serotonin 5-HT_{2A} receptors compared with the D_1 receptor and a high uptake in striatum and neocortex (Halldin et al. 1998). It has been successfully used to image striatal and extrastriatal D_1 receptors in humans (Abi Dargham et al. 2000) and was shown to give relatively modest radiation doses (Cropley et al. 2006).

Because many pathological and non-pathological conditions involve changes in D_2 receptor density, and many antipsychotic and anti-Parkinsonian drugs affect this DA receptor sub-type, considerable effort has been dedicated to the production of D_2-specific imaging agents. The first class of imaging tracers widely used to study the D_2 receptor was based on spiperone, a butyrophenone DA antagonist used as neuroleptic drug (Burns et al. 1984; Arnett et al. 1986; Coenen et al. 1987; Nakatsuka et al. 1987; Lever et al. 1990; Suehiro et al. 1990; Moerlein et al. 1997). However, since [^{11}C]N-methylspiperone and the other butyrophenone derivatives exhibited high affinity also for the serotonergic 5-HT$_2$ receptors (Frost et al. 1987; Andree et al. 1998), current ligands of choice for detection of D_2/D_3 receptors are benzamide derivatives.

[^{11}C]Raclopride (Farde et al. 1985) and [^{123}I]iodobenzamide (Kung et al. 1989) are selective ligands with a moderate affinity for the D_2/D_3 receptors, and they have been proven to be useful tracers for the imaging of brain regions with high DA receptor density and in receptor occupancy studies for drug development (Laruelle 2000). However, ligands with higher receptor affinity are required to image the extrastriatal regions of the human brain, since D_2 receptor density in such regions (nucleus occumbens, olfactory tubercles, thalamus, hypothalamus, cortical region, etc.) can be 10- to 100-times lower than in the striatal region. The iodine-containing benzamide epidepride, its bromine analogue isoremoxipride, and the fluorine-containing fallypride have been labelled with PET and SPECT radionuclides and have shown considerable extrastriatal uptake both in non-human primates and in human brains (Kessler et al. 1992; Halldin et al. 1995; Loc'h et al. 1996; Langer et al. 1999; Bradley et al. 2000; Mukherjee et al. 2004b).

The D_2 imaging tracers mentioned so far are antagonists and bind to the receptor in both high-affinity (G protein-coupled) and low-affinity (uncoupled with G protein) states (Sibley et al. 1982), whereas agonists have different affinities for the two states. Since the high-affinity state is believed to be the functional state of the D_2 receptor, labelled DA agonists are expected to be highly sensitive to endogenous competition and to be superior imaging tools for probing fluctuations in endogenous DA levels (Laruelle 2000). Distribution studies with ^{11}C-labelled agonists such as [^{11}C]aminotetralin (Mukherjee et al. 2000), [^{11}C]PPHT and [^{11}C]ZYY-339 (Mukherjee et al. 2004a), [^{11}C]norapomorphine (Hwang et al. 2004), and others (Wilson et al. 2005; Elsinga et al. 2006) have been carried out both in vivo and ex vivo. They all confirmed tracer uptake in the D_2 receptors-rich brain regions, but the interaction with the high-affinity state of the receptor requires further study.

3.2 The Serotonergic System

The monoamine serotonin (SER) is a neurotransmitter involved in the pathophysiology and therapy of several neurological and psychiatric disorders such as depression (Stockmeier 2003), Parkinson's disease (Kerenyi et al. 2003), Alzheimer's disease (Palmer et al. 1987), schizophrenia (Dean 2003) and eating disorders (Stamatakis and Hetherington 2003). The serotonergic function in the human brain is imaged mainly with radiotracers for the SER transporter (SERT) and for the SER receptors 5-HT$_{1A}$ and 5-HT$_{2A}$.

SERT, a protein located on the pre-synaptic serotonergic neurons, is the target of a widely used class of antidepressant drugs (Owens 1996/1997). For this reason, its expression in the human brain has been widely studied using nuclear imaging (Hesse et al. 2004). Recently, some ^{123}I-labelled and ^{11}C-labelled tropane derivatives have been proposed as candidate imaging agents with high specificity for SERT over DAT, but have shown either low brain uptake (Quinlivan et al. 2003) or high brain uptake with non SERT-specific binding (Plisson et al. 2004). However, the most promising SERT tracers belong to a class of diphenylsulphide derivatives (Li et al. 2004). The short-lived $[^{11}$C]DASB was found to be highly suitable for mapping SER reuptake sites in humans (Frankle et al. 2004) and showed reduced SERT density in some recreational MDMA users (Lingford 2005; McCann et al. 2005). Finally, since in vivo measurements on other ^{11}C-labelled diphenylsulphide derivatives revealed lower specific to non-specific partition coefficients than $[^{11}$C]DASB (Huang et al. 2004; Zhu et al. 2004) new candidate SERT tracers are under investigation (Zessin et al. 2006).

The density of SER 1A receptors (5-HT$_{1A}$) is high in the limbic forebrain and low in basal ganglia, substantia nigra and adult cerebellum. Several radioligands for the 5-HT$_{1A}$ based on the agonist 9-OH-DPAT and on apomorphine derivatives have been developed but, to date, the most diffused imaging tracers are based on the potent and selective antagonist WAY-100635 (Passchier and van Waarde 2001). For PET imaging, WAY-100635 (Houle et al. 2000) has been labelled with ^{11}C both in the methyl $\{[$O-methyl-^{11}C]WAY-100635 (Mathis et al. 1994)$\}$ and in the carbonyl position $\{[^{11}$C]WAY-100635 (Pike et al. 1996)$\}$. Both radiotracers showed fast metabolism in plasma, but $[^{11}$C]WAY-100635 was deemed the most useful derivative, due to its better metabolic profile with no radioactive lipophilic species entering the human brain (Osman et al. 1998). Several derivatives of WAY-100635 labelled with ^{18}F have also been synthesized (Karramkam et al. 2003) and evaluated in rats (Tipre et al. 2006) and humans (Derry et al. 2006). However, in humans these compounds suffered from metabolism problems and a search for more stable tracers is ongoing (Defraiteur et al. 2006; Saigal et al. 2006). Recently, a new agonist was produced that may provide more information on signal transduction capacity. This ^{11}C-labelled tracer (MPT) exhibited high affinity and selectivity for the 5-HT$_{1A}$ in baboons (Kumar et al. 2006).

For SPECT imaging of the 5-HT$_{1A}$ receptors, ^{123}I-iodinated derivatives of WAY-100635 and Org 13063 were evaluated and resulted in poor brain uptake in rodents (Vandecapelle et al. 2001) and humans (Kung et al. 1996). Potential ^{99m}Tc-labelled 5-HT$_{1A}$ tracers have also been developed and are under investigation (Heimbold et al. 2002; Leon et al. 2002; Tsoukalas et al. 2003).

In the human brain, SER 2A receptors (5-HT$_{2A}$) are present in high concentration in the entire cortex and in subcortical structures (Forutan et al. 2002). Although initial imaging of 5-HT$_{2A}$ distribution in the human brain was performed with the PET tracers $[^{11}$C]methylspiperone (Andree et al. 1998) and $[^{18}$F]setoperone (Blin et al. 1990), ligands with affinity for both the DA and SER receptors, more selective SER tracers have been developed since (Westkaemper and Glennon 2002). To date, the most used PET tracer for 5-HT$_{2A}$ imaging in the human brain is the alkyl-piperidine compound [^{18}F]altanserin (Lemaire et al. 1991). [^{18}F]Altanserin is a potent antagonist exhibiting a high selectivity for the 5-HT$_{2A}$ over the D2 receptors, yet with a residual affinity for α_1-adrenoreceptors and histamine H$_1$ receptors. Despite plasma metabolism leading to radioactive lipophilic species, the feasibility of [^{18}F]altanserin PET in human brain has been confirmed (Tan et al. 1999; Forutan et al. 2002), but more selective and more stable 5-HT$_{2A}$ PET tracers, labelled with both ^{18}F and ^{11}C, have been developed (Lundkvist et al. 1996; Sobrio et al. 2000; Fu et al. 2002).

In the late 1980s, [^{123}I]ketanserin was developed as a potential 5-HT$_{2A}$ SPECT tracer and was evaluated in depressed patients (D'haenen et al. 1992), but it displayed rather poor brain penetration and high affinity for the α_1-adrenoreceptors. ^{123}I-Iodinated derivatives of spiperone, which have high selectivity but moderate affinity for the 5-HT$_{2A}$ receptors in vitro, were evaluated in mice and showed relatively high brain uptake with regional distribution consistent with the known 5-HT$_{2A}$ distribution (Samnick et al. 1998). Recently, a new ^{123}I-labelled ligand with a slight modification in the piperidine ring of the spiperone showed good brain uptake in mice (Blanckaert et al. 2005). However, further evaluation is needed to confirm specific binding to the 5-HT$_{2A}$ receptors. To date, the labelled antagonist [^{123}I]-5-I-R91150 (Mertens et al. 1994) is the most promising 5-HT$_{2A}$ imaging agent for SPECT, and has been used to map these receptors in healthy subjects (Baeken et al. 1998) and patients with depression (Schins et al. 2005), Alzheimer's disease (Versijpt et al. 2003a) and other neurological disorders (Peremans et al. 2005; Catafau et al. 2006).

3.3 Benzodiazepine Receptors

Benzodiazepines are drugs with anxiolitic, anticonvulsant, muscle relaxant and hypnotic properties, and their binding sites have been separated in two main classes: central and peripheral receptors. The central benzodiazepine receptor (BR) is expressed exclusively in the central nervous system and is located on the extracellular domain of the γ-aminobutyric acid (GABA) receptor (Zisterer and Williams 1997; Nutt and Malizia 2001). Various neurological and psychiatric diseases (epilepsy, Huntington's disease, Alzheimer's disease, schizophrenia, hepatic encephalopathy, anxiety disorders) can be caused by alterations of the GABA$_A$-BRs (Katsifis et al. 2003; Mitterhauser et al. 2004).

Flumazenil is a potent BR antagonist suggested as an antidote to benzodiazepine overdoses. The PET tracer [^{11}C]flumazenil (Maziere et al. 1984) has been the tracer of choice for imaging the GABA$_A$-BR so far, along with the iodinated analogue [^{123}I]iomazenil for SPECT imaging (Beer et al. 1990; Heiss and Herholz 2006). Despite their usefulness in imaging brain regions with elevated receptor density, [^{11}C]flumazenil and [^{123}I]iomazenil exhibit fast tissue uptake and wash-out, and rapid plasma metabolism in vivo. To overcome these problems, the imidazole ring was modified in [^{76}Br]NNC 13-8199, [^{11}C]NNC 13-8199 (Foged et al. 1997) and in a ^{123}I-derivative of bretazenil (Katsifis et al. 2003), which resulted in improved plasma stability for each compound. Due to the short half-life of ^{11}C, ^{18}F-labelled derivatives of flumazenil, 5-(2'-[^{18}F]fluoroethyl)flumazenil ([^{18}F]FEF) (Moerlein and Perlmutter 1992) and 2'-[^{18}F]fluoroflumazenil ([^{18}F]FFMZ) (Mitterhauser et al. 2004) have been produced as a potential GABA$_A$ ligands for PET evaluation of BRs. Evaluation of [^{18}F]FFMZ in monkeys (Ryzhikov et al. 2005) and humans (Chang et al. 2005) showed selective uptake in areas with high receptor density, similar to that of the ^{11}C analogue. However, [^{18}F]FEF showed lower affinity, a rapid kinetics in the brain and faster metabolism than [^{11}C]flumazenil (Gründer et al. 2001).

The peripheral BR is ubiquitously distributed in peripheral tissues as well as in glial cells of the central nervous system (Zisterer and Williams 1997). Recent studies have shown that increased levels of receptor are associated with neuronal cell death and could be indicative of neurodegenerative disorders, including Alzheimer's disease, Huntington's disease, Wernicke's encephalopathy, multiple sclerosis and epilepsy (Zhang et al. 2003a). The radiopharmaceutical, [^{11}C]PK11195 was initially developed as a potential PET tracer to characterize the peripheral BRs (Camsonne et al. 1984) but suffered from poor brain uptake. The enantiomer [^{11}C](R)-PK11195 has been used as a marker of in vivo microglial activation in degenerative brain lesions disease (Banati et al. 2000; Henkel et al. 2004; Turner et al. 2004; Gerhard et al. 2005, 2006). In addition, a ^{123}I-labelled analogue of PK11195 exhibited increased brain uptake compared with the ^{11}C-labelled analogue, probably because of its higher lipophilicity, and was able to detect inflammatory pathology in Alzheimer's disease patients (Versijpt et al. 2003b).

New promising PET tracers for in vivo imaging of the peripheral BRs have been developed by labelling DAA1106, a potent and selective receptor ligand, with ^{11}C and ^{18}F (Zhang et al. 2003a, 2003b). In vivo results in rodents showed high radioactivity uptakes in high peripheral BR density regions in the brain, with high selectivity and specificity for the receptor. Recently, a ^{11}C-labelled derivative of quinoline 2-carboxamide was also synthesized and evaluated ex vivo and in vivo, and showed specific accumulation in peripheral BR-rich tissues (Cappelli et al. 2006).

3.4 Opioid Receptors

In the brain, the three major opioid receptors (OR) types (μ, δ, and κ) mediate the effects of endogenous and exogenous opioids such as depression, sedation and reward. The central opioid system plays a key role in drug and alcohol addiction and in perception and emotional processing of pain (Sprenger et al. 2005).

At first, morphine, codeine and heroine were labelled with ^{11}C for PET imaging of the OR function, but they were not suited for imaging studies due to non-specific binding and fast metabolism. [^{11}C]Carfentanil, a ligand with high affinity for the μ-OR, was the first radiotracer used to image OR in the human brain (Frost et al. 1985) and was utilized to evaluate the role of μ-OR and its endogenous ligands in eating disorders (Zubieta et al. 2001; Bencherif et al. 2005). Experiments with [^{11}C]carfentanil in alcohol- or cocaine-addicted patients also showed increased availability of μ-OR in a neural network that has been associated with drug crav-ing (Zubieta et al. 1996; Heinz et al. 2005). In addition, a decrease in μ-OR availability was observed in heroin-dependent humans maintained with buprenor-phine (Greenwald et al. 2003). Analogues of carfentanil were also labelled with ^{11}C and ^{18}F as alternative tracers for PET imaging of μ-OR (Jewett and Kilbourn 2004; Shiue and Welch 2004; Henriksen et al. 2005). ^{11}C-Labelled diprenorphine, a non-selective opioid antagonist, and buprenorphine, an approved analgesic drug with a mixed agonist/antagonist behaviour, were evaluated in baboons pretreated with naloxone, a μ-OR antagonist used to counter the effects of opioid over-dose. They both showed specific binding in the striatum, with better results for [^{11}C]diprenorphine over [^{11}C]buprenorphine due to faster clearance from the cere-bellum (Shiue et al. 1991). Sex-related differences in μ- and κ-OR avidity in el-derly people (healthy volunteers and Alzheimer's patients) were shown by using [^{18}F]cyclofoxy, a naltrexone analogue with high affinity to both μ- and κ-OR (Cohen et al. 2000).

Beside addiction, the κ-OR has also been implicated in several brain disorders, including Alzheimer's disease, epilepsy and Tourette's syndrome, and κ-OR activa-tion has shown neuroprotective effects in ischemic rats (Machulla and Heinz 2005). Therefore, the development of specific tracers for this receptor type would provide the unique opportunity to assess the κ-OR availability and functional state. To this aim, the high-affinity agonist [^{11}C]GR103545 holds promise for κ-OR PET imag-ing in humans. In fact, pre-clinical evaluation in mouse and baboon brains showed specific and selective binding to the receptor, moderate metabolism and appropriate kinetics (Ravert et al. 2002; Talbot et al. 2005).

The naltrindole derivative [^{11}C]MeNTI, a selective δ-opioid antagonist, was used for PET imaging of δ-OR in the human brain (Smith et al. 1999), while other nal-trindole analogues were evaluated in vitro and in brain homogenates as potential radioligands (Clayson et al. 2001; Tyacke et al. 2002). The development of δ-OR-specific PET imaging tracers holds promise in the clinical evaluation of depressive states, as the association between this OR and depression has been shown recently in animal models (Jutkiewicz 2006).

4 Heart and Lung Neuroreceptors

Cardiovascular and respiratory problems are of major socio-economic impact and in 2003 heart and respiratory diseases were the first and fourth cause of death in the United States, respectively (Pleis and Lethbridge 2006). Therefore, imaging the concentration, distribution and occupancy of the receptors involved in respiratory and cardiovascular disorders is a very attractive research area as it can provide new insights in the aetiology of these diseases as well as the means to diagnose them, monitor the treatment outcomes, and test new drug candidates. The following sec-tions will discuss some of the radiotracers for two of the main postsynaptic receptors of the heart and lung: the adrenergic and the muscarinic/cholinergic receptors.

4.1 Adrenergic Receptors

The adrenergic system is an essential regulator of neuronal, vegetative, endocrine, cardiovascular, and metabolic functions. The adrenergic receptors or adrenoceptors (AdRs), a class of G protein-coupled receptors, are the targets of adrenalin and noradrenalin, and can be classified into two major families, α and β (Guimaraes and Moura 2001). Changes in the number of AdRs are associated with various cardiovascular diseases, such as myocardial ischemia (Corr and Crafford 1981), congestive heart failure (Sucharov 2007) and hypertension (Yamada et al. 1984). Furthermore, β_2-AdR agonists are the most widely used drugs in the short- and long-term treatment of asthma and chronic obstructive pulmonary disease (COPD), even though the molecular mechanism responsible for the bronchodilation effect is not completely defined and serious adverse effects can occur (Giembycz and Newton 2006). For these reasons, several specific and non-specific radiotracers have been developed to monitor the distribution and occupancy of AdRs (Pike et al. 2000; Elsinga et al. 2004; Kopka et al. 2005).

The α-AdRs are divided in two sub-groups, the α_1- and α_2-AdRs (Starke 1981; Hein 2006). In the heart, they are implicated in ventricular hypertrophy, ischemia and arrhythmogenesis and regulate cardiovascular functions such as noradrenaline release and coronary vasoconstriction (Drew 1976; Yamaguchi and Kopin 1980). Furthermore, α-AdRs are considered to act as a backup for β_1-AdRs. In fact, an increase in α_1-AdRs is observed when a decrease in β_1-AdRs occurs as a result of disease (Bristow et al. 1988; Heusch 1990). The role of α-AdRs in the lung is less clear, even though mediation in bronchoconstriction has been shown (Elsinga et al. 2004).

To the best of our knowledge, the only radiotracer used in humans for imaging the α_1-AdRs is [11C]GB67, an analogue of the antagonist prazosin (Law et al. 2000), and this exhibited high and specific myocardial uptake both in rodents and in two male healthy volunteers and is considered to be a promising PET tracer for the α_1-AdR. Attempts to directly label prazosin with 11C resulted in high non-specific myocardial uptake in dogs (Ehrin et al. 1988). Another promising α_1-AdR ligand, [11C]RN5, exhibited high accumulation in heart, spleen and lung in rats and blocking studies confirmed α_1-AdRs mediated uptake (Matarrese et al. 2002). More recently, two derivatives of the antipsychotic sertindole were labelled with 11C and evaluated in monkey brains but resulted in low uptake in regions known to contain α_1-AdRs (Balle et al. 2004).

A few radioligands for the α_2-AdRs have been developed and evaluated in vivo for brain imaging but they all suffered from low uptake and non specific binding in lung or heart (Hume et al. 1996, 2000; Shiue et al. 1998; Jakobsen et al. 2006; Van der Mey et al. 2006).

The β-AdR family include four different receptor sub-types, β_1–β_4. The β_1 and β_2 sub-types exert a major role in controlling cardiac function. In heart diseases such as ischemia, heart failure and hypertension, the total amount of β_1- and β_2-AdRs is reduced (Khamssi and Brodde 1990; Yamada et al. 1996; Castellano and Bohm 1997; Anthonio et al. 2000), while a reduction of the normal β_1/β_2 ratio (4:1) is sometimes observed in failing human heart without any change in the β_2-AdRs (Brodde 1991). In the human lung, the β_2-AdR sub-type predominates, whereas the β_1-AdR distribution is limited (7:3 ratio) (Barnes 2004), and a diminished functionality of the β_2 receptor was observed in severely asthmatic patients (Nijkamp and Henricks 1990).

In humans, the non-sub-type selective antagonist (S)-[^{11}C]CGP 12177 was used to determine cardiac and pulmonary receptor density (Ueki et al. 1993; Qing et al. 1997) and to evaluate the pre- and post-synaptic autonomic dysfunction of the heart (Wichter et al. 2000; Schafers et al. 2001). Furthermore, by using (S)-[^{11}C]CGP 12177, a decrease in β-AdRs was observed in patients with heart failure (Merlet et al. 1993), hypertrophic cardiomyopathy (Lefroy et al. 1993; Choudhury et al. 1996) and Brugada syndrome (Kies et al. 2004). To overcome the cumbersome synthesis of (S)-[^{11}C]CGP 12177, which involves the use of [^{11}C]phosgene, the isopropyl analogue (S)-[^{11}C]CGP 12388 was developed for clinical use. (S)-[^{11}C]CGP 12388 proved to be as potent as (S)-[^{11}C]CGP 12177 in vitro (Elsinga et al. 1997) and β-AdR specific binding was confirmed in vivo (van Waarde et al. 1998). In humans, this compound was used to measure β-AdR cardiac density in healthy subjects (Doze et al. 2002a) and patients with idiopathic dilated cardiomyopathy (De Jong et al. 2005). (S)-[^{11}C]CGP 12388 was also used to evaluate the mechanism of action of inhaled β-adrenergic drugs in healthy volunteers (van Waarde et al. 2005). Several ^{18}F radiolabelled ligands were also developed for non-sub-type selective β-AdR PET imaging of the lung and heart (Elsinga et al. 1997; Tewson et al. 1999). Among these, (S)-[^{18}F]fluorocarazolol was used to image myocardial and pulmonary β-AdRs in animals (Elsinga et al. 1996) and humans (Visser et al. 1997b) and was suggested as a possible brain β-AdR imaging tracer (van Waarde et al. 1997; Doze et al. 2002b).

Selective ligands for the β_1-AdRs may be of better use for cardiac imaging, since heart disease affects mainly the myocardial density of β_1-AdRs (Bristow et al. 1986; Brodde 1991). To this aim, several β_1-selective ligands were labelled with ^{11}C (Antoni et al. 1989; Elsinga et al. 1994; Valette et al. 1999; Soloviev et al. 2001; Kopka et al. 2003) and ^{18}F (De Groot et al. 1993) and evaluated in vitro and in vivo but suffered from high non-specific binding. The selective β_1-antagonist ICI 89406 was labelled also with ^{123}I and evaluated for SPECT imaging of β_1-AdRs. Despite high in vitro selectivity for the β_1-AdR, this tracer exhibited fast dehalogenation in rats and was not considered suitable for human studies (Wagner et al. 2004).

Specific binding to β_2-AdR in the lung in vivo was observed for the first time with the racemic agonist [^{11}C]formoterol (Visser et al. 1998). Later, a ^{11}C-labelled derivative of the potent β_2-antagonist ICI 118551 was evaluated in rats and monkeys. However, despite high lung and heart uptake, blocking studies revealed non-β_2-specific binding (Moresco et al. 2000). More recently, [^{18}F]FEFE was obtained by radiolabelling feneterol, a β_2-AdR agonist widely used to treat bronchoconstriction, and showed sub-type specific binding in the lung of guinea pigs (Schirrmacher et al. 2003).

4.2 Muscarinic Receptors

The muscarinic acetylcholine receptor (mAChR) is selectively activated by muscarine and blocked by atropine. Five mAChR sub-types (M_1–M_5) has been identified by means of molecular cloning techniques, and all have distinct distributions, pharmacological profiles and physiological functions (Caulfield and Birdsall 1998). Due to the relationship between mAChRs and schizophrenia, dementia, Parkinson's and Alzheimer's disease, a variety of radiotracers has been investigated for mAChR imaging in the central nervous system (Eckelman 2006). The M_2 and M_2/M_3 mAChR sub-types are widely distributed throughout heart and lung, respectively. In the heart, the release of the neurotransmitter acetylcholine leads to activation of the M_2 mAChRs, which mediates changes in ion channel activity (Harvey and Belevych 2003). In the lung, acetylcholine acting on mAChRs plays a regulatory role in airway remodelling associated with chronic airway inflammation (asthma and COPD) (Gosens et al. 2006).

A few derivatives of the antagonist quinuclidinyl benzylate (QNB) were developed as potential mAChR brain imaging agents (Gibson et al. 1984; Luo et al. 1996). Among these, [^{11}C]MQNB was shown to bind specifically to the cardiac mAChRs in baboons (Maziere et al. 1981) and dogs (Delforge et al. 1990). In patients with congestive heart failure (Le Guludec et al. 1997) and familial amyloidpolyneuropathy (Delahaye et al. 2001), [^{11}C]MQNB PET imaging showed increased mAChR density respect to control subjects. On the contrary, no change in myocardial mAChRs was seen with [^{11}C]MQNB PET in orthotopic transplantation patients when compared with control subjects (Le Guludec et al. 1994).

Several iodinated ligands have also been investigated as potential mAChR imaging agents (Matsumura et al. 1991; McPherson et al. 2000). Among these, [^{123}I]N-methyl-4-iododexetimide seams promising as an imaging agent for cardiac mAChR SPECT imaging as it showed rapid and high myocardial uptakes and high heart to lung ratios (Hicks et al. 1995).

To date, (R)-[^{11}C]VC-002 is the only radiotracer used in humans to image lung mAChRs (Visser et al. 1997a). In a study performed in two healthy volunteers, constant (R)-[^{11}C]VC-002 levels in the lung up to 60 min post-injection together with a rapid plasma clearance allowed the acquisition of clear lung PET images. Furthermore, the lung uptake was competitively blocked with glycopyrronium bromide, thus confirming specific mAChR binding (Visser et al. 1999). Recently, two mAChR antagonists used in the treatment of COPD and asthma (ipratroprium and tiotropium), have been labelled with ^{11}C (Issa et al. 2006) and will be used to study inhaled drug deposition in human lung by PET.

5 Conclusions

The binding interaction between radiolabelled ligands and their receptors allows physicians and scientists to detect and investigate disease states non-invasively by means of nuclear imaging techniques. This chapter has discussed a broad variety of small molecule radiotracers developed for molecular imaging of tumours, brain, heart and lung. Similar agents can be developed for new molecular targets as they are identified.

References

Abi Dargham A, Martinez D, Mawlawi O, Simpson N, Hwang DR, Slifstein M, Anjilvel, S, Pidcock J, Guo NN, Lombardo I, Mann JJ, Van Heertum R, Foged C, Halldin C, Laruelle M (2000) Measurement of striatal and extrastriatal dopamine D1 receptor binding potential with [^{11}C]NNC 112 in humans: validation and reproducibility. J Cereb Blood Flow Metab 20: 225–243

Ali H, Rousseau J, van Lier JE (1994) Synthesis of (17α,20E/Z)Iodovinyl testosterone and 19-nortestosterone derivatives as potential radioligands for androgen and progesterone receptors. J Steroid Biochem Mol Biol 49:15–29

Ali H, Rousseau J, Ahmed N, Guertin V, Hochberg RB, van Lier JE (2003a) Synthesis of the 7α-cyano-(17α,20E/Z)-[^{125}I]iodovinyl-19-nortestosterones: potential radioligands for androgen and progesterone receptors. Steroids 68:1163–1171

Ali H, Rousseau J, Paquette B, Dube C, Marko B, van Lier JE (2003b) Synthesis and biological properties of 7α-cyano derivatives of the (17α,20E/Z)-[^{125}I]iodovinyl- and 16α-[^{125}I]iodoestradiols. Steroids 68:1189–1200

Andree B, Nyberg S, Ito H, Ginovart N, Brunner F, Jaquet F, Halldin C, Farde L (1998) Positron emission tomographic analysis of dose-dependent MDL 100,907 binding to 5-hydroxytryptamine-2A receptors in the human brain. J Clin Psychopharmacol 18:317–323

Anthonio RL, Brodde O-E, van Veldhuisen DJ, Scholtens E, Crijns HJGM, van Gilst WH (2000) β-Adrenoceptor density in chronic infarcted myocardium: a subtype specific decrease of β$_1$-adrenoceptor density. Int J Cardiol 72:137–141

Antoni G, Ulin J, Langstrom B (1989) Synthesis of the ^{11}C-labelled β-adrenergic receptor ligands atenolol, metoprolol and propranolol. Appl Radiat Isot 40:561–564

Antony AC (1996) Folate receptors. Annu Rev Nutr 16:501–521

Arnett CD, Wolf AP, Shiue CY, Fowler JS, MacGregor RR, Christman DR, Smith MR (1986) Improved delineation of human dopamine receptors using [^{18}F]-N-methylspiroperidol and PET. J Nucl Med 27:1878–1882

Arterburn JB, Corona C, Rao KV, Carlson KE, Katzenellenbogen JA (2003) Synthesis of 17-α-substituted estradiol-pyridin-2-yl hydrazine conjugates as effective ligands for labeling with Alberto's complex fac-[Re(OH$_2$)$_3$(CO)$_3$]$^+$ in water. J Org Chem 68:7063–7070

Asselin MC, Amano S, Chirakal R, Thompson M, Nahmias C (2002) Patterns of distribution of [^{18}F]6-fluoro-L-m-tyrosine in PET images of patients with movement disorders. In: Senda M, Kimura Y, Herscovitch P (eds) Brain imaging with PET. Academic Press, San Diego

Baeken C, D'haenen H, Flamen P, Mertens J, Terriere D, Chavatte K, Boumon R, Bossuyt A (1998) ^{123}I-5-I-R91150, a new single-photon emission tomography ligand for 5-HT$_{2A}$ receptors: influence of age and gender in healthy subjects. Eur J Nucl Med Mol Imaging 25:1617–1622

Balle T, Halldin C, Andersen L, Hjorth Alifrangis L, Badolo L, Gjervig Jensen K, Chou Y-W, Andersen K, Perregaard J, Farde L (2004) New α$_1$-adrenoceptor antagonists derived from the antipsychotic sertindole-carbon-11 labelling and pet examination of brain uptake in the cynomolgus monkey. Nucl Med Biol 31:327–336

Banati RB, Newcombe J, Gunn RN, Cagnin A, Turkheimer F, Heppner F, Price G, Wegner F, Giovannoni G, Miller DH, Perkin GD, Smith T, Hewson AK, Bydder G, Kreutzberg GW, Jones T, Cuzner ML, Myers R (2000) The peripheral benzodiazepine binding site in the brain in multiple sclerosis: quantitative in vivo imaging of microglia as a measure of disease activity. Brain 123:2321–2337

Barnes PJ (2004) Distribution of receptor targets in the lung. Proc Am Thorac Soc 1:345–351

Barrio JR, Huang SC, Phelps ME (1997) Biological imaging and the molecular basis of dopaminergic diseases. Biochem Pharmacol 54:341–348

Barthel H, Cleij MC, Collingridge DR, Hutchinson OC, Osman S, He Q, Luthra SK, Brady F, Price PM, Aboagye EO (2003) 3′-Deoxy-3′-[^{18}F]fluorothymidine as a new marker for monitoring tumor response to antiproliferative therapy in vivo with positron emission tomography. Cancer Res 63:3791–3798

Beer HF, Blauenstein PA, Hasler PH, Delaloye B, Riccabona G, Banger I, Hunkeler W, Bonetti EP, Pieri L, Richards JG, Schubiger PA (1990) In vitro and in vivo evaluation of iodine-123-Ro 16-0154: a new imaging agent for SPECT investigations of benzodiazepine receptors. J Nucl Med 31:1007–1014

Bencherif B, Guarda AS, Colantuoni C, Ravert HT, Dannals RF, Frost JJ (2005) Regional μ-opioid receptor binding in insular cortex is decreased in bulimia nervosa and correlates inversely with fasting behavior. J Nucl Med 46:1349–1351

Bennink RJ, Rijks LJ, van Tienhoven G, Noorduyn LA, Janssen AG, Sloof GW (2001) estrogen receptor status in primary breast cancer: iodine 123-labeled cis-11β-methoxy-17α-iodovinyl estradiol scintigraphy. Radiology 220:774–779

Bennink RJ, van Tienhoven G, Rijks LJ, Noorduyn AL, Janssen AG, Sloof GW (2004) In vivo prediction of response to antiestrogen treatment in estrogen receptor-positive breast cancer. J Nucl Med 45:1–7

Berardi F, Ferorelli S, Abate C, Colabufo NA, Contino M, Perrone R, Tortorella V (2004) 4-(Tetralin-1-yl)- and 4-(naphthalen-1-yl)alkyl derivatives of 1-cyclohexylpiperazine as σ receptor ligands with agonist σ_2 activity. J Med Chem 47:2308–2317

Berardi F, Ferorelli S, Abate C, Pedone MP, Colabufo NA, Contino M, Perrone R (2005) methyl substitution on the piperidine ring of N-[-(6-methoxynaphthalen-1-yl)alkyl] derivatives as a probe for selective binding and activity at the σ_1 receptor. J Med Chem 48:8237–8244

Bettio A, Honer M, Muller C, Bruhlmeier M, Muller U, Schibli R, Groehn V, Schubiger AP, Ametamey SM (2006) Synthesis and preclinical evaluation of a folic acid derivative labeled with ^{18}F for PET imaging of folate receptor-positive tumors. J Nucl Med 47:1153–1160

Bigott HM, Parent E, Luyt LG, Katzenellenbogen JA, Welch MJ (2005) design and synthesis of functionalized cyclopentadienyl tricarbonylmetal complexes for technetium-94m PET imaging of estrogen receptors. Bioconjugate Chem 16:255–264

Billings JJ, Kung M-P, Chumpradit S, Mozley D, Alavi A, Kung HF (1992) Characterization of radioiodinated TISCH: a high-affinity and selective ligand for mapping CNS D_1 dopamine receptor. J Neurochem 58:227–236

Blanckaert P, Burvenich I, Staelens L, Dierckx RA, Slegers G (2005) Synthesis, radiosynthesis and in vivo evaluation in mice of [^{123}I]-(4-fluorophenyl){1-[2-(4-iodophenyl)ethyl]piperidin-4-yl}methanone for visualization of the 5-HT$_{2A}$ receptor with SPECT. Appl Radiat Isot 62:737–743

Blin J, Sette G, Fiorelli M, Bletry O, Elghozi JL, Crouzel C, Baron JC (1990) A method for the in vivo investigation of the serotonergic 5-HT$_2$ receptors in the human cerebral cortex using positron emission tomography and ^{18}F-labeled setoperone. J Neurochem 54:1744–1754

Boja JW, Patel A, Ivy Carroll F, Abdur Rahman M, Philip A, Lewin AH, Kopajtic TA, Kuhar MJ (1991) [^{125}I]RTI-55: a potent ligand for dopamine transporters. Eur J Pharmacol 194:133–134

Bonasera TA, O'Neil JP, Xu M, Dobkin JA, Cutler PD, Lich LL, Choe YS, Katzenellenbogen JA, Welch MJ (1996) preclinical evaluation of fluorine-18-labeled androgen receptor ligands in baboons. J Nucl Med 37:1009–1015

Bradley TC, Tanjore KN, Bingzhi S, Jogeshwar M (2000) Quantitation of striatal and extrastriatal D-2 dopamine receptors using PET imaging of [^{18}F]fallypride in nonhuman primates. Synapse 38:71–79

Bristow MR, Ginsburg R, Umans V, Fowler M, Minobe W, Rasmussen R, Zera P, Menlove R, Shah P (1986) β_1 and β_2-adrenergic subpopulations in non-failing and failing human ventricle myocardium: coupling of both receptor subtypes to muscle contraction and selective β_1 receptor downregulation in heart failure. Circ Res 59:297–309

Bristow MR, Minobe W, Rasmussen R, Hershberger RE, Hoffman BB (1988) α_1 adrenergic receptors in the nonfailing and failing human heart. J Pharmacol Exp Ther 247:1039–1045

Brodde OE (1991) β_1 and β_2 adrenoceptors in the human heart: properties, function, and alterations in chronic heart failure. Pharmacol Rev 43:203–242

Burn DJ, O'Brien JT (2003) Use of functional imaging in Parkinsonism and dementia. Mov Disord 18:S88–S95

Burns HD, Dannals RF, Langstrom B, Ravert HT, Zemyan SE, Duelfer T, Wong DF, Frost JJ, Kuhar MJ, Wagner HN Jr, (1984) (3-N-[11C]methyl)spiperone, a ligand binding to dopamine receptors: radiochemical synthesis and biodistribution studies in mice. J Nucl Med 25: 1222–1227

Camargo EE (2001) Brain SPECT in neurology and psychiatry. J Nucl Med 42:611–623

Camsonne R, Crouzel C, Comar D, Mazière M, Prenant C, Sastre J, Moulin M, Syrota A (1984) Synthesis of N-([11C]) methyl, N-(methyl-1 propyl), (chloro-2 phenyl)-1 isoquinoleine carboxamide-3 (PK 11195): a new ligand for peripheral benzodiazepine receptors. J Labelled Comp Radiopharm 21:985–991

Cappelli A, Matarrese M, Moresco RM, Valenti S, Anzini M, Vomero S, Turolla EA, Belloli S, Simonelli P, Filannino MA (2006) Synthesis, labeling, and biological evaluation of halogenated 2-quinolinecarboxamides as potential radioligands for the visualization of peripheral benzodiazepine receptors. Bioorg Med Chem 14:4055–4066

Castellano M, Bohm M (1997) The cardiac β-adrenoceptor-mediated signaling pathway and its alterations in hypertensive heart disease. Hypertension 29:715–722

Catafau AM, Danus M, Bullich S, Nucci G, Llop J, Abanades S, Cunningham VJ, Eersels JLH, Pavia J, Farre M (2006) Characterization of the SPECT 5-HT$_{2A}$ receptor ligand ^{123}I-R91150 in healthy volunteers: part 2 – ketanserin displacement. J Nucl Med 47:929–937

Caulfield MP, Birdsall NJM (1998) International Union of Pharmacology. XVII. Classification of muscarinic acetylcholine receptors. Pharmacol Rev 50:279–290

Caveliers V, Everaert H, Lahoutte T, Dierickx LO, John CS, Bossuyt A (2001) Labelled sigma receptor ligands: can their role in neurology and oncology be extended? Eur J Med Chem 28:133–135

Caveliers V, Everaert H, John CS, Lahoutte T, Bossuyt A (2002) Sigma receptor scintigraphy with N-[2-(1'-piperidinyl)ethyl]-3-^{123}I-iodo-4-methoxybenzamide of patients with suspected primary breast cancer: first clinical results. J Nucl Med 43:1647–1649

Chang YS, Jeong JM, Yoon YH, Kang WJ, Lee SJ, Lee DS, Chung J–K, Lee MC (2005) Biological properties of 2'-[18F]fluoroflumazenil for central benzodiazepine receptor imaging. Nucl Med Biol 32:263–268

Choe YS, Katzenellenbogen JA (1995a) Synthesis of C-6 fluoroandrogens: evaluation of ligands for tumor receptor imaging. Steroids 60:414–422

Choe YS, Lidstrom PJ, Chi DY, Bonasera TA, Welch MJ, Katzenellenbogen JA (1995b) Synthesis of 11 β-[18F]fluoro-5 α-dihydrotestosterone and 11 β-[18F]fluoro-19-nor-5 α-dihydrotestosterone: preparation via halofluorination-reduction, receptor binding, and tissue distribution. J Med Chem 38:816–825

Choi SR, Yang B, Plossl K, Chumpradit S, Wey SP, Acton PD, Wheeler K, Mach RH, Kung HF (2001) Development of a Tc-99m labeled σ_2 receptor-specific ligand as a potential breast tumor imaging agent. Nucl Med Biol 28:657–666

Choudhury L, Guzzetti S, Lefroy DC, Nihoyannopoulos P, McKenna WJ, Oakley CM, Camici PG (1996) Myocardial β adrenoceptors and left ventricular function in hypertrophic cardiomyopathy. Heart 75:50–54

Clark GM, Sledge GW Jr, Osborne CK, McGuire WL (1987) Survival from first recurrence: relative importance of prognostic factors in 1,015 breast cancer patients. J Clin Oncol 5:55–61

Clayson J, Jales A, Tyacke RJ, Hudson AL, Nutt DJ, Lewis JW, Husbands SM (2001) Selective δ–opioid receptor ligands:potential PET ligands based on naltrindole. Bioorg Med Chem Lett 11:939–943

Coenen HH, Laufer P, Stocklin G, Wienhard K, Pawlik G, Bocher-Schwarz HG, Heiss WD (1987) 3-N-(2-[^{18}F]-fluoroethyl)-spiperone: a novel ligand for cerebral dopamine receptor studies with pet. Life Sci 40:81–88

Cohen RM, Carson RE, Sunderl T (2000) Opiate receptor avidity in the thalamus is sexually dimorphic in the elderly. Synapse 38:226–229

Colabufo NA, Berardi F, Contino M, Fazio F, Matarrese M, Moresco RM, Niso M, Perrone R, Tortorella V (2005) Distribution of sigma receptors in EMT-6 cells: preliminary biological evaluation of PB167 and potential for in vivo PET. J Pharm Pharmacol 57:1453–1460

Corr PB, Crafford WA (1981) Enhanced α–adrenergic responsiveness in ischemic myocardium: role of α-adrenergic blockade. Am Heart J 102:605–612

Cropley VL, Fujita M, Musachio JL, Hong J, Ghose S, Sangare J, Nathan PJ, Pike VW, Innis RB (2006) Whole-body biodistribution and estimation of radiation-absorbed doses of the dopamine D$_1$ receptor radioligand ^{11}C-NNC 112 in humans. J Nucl Med 47:100–104

Cui X, Schiff R, Arpino G, Osborne CK, Lee AV (2005) Biology of progesterone receptor loss in breast cancer and its implications for endocrine therapy. J Clin Oncol 23:7721–7735

D'haenen H, Bossuyt A, Mertens J, Bossuyt–Piron C, Gijsemans M, Kaufman L (1992) SPECT imaging of serotonin 2 receptors in depression. Psychiatry Res 45:227–237

DaSilva JN, Kilbourn MR (1992) In vivo binding of [^{11}C]tetrabenazine to vesicular monoamine transporters in mouse brain. Life Sci 51:593–600

DaSilva JN, Wilson AA, Nobrega JN, Jiwa D, Houle S (1996) Synthesis and autoradiographic localization of the dopamine D-1 agonists [^{11}C]SKF 75670 and [^{11}C]SKF 82957 as potential PET radioligands. Appl Radiat Isot 47:279–284

De Groot TJ, van Waarde A, Elsinga PH, Visser GM, Brodde OE, Vaalburg W (1993) Synthesis and evaluation of 1'-[^{18}F]fluorometoprolol as a potential tracer for the visualization of β-adrenoceptors with PET. Nucl Med Biol 20:637–642

De Groot TJ, Braker AH, Elsinga PH, Visser GM, Vaalburg W (1994) Synthesis of 6 α-[^{18}F]fluoroprogesterone: a first step towards a potential receptor-ligand for PET. Appl Radiat Isot 45:811–813

De Jong RM, Willemsen AT, Slart RH, Blanksma PK, van Waarde A, Cornel JH, Vaalburg W, van Veldhuisen DJ, Elsinga PH (2005) Myocardial β-adrenoceptor downregulation in idiopathic dilated cardiomyopathy measured in vivo with PET using the new radioligand (S)-[^{11}C]CGP12388. Eur J Nucl Med Mol Imaging 32:443–447

De La Fuente-Fernández R, Furtado S, Guttman M, Furukawa Y, Lee CS, Calne DB, Ruth TJ, Stoessl AJ (2003) VMAT2 binding is elevated in dopa-responsive dystonia: visualizing empty vesicles by PET. Synapse 49:20–28

Dean B (2003) The cortical serotonin$_{2A}$ receptor and the pathology of schizophrenia: a likely accomplice. J Neurochem 85:1–13

Defraiteur C, Lemaire C, Luxen A, Plenevaux A (2006) Radiochemical synthesis and tissue distribution of p-[^{18}F]DMPPF, a new 5 – HT$_{1A}$ ligand for PET, in rats. Nucl Med Biol 33:667–675

Dehdashti F, McGuire AH, Van Brocklin HF, Siegel BA, Andriole DP, Griffeth LK, Pomper MG, Katzenellenbogen JA, Welch MJ (1991) Assessment of 21-[^{18}F]fluoro-16 α-ethyl-19-norprogesterone as a positron-emitting radiopharmaceutical for the detection of progestin receptors in human breast carcinomas. J Nucl Med 32:1532–1537

Dehdashti F, Mortimer JE, Siegel BA, Griffeth LK, Bonasera TJ, Fusselman MJ, Detert DD, Cutler PD, Katzenellenbogen JA, Welch MJ (1995) Positron tomographic assessment of estrogen receptors in breast cancer: comparison with FDG-PET and in vitro receptor assays. J Nucl Med 36:1766–1774

Dehdashti F, Picus J, Michalski JM, Dence CS, Siegel BA, Katzenellenbogen JA, Welch MJ (2005) Positron tomographic assessment of androgen receptors in prostatic carcinoma. Eur J Nucl Med Mol Imaging 32:344–350

Delahaye N, Le Guludec D, Dinanian S, Delforge J, Slama MS, Sarda L, Dolle F, Mzabi H, Samuel D, Adams D, Syrota A, Merlet P (2001) Myocardial muscarinic receptor upregulation and normal response to isoproterenol in denervated hearts by familial amyloid polyneuropathy. Circulation 104:2911–2916

Delforge J, Janier M, Syrota A, Crouzel C, Vallois JM, Cayla J, Lancon JP, Mazoyer BM (1990) Noninvasive quantification of muscarinic receptors in vivo with positron emission tomography in the dog heart. Circulation 82:1494–1504

Dence CS, John CS, Bowen WD, Welch MJ (1997) Synthesis and evaluation of [18F] labeled benzamides: high affinity sigma receptor ligands for PET imaging. Nucl Med Biol 24: 333–340

Denis LJ, Griffiths K (2000) Endocrine treatment in prostate cancer. Semin Surg Oncol 18:52–74

Derry C, Benjamin C, Bladin P, le Bars D, Tochon-Danguy H, Berkovic SF, Zimmer L, Costes N, Mulligan R, Reutens D (2006) Increased serotonin receptor availability in human sleep:Evidence from an [18F]MPPF PET study in narcolepsy. Neuroimage 30:341–348

Dixit V, VandenBossche J, Sherman DM, Thompson DH, Andres RP (2006) Synthesis and grafting of thioctic acid-PEG-folate conjugates onto Au nanoparticles for selective targeting of folate receptor-positive tumor cells. Bioconjugate Chem 17:603–609

Doze P, Elsinga PH, van Waarde A, Pieterman RM, Pruim J, Vaalburg W, Willemsen AT (2002a) Quantification of β-adrenoceptor density in the human heart with (S)-[11C]CGP 12388 and a tracer kinetic model. Eur J Nucl Med Mol Imaging 29:295–304

Doze P, van Waarde A, Tewson TJ, Vaalburg W, Elsinga PH (2002b) Synthesis and evaluation of (S)-[18F]-fluoroethylcarazolol for in vivo β-adrenoceptor imaging in the brain. Neurochem Int 41:17–27

Drew GM (1976) Effects of α-adrenoceptor agonists and antagonists on pre- and postsynaptically located α-adrenoceptors. Eur J Pharmacol 36:313–320

Drummond AE (2006) The role of steroids in follicular growth. Reprod Biol Endocrinol 10:4–16

Eckelman WC (2006) Imaging of muscarinic receptors in the central nervous system. Curr Pharm Des 12:3901–3913

Ehrin E, Luthra SK, Crouzel C, Pike VW (1988) Preparation of carbon-11 labelled prazosin, a potent and selective 1-adrenoreceptor antagonist. J Labelled Comp Radiopharm 25:177–183

Elsinga PH, Van Waarde A, Visser GM, Vaalburg W (1994) Synthesis and preliminary evaluation of (R,S)-1-[2-((Carbamoyl-4-hydroxy)phenoxy)-ethylamino]-3-[4-(1-[11C]-methyl-4-trifluoromethyl-2-imidazolyl)phenoxy]-2-propanol ([11C]CGP 20712A) as a selective β1-adrenoceptor ligand for PET. Nucl Med Biol 21:211–217

Elsinga PH, Vos MG, van Waarde A, Braker AH, de Groot TJ, Anthonio RL, Weemaes A-MA, Brodde O-E, Visser GM, Vaalburg W (1996) (S,S)- and (S,R)-1' − [18F]fluorocarazolol, ligands for the visualization of pulmonary β-adrenergic receptors with PET. Nucl Med Biol 23: 159–167

Elsinga PH, van Waarde A, Jaeggi KA, Schreiber G, Heldoorn M, Vaalburg W (1997) Synthesis and Evaluation of (S)-4-(3-(2' − [11C]Isopropylamino)-2-hydroxypropoxy)-2H-benzimidazol-2-one ((S)-[11C]CGP 12388) and (S)-4 − (3 − ((1' − [18F]Fluoroisopropyl)amino)-2-hydroxypropoxy)-2H-benzimidazol-2-one ((S)-[18F]Fluoro-CGP 12388) for visualization of β-adrenoceptors with positron emission tomography. J Med Chem 40:3829–3835

Elsinga PH, van Waarde A, Vaalburg W (2004) Receptor imaging in the thorax with PET. Eur J Pharmacol 499:1–13

Elsinga HP, Hatano K, Ishiwata K (2006) PET tracers for imaging of the dopaminergic system. Curr Med Chem 13:2139–2153

Farde L, Ehrin E, Eriksson L, Greitz T, Hall H, Hedstrom CG, Litton JE, Sedvall G (1985) Substituted benzamides as ligands for visualization of dopamine receptor binding in the human brain by positron emission tomography. Proc Natl Acad Sci U S A 82:3863–3867

Farde L, Halldin C, Stone-Elander S, Sedvall G (1987) PET analysis of human dopamine receptor subtypes using 11C-SCH 23390 and 11C-raclopride. Psychopharmacology (Berl) 92:278–284

Ferris CD, Hirsch DJ, Brooks BP, Snyder SH (1991) Sigma receptors: from molecule to man. J Neurochem 57:729–737

Fischman AJ (2005) Role of [18F]-dopa-PET imaging in assessing movement disorders. Radiol Clin North Am 43:297–304

Foged C, Halldin C, Loc'h C, Maziere B, Karlsson P, Maziere M, Swahn C-G, Farde L (1996) 11C- and 76Br-labelled NNC 22-0010, selective dopamine D1 receptor radioligands for PET. Nucl Med Biol 23:837–844

Foged C, Halldin C, Loc'h C, Mazière B, Pauli S, Maziére M, Hansen HC, Suhara T, Swahn CG, Karlsson P, Farde L (1997) Bromine-76 and carbon-11 labelled NNC 13-8199, metabolically stable benzodiazepine receptor agonists as radioligands for positron emission tomography (PET). Eur J Nucl Med Mol Imaging 24:1261–1267

Foged C, Halldin C, Swahn CG, Ginovart N, Karlsson P, Lundkvist C, Farde L (1998) [^{11}C]NNC 22-0215, a metabolically stable dopamine D_1 radioligand for PET. Nucl Med Biol 25:503–508

Forbes JF (1997) The incidence of breast cancer: the global burden, public health considerations. Semin Oncol 24:S1-20–S21-35

Forutan F, Estalji S, Beu M, Nikolaus S, Hamacher K, Coenen NN, Vosberg V (2002) Distribution of 5HT$_{2A}$ receptors in the human brain: comparison of data in vivo and post mortem. Nuklearmedizin 41:197–201

Frankle WG, Huang Y, Hwang D-R, Talbot PS, Slifstein M, Van Heertum R, Abi-Dargham A, Laruelle M (2004) Comparative evaluation of serotonin transporter radioligands ^{11}C-DASB and ^{11}C-McN 5652 in healthy humans. J Nucl Med 45:682–694

Frost JJ, Wagner HN Jr, Dannals RF, Ravert HT, Links JM, Wilson AA, Burns HD, Wong DF, McPherson RW, Rosembaum AE, Kuhar MJ, Snyder SH (1985) Imaging opiate receptors in the human brain by positron emission tomography. J Comput Assist Tomogr 9:231–236

Frost JJ, Smith AC, Kuhar MJ, Dannals RF, Wagner HN Jr (1987) In vivo binding of ^{3}H-N-methylspiperone to dopamine and serotonin receptors. Life Sci 40:987–995

Fu X, Tan PZ, Kula NS, Baldessarini R, Tamagnan G, Innis RB, Baldwin RM (2002) Synthesis, Receptor Potency, and Selectivity of Halogenated Diphenylpiperidines as Serotonin 5-HT$_{2A}$ Ligands for PET or SPECT Brain Imaging. J Med Chem 45:2319–2324

Furukawa T, Lohith TG, Takamatsu S, Mori T, Tanaka T, Fujibayashi Y (2006) Potential of the FES-hERL PET reporter gene system – Basic evaluation for gene therapy monitoring. Nucl Med Biol 33:145–151

Gabizon A, Shmeeda H, Horowitz AT, Zalipsky S (2004) Tumor cell targeting of liposome-entrapped drugs with phospholipid-anchored folic acid-PEG conjugates. Adv Drug Deliv Rev 56:1177–1192

Garg PK, Labaree DC, Hoyte RM, Hochberg RB (2001) 7α-[^{18}F]fluoro-17α-methyl-5α-dihydrotestosterone: a ligand for androgen receptor-mediated imaging of prostate cancer. Nucl Med Biol 28:85–90

Garnett ES, Firnau G, Nahmias C (1983) Dopamine visualized in the basal ganglia of living man. Nature 305:137–138

Gerhard A, Schwarz J, Myers R, Wise R, Banati RB (2005) Evolution of microglial activation in patients after ischemic stroke: a [^{11}C](R)-PK11195 PET study. Neuroimage 24:591–595

Gerhard A, Pavese N, Hotton G, Turkheimer F, Es M, Hammers A, Eggert K, Oertel W, Banati RB, Brooks DJ (2006) In vivo imaging of microglial activation with [^{11}C](R)-PK11195 PET in idiopathic Parkinson's disease. Neurobiol Dis 21:404–412

Gibson RE, Weckstein DJ, Jagoda EM, Rzeszotarski WJ, Reba RC, Eckelman WC (1984) The characteristics of I-125 4-IQNB and H-3 QNB in vivo and in vitro. J Nucl Med 25:214–222

Giembycz MA, Newton R (2006) Beyond the dogma: novel $β_2$-adrenoceptor signalling in the airways. Eur Respir J 27:1286–1306

Göran S, Lars F, Allen B, Hakan H, Christer H (1991) ^{11}C-SCH 39166, a selective ligand for visualization of dopamine-D_1 receptor binding in the monkey brain using PET. Psychopharmacology (Berl) 103:150–153

Gosens R, Zaagsma J, Meurs H, Halayko AJ (2006) Muscarinic receptor signaling in the pathophysiology of asthma and COPD. Respir Res 7:73

Goswami R, Ponde DE, Kung M-P, Hou C, Kilbourn MR, Kung HF (2006) Fluoroalkyl derivatives of dihydrotetrabenazine as positron emission tomography imaging agents targeting vesicular monoamine transporters. Nucl Med Biol 33:685–694

Greenwald M, K., Johanson CE, Moody DE, Woods J, H., Kilbourn MR, Koeppe RA, Schuster CR, Zubieta JK (2003) Effects of buprenorphine maintenance dose on μ-opioid receptor availability, plasma concentrations, and antagonist blockade in heroin-dependent volunteers. Neuropsychopharmacology 28:2000–2009

Gründer G, Siessmeier T, Lange-Asschenfeldt C, Vernaleken I, Buchholz HG, Stoeter P, Drzezga A, Lüddens H, Rösch F, Bartenstein P (2001) [18F]Fluoroethylflumazenil: a novel tracer for PET imaging of human benzodiazepine receptors. Eur J Nucl Med Mol Imaging 28: 1463–147

Guimaraes S, Moura D (2001) Vascular adrenoceptors: an update. Pharmacol Rev 53:319–356

Guo W, Hinkle GH, Lee RJ (1999) 99mTc-HYNIC-folate: a novel receptor-based targeted radio-pharmaceutical for tumor imaging. J Nucl Med 40:1563–1569

Halldin C, Stone-Elander S, Farde L, Ehrin E, Fasth KJ, Langstrom B, Sedvall G (1986) Preparation of 11C-labelled SCH 23390 for the in vivo study of dopamine D-1 receptors using positron emission tomography. Int J Rad Appl Instrum [A] 37:1039–1043

Halldin C, Farde L, Hogberg T, Mohell N, Hall H, Suhara T, Karlsson P, Nakashima Y, Swahn CG (1995) Carbon-11-FLB 457: a radioligand for extrastriatal D_2 dopamine receptors. J Nucl Med 36:1275–1281

Halldin C, Foged C, Chou YH, Karlsson P, Swahn CG, Sandell J, Sedvall G, Farde L (1998) Carbon-11-NNC 112: a radioligand for PET examination of striatal and neocortical D_1-dopamine receptors. J Nucl Med 39:2061–2068

Harvey RD, Belevych AE (2003) Muscarinic regulation of cardiac ion channels. Br J Pharmacol 139:1074–1084

Hashimoto K, Ishiwata K (2006) sigma receptor ligands: possible application as therapeutic drugs and as radiopharmaceuticals. Curr Pharm Des 12:3857–3876

Heimbold I, Drews A, Syhre R, Kretzschmar M, Pietzsch H-J, Johannsen B (2002) A novel technetium-99m radioligand for the 5-HT$_{1A}$ receptor derived from desmethyl-WAY-100635 (DWAY). Eur J Nucl Med Mol Imaging 29:82–87

Hein L (2006) Adrenoceptors and signal transduction in neurons. Cell Tissue Res 326:541–551

Heinlein AC, Chang C (2004) Androgen receptor in prostate cancer. Endocr Rev 25:276–308

Heinz A, Reimold M, Wrase J, Hermann D, Croissant B, Mundle G, Dohmen BM, Braus DH, Schumann G, Machulla H-J, Bares R, Mann K (2005) Correlation of stable elevations in striatal μ-opioid receptor availability in detoxified alcoholic patients with alcohol craving: a positron emission tomography study using carbon 11-labeled carfentanil. Arch Gen Psychiatry 62: 57–64

Heiss WD, Herholz K (2006) Brain receptor imaging. J Nucl Med 47:302–312

Henkel K, Karitzky J, Schmid M, Mader I, Glatting G, Unger JW, Neumaier B, Ludolph AC, Reske SN, Landwehrmeyer GB (2004) Imaging of activated microglia with PET and [11C]PK 11195 in corticobasal degeneration. Mov Disord 19:817–821

Henriksen G, Platzer S, Marton J, Hauser A, Berthele A, Schwaiger M, Marinelli L, Lavecchia A, Novellino E, Wester HJ (2005) Syntheses, biological evaluation, and molecular modeling of 18F-labeled 4-anilidopiperidines as μ-opioid receptor imaging agents. J Med Chem 48: 7720–7732

Hesse S, Barthel H, Schwarz J, Sabri O, Muller U (2004) Advances in in vivo imaging of serotonergic neurons in neuropsychiatric disorders. Neurosci Biobehav Rev 28:547–563

Heusch G (1990) α–Adrenergic mechanisms in myocardial ischemia. Circulation 81:1–13

Hicks RJ, Kassiou M, Eu P, Katsifis AG, Garra M, Power J, Najdovski L, Lambrecht RM (1995) Iodine-123 N-methyl-4-iododexetimide:a new radioligand for single-photon emission tomographic imaging of myocardial muscarinic receptors. Eur J Nucl Med 22:339–345

Hilgenbrink AR, Low PS (2005) Folate receptor-mediated drug targeting: from therapeutics to diagnostics. J Pharm Sci 94:2135–2146

Hopp TA, Weiss HL, Hilsenbeck SG, Cui Y, Allred DC, Horwitz KB, Fuqua SAW (2004) Breast cancer patients with progesterone receptor PR-A-rich tumors have poorer disease-free survival rates. Clin Cancer Res 10:2751–2760

Hostetler ED, Jonson SD, Welch MJ, Katzenellenbogen JA (1999) Synthesis of 2-[18F]fluoroestradiol, a potential diagnostic imaging agent for breast cancer: strategies to achieve nucleophilic substitution of an electron–rich aromatic ring with [18F]F−. J Org Chem 64:178–185

Hou C, Tu Z, Mach R, Kung HF, Kung M–P (2006) Characterization of a novel iodinated σ_2 receptor ligand as a cell proliferation marker. Nucl Med Biol 33:203–209

Houle S, DaSilva JN, Wilson AA (2000) Imaging the 5-HT$_{1A}$ receptors with PET: WAY-100635 and analogues. Nucl Med Biol 27:463–466

Huang Y, Hammond PS, Whirrett BR, Kuhner RJ, Wu L, Childers SR, Mach RH (1998) synthesis and quantitative structure-activity relationships of N-(1-benzylpiperidin-4-yl)phenylacetamides and related analogues as potent and selective σ_1 receptor ligands. J Med Chem 41:2361–2370

Huang Y, Narendran R, Bae SA, Erritzoe D, Guo N, Zhu Z, Hwang DR, Laruelle M (2004) A PET imaging agent with fast kinetics: synthesis and in vivo evaluation of the serotonin trans-porter ligand [^{11}C]2-[2-dimethylaminomethylphenylthio)]-5-fluorophenylamine ([^{11}C]AFA). Nucl Med Biol 31:727–738

Hume SP, Ashworth S, Lammertsma AA, Opacka-Juffry J, Law MP, McCarron JA, Clark RD, Nutt DJ, Pike VW (1996) Evaluation in rat of RS-79948-197 as a potential PET ligand for central α_2-adrenoceptors. Eur J Pharmacol 317:67–73

Hume SP, Hirani E, Opacka-Juffry J, Osman S, Myers R, Gunn RN, McCarron JA, Clark RD, Melichar J, Nutt DJ, Pike VW (2000) Evaluation of [O-methyl-[^{11}C]RS-15385-197 as a positron emission tomography radioligand for central α_2-adrenoceptors. Eur J Nucl Med 27:475–484

Hwang DR, Narendran R, Huang Y, Slifstein M, Talbot PS, Sudo Y, Van Berckel BN, Kegeles LS, Martinez D, Laruelle M (2004) Quantitative analysis of (–)-N-^{11}C-propyl-norapomorphine in vivo binding in nonhuman primates. J Nucl Med 45:338–346

Issa F, Kassiou M, Chan H, McLeod MD (2006) Synthesis and radiolabelling of ipratropium and tiotropium for use as pet ligands in the study of inhaled drug deposition. Aust J Chem 59:53–58

Jacobson O, Bechor Y, Icar A, Novak N, Birman A, Marom H, Fadeeva L, Golan E, Leibovitch I, Gutman M (2005) Prostate cancer PET bioprobes: synthesis of [^{18}F]-radiolabeled hydroxyflu-tamide derivatives. Bioorg Med Chem 13:6195–6205

Jacobson O, Laky D, Carlson KE, Elgavish S, Gozin M, Even-Sapir E, Leibovitc I, Gutman M, Chisin R, Katzenellenbogen JA, Mishani E (2006) Chiral dimethylamine flutamide derivatives–modeling, synthesis, androgen receptor affinities and carbon-11 labeling. Nucl Med Biol 33:695–704

Jakobsen S, Pedersen K, Smith DF, Jensen SB, Munk OL, Cumming P (2006) Detection of α_2-adrenergic receptors in brain of living pig with ^{11}C-yohimbine. J Nucl Med 47:2008–2015

Jemal A, Siegel R, Ward E, Murray T, Xu J, Smigal C, Thun MJ (2006) Cancer statistics, 2006. CA Cancer J Clin 56:106–130

Jewett DM, Kilbourn MR (2004) In vivo evaluation of new carfentanil-based radioligands for the µ-opiate receptor. Nucl Med Biol 31:321–325

John CS, Vilner BJ, Gulden ME, Efange SM, Langason RB, Moody TW, Bowen WD (1995) Synthesis and pharmacological characterization of 4-[^{125}I]-N-(N-benzylpiperidin-4-yl)-4-iodobenzamide: a high affinity sigma receptor ligand for potential imaging of breast cancer. Cancer Res 55:3022–3027

John CS, Bowen WD, Fisher SJ, Lim BB, Geyer BC, Vilner BJ, Wahl RL (1999a) Synthesis, in vitro pharmacologic characterization, and preclinical evaluation of N-[2-(1′-piperidinyl)ethyl]-3-[^{125}I]iodo-4-methoxybenzamide (P[^{125}I]MBA) for imaging breast cancer. Nucl Med Biol 26:377–382

John CS, Vilner BJ, Geyer BC, Moody T, Bowen WD (1999b) Targeting sigma receptor-binding benzamides as in vivo diagnostic and therapeutic agents for human prostate tumors. Cancer Res 59:4578–4583

Johnston SRD, Saccani-Jotti G, Smith IE, Salter J, Newby J, Coppen M, Ebbs SR, Dowsett M (1995) Changes in estrogen receptor, progesterone receptor, and ps2 expression in tamoxifen-resistant human breast cancer. Cancer Res 55:3331–3338

Jonson SD, Bonasera TA, Dehdashti F, Cristel ME, Katzenellenbogen JA, Welch MJ (1999) Comparative breast tumor imaging and comparative in vitro metabolism of 16α-[^{18}F]fluoroestradiol-17β and 16β-[^{18}F]fluoromoxestrol in isolated hepatocytes. Nucl Med Biol 26:123–130

Jutkiewicz EM (2006) The antidepressant -like effects of δ-opioid receptor agonists. Mol Interv 6:162–169

Karlsson P, Farde L, Halldin C, Swahn CG, Sedvall G, Foged C, Hansen KT, Skrumsager B (1993) PET examination of [^{11}C]NNC 687 and [^{11}C]NNC 756 as new radioligands for the D$_1$-dopamine receptor. Psychopharmacology (Berl) 113:149–156

Karramkam M, Hinnen F, Berrehouma M, Hlavacek C, Vaufrey F, Halldin C, McCarron JA, Pike VW, Dolle F (2003) Synthesis of a [6-Pyridinyl-^{18}F]-labelled fluoro derivative of WAY-100635 as a candidate radioligand for brain 5-HT$_{1A}$ receptor imaging with PET. Bioorg Med Chem 11:2769–2782

Kassiou M, Scheffel U, Ravert HT, Mathews WB, Musachio JL, Lambrecht RM, Dannals RF (1995) [^{11}C]A–69024: a potent and selective non-benzazepine radiotracer for in vivo studies of dopamine D$_1$ receptors. Nucl Med Biol 22:221–226

Kassiou M, Mardon K, Mattner F, Katsifis A, Dikic B (2001) Pharmacological evaluation of (+)-2-[^{123}I]A-69024 A radioligand for in vivo studies of dopamine D$_1$ receptors. Life Sci 69:669–675

Katchen B, Buxbaum S (1975) Disposition of a new, nonsteroid, antiandrogen α, α, α trifluoro 2 methyl 4′ nitro m propionotoluidide (Flutamide), in men following a single oral 200 mg dose. J Clin Endocrinol Metab 41:373–379

Katsifis A, Mardon K, Mattner F, Loc'h C, McPhee ME, Dikic B, Kassiou M, Ridley DD (2003) Pharmacological evaluation of (S)-8-[^{123}I]iodobretazenil: a radioligand for in vivo studies of central benzodiazepine receptors. Nucl Med Biol 30:191–198

Kawamura K, Elsinga PH, Kobayashi T, Ishii SI, Wang WF, Matsuno K, Vaalburg W, Ishiwata K (2003) Synthesis and evaluation of ^{11}C- and ^{18}F-labeled 1-[2-(4-alkoxy-3-methoxyphenyl)ethyl]-4-(3-phenylpropyl)piperazines as sigma receptor ligands for positron emission tomography studies. Nucl Med Biol 30:273–284

Kawamura K, Kubota K, Kobayashi T, Elsinga PH, Ono M, Maeda M, Ishiwata K (2005) Evaluation of [^{11}C]SA5845 and [^{11}C]SA4503 for imaging of sigma receptors in tumors by animal PET. Ann Nucl Med 19:701–709

Ke CY, Mathias CJ, Yang Z–F, Luo J, Waters DJ, Low PS, Green MA (1999) Synthesis and evaluation of folate-bis(thiosemicarbazone) and folate-CYCLAM conjugates for possible use as folate-receptor-targeted copper radiopharmaceuticals. J Labelled Comp Radiopharm 42:S821–S823

Ke CY, Mathias CJ, Green MA (2004) Folate-receptor-targeted radionuclide imaging agents. Adv Drug Deliv Rev 56:1143–1160

Kerenyi L, Ricaurte GA, Schretlen DJ, McCann U, Varga J, Mathews WB, Ravert HT, Dannals RF, Hilton J, Wong DF, Szabo Z (2003) Positron emission tomography of striatal serotonin transporters in Parkinson disease. Arch Neurol 60:1223–1229

Kessler RM (2003) Imaging methods for evaluating brain function in man. Neurobiol Aging 24:S21–S35

Kessler RM, Mason NS, Votaw JR, De Paulis T, Clanton JA, Ansari MS, Schmidt DE, Manning RG, Bell RL (1992) Visualization of extrastriatal dopamine D$_2$ receptors in the human brain. Eur J Pharmacol 223:105–107

Khamssi M, Brodde OE (1990) The role of cardiac β$_1$- and β$_2$-adrenoceptor stimulation in heart failure. J Cardiovasc Pharmacol 16:S133–S137

Kies P, Wichter T, Schafers M, Paul M, Schafers KP, Eckardt L, Stegger L, Schulze–Bahr E, Rimoldi O, Breithardt G, Schober O, Camici PG (2004) abnormal myocardial presynaptic norepinephrine recycling in patients with brugada syndrome. Circulation 110:3017–3022

Kopka K, Wagner S, Riemann B, Law MP, Puke C, Luthra SK, Pike VW, Wichter T, Schmitz W, Schober O, Schafers M (2003) Design of new β$_1$-selective adrenoceptor ligands as potential radioligands for in vivo imaging. Bioorg Med Chem 11:3513–3527

Kopka K, Law MP, Breyholz HJ, Faust A, Holtke C, Riemann B, Schober O, Schafers M, Wagner S (2005) Non-invasive molecular imaging of β-adrenoceptors in vivo:perspectives for PET-radioligands. Curr Med Chem 12:2057–2074

Kuiper GG, Enmark E, Pelto-Huikko M, Nilsson S, Gustafsson JA (1996) Cloning of a novel estrogen receptor expressed in rat prostate and ovary. Proc Natl Acad Sci U S A 93:5925–5930

Kumar JSD, Majo VJ, Hsiung SC, Millak MS, Liu KP, Tamir H, Prabhakaran J, Simpson NR, VanHeertum RL, Mann JJ, Parsey RV (2006) Synthesis and in vivo validation of [o-methyl-^{11}C]2-{4-[4-(7-methoxynaphthalen-1-yl)piperazin-1-yl]butyl}-4-methyl-2h-[1,2,4]triazine-3,5-dione: a novel 5-HT$_{1A}$ receptor agonist positron emission tomography ligand. J Med Chem 49:125–134

Kung HF (2001) Development of Tc-99m labeled tropanes: TRODAT-1, as a dopamine transporter imaging agent. Nucl Med Biol 28:505–508

Kung HF, Guo YZ, Billings J, Xu X, Mach RH, Blau M, Ackerhalt RE (1988) Preparation and biodistribution of [^{125}I]IBZM: a potential CNS D-2 dopamine receptor imaging agent. Int J Rad Appl Instrum B 15:195–201

Kung HF, Pan S, Kung MP, Billings J, Kasliwal R, Reilley J, Alavi A (1989) In vitro and in vivo evaluation of [^{123}I]IBZM:a potential CNS D-2 dopamine receptor imaging agent. J Nucl Med 30:88–92

Kung HF, Frederick D, Kim HJ, McElgin W, Kung MP, Mu M, Mozley DP, Vessotskie JM, Stevenson AD, Kushner SA, Zhuang ZP (1996) In vivo SPECT imaging of 5-HT$_{1A}$ receptors with [^{123}I] p-MPPI in nonhuman primates. Synapse 24:273–281

Kung HF, Kung MP, Choi SR (2003) Radiopharmaceuticals for single-photon emission computed tomography brain imaging. Semin Nucl Med 33:2–13

Labaree DC, Brown TJ, Hoyte RM, Hochberg RB (1997) 7α-iodine-125-iodo-5α-dihydrotestosterone: a radiolabeled ligand for the androgen receptor. J Nucl Med 38:402–409

Labaree DC, Hoyte RM, Nazareth LV, Weigel NL, Hochberg RB (1999) 7α-Iodo and 7α-fluoro steroids as androgen receptor-mediated imaging agents. J Med Chem 42:2021–2034

Landel CC, Potthoff SJ, Nardulli AM, Kushner PJ, Greene GL (1997) Estrogen receptor accessory proteins augment receptor–DNA interaction and DNA bending. J Steroid Biochem Mol Biol 63:59–73

Langer O, Halldin C, Dolle F, Swahn CG, Olsson H, Karlsson P, Hall H, Sandell J, Lundkvist C, Vaufrey F, Loc'h C, Crouzel C, Maziere B, Farde L (1999) Carbon-11 epidepride: a suitable radioligand for PET investigation of striatal and extrastriatal dopamine D$_2$ receptors. Nucl Med Biol 26:509–518

Larson SM, Morris M, Gunther I, Beattie B, Humm JL, Akhurst TA, Finn RD, Erdi Y, Pentlow K, Dyke J, Squire O, Bornmann W, McCarthy T, Welch M, Scher H (2004) Tumor localization of 16β-^{18}F-fluoro-5α-dihydrotestosterone versus ^{18}F-FDG in patients with progressive, metastatic prostate cancer. J Nucl Med 45:366–373

Laruelle M (2000) Imaging synaptic neurotransmission with in vivo binding competition techniques: a critical review. J Cereb Blood Flow Metab 20:423–451

Law MP, Osman S, Pike VW, Davenport RJ, Cunningham VJ, Rimoldi O, Rhodes CG, Giardinà D, Camici PG (2000) Evaluation of [^{11}C]GB67, a novel radioligand for imaging myocardial α$_1$-adrenoceptors with positron emission tomography. Eur J Nucl Med 27:7–17

Le Guludec D, Delforge J, Syrota A, Desruennes M, Valette H, Gandjbakhch I, Merlet P (1994) In vivo quantification of myocardial muscarinic receptors in heart transplant patients. Circulation 90:172–178

Le Guludec D, Cohen-Solal A, Delforge J, Delahaye N, Syrota A, Merlet P (1997) increased myocardial muscarinic receptor density in idiopathic dilated cardiomyopathy: an in vivo PET study. Circulation 96:3416–3422

Leamon CP, Low PS (1991) Delivery of macromolecules into living cells: a method that exploits folate receptor endocytosis. Proc Natl Acad Sci U S A 88:5572–5576

Leamon CP, Reddy JA (2004) Folate-targeted chemotherapy. Adv Drug Deliv Rev 56:1127–1141

Leamon CP, Parker MA, Vlahov IR, Xu LC, Reddy JA, Vetzel M, Douglas N (2002) synthesis and biological evaluation of EC20: a new folate-derived, ^{99m}Tc-based radiopharmaceutical. Bioconjugate Chem 13:1200–1210

Lefroy DC, De Silva R, Choudhury L, Uren NG, Crake T, Rhodes CG, Lammertsma AA, Boyd H, Patsalos PN, Nihoyannopoulos P, Oakley CM, Jones T, Camici PG (1993) Diffuse reduction of myocardial β-adrenoceptors in hypertrophic cardiomyopathy:a study with positron emission tomography. J Am Coll Cardiol 22:1653–1660

Lemaire C, Cantineau R, Guillaume M, Plenevaux A, Christiaens L (1991) Fluorine-18-altanserin: a radioligand for the study of serotonin receptors with PET: radiolabeling and in vivo biologic behavior in rats. J Nucl Med 32:2266–2272

Leon A, Rey A, Mallo L, Pirmettis I, Papadopoulos M, Leon E, Pagano M, Manta E, Incerti M, Raptopoulou C (2002) Novel mixed ligand technetium complexes as 5-HT$_{1A}$ receptor imaging agents. Nucl Med Biol 29:217–226

Lever JR, Scheffel UA, Stathis M, Musachio JL, Wagner HN Jr (1990) In vitro and in vivo binding of (E)- and (Z)-N-(iodoallyl)spiperone to dopamine D$_2$ and serotonin 5-HT$_2$ neuroreceptors. Life Sci 46:1967–1976

Li Q, Ma L, Innis RB, Seneca N, Ichise M, Huang H, Laruelle M, Murphy DL (2004) Pharmacological and genetic characterization of two selective serotonin transporter ligands: 2-[2-(dimethylaminomethylphenylthio)]-5-fluoromethylphenylamine (AFM) and 3-amino-4-[2-(dimethylaminomethyl-phenylthio)]benzonitrile (DASB). J Pharmacol Exp Ther 308: 481–486

Linden HM, Stekhova SA, Link JM, Gralow JR, Livingston RB, Ellis GK, Petra PH, Peterson LM, Schubert EK, Dunnwald LK, Krohn KA, Mankoff DA (2006) quantitative fluoroestradiol positron emission tomography imaging predicts response to endocrine treatment in breast cancer. J Clin Oncol 24:2793–2799

Lingford HA (2005) Human brain imaging and substance abuse. Curr Opin Pharmacol 5:42–46

Liu A, Dence CS, Welch MJ, Katzenellenbogen JA (1992) Fluorine-18-labeled androgens: radiochemical synthesis and tissue distribution studies on six fluorine-substituted androgens, potential imaging agents for prostatic cancer. J Nucl Med 33:724–734

Liu AJ, Katzenellenbogen JA, VanBrocklin HF, Mathias CJ, Welch MJ (1991) 20-[^{18}F]fluoromibolerone, a positron-emitting radiotracer for androgen receptors: synthesis and tissue distribution studies. J Nucl Med 32:81–88

Liu M, Xu W, Xu Lj, Zhong Gr, Chen Sl, Lu Wy (2005) Synthesis and biological evaluation of diethylenetriamine pentaacetic acid-polyethylene glycol-folate: a new folate-derived, ^{99m}Tc-based radiopharmaceutical. Bioconjugate Chem 16:1126–1132

Loc'h C, Halldin C, Bottlaender M, Swahn C-G, Moresco R–M, Maziere M, Farde L, Maziere B (1996) Preparation of [^{76}Br]FLB 457 and [^{76}Br]FLB 463 for examination of striatal and extrastriatal dopamine D-2 receptors with PET. Nucl Med Biol 23:813–819

Lundkvist C, Halldin C, Ginovart N, Nyberg S, Swahn C-G, Carr AA, Brunner F, Farde L (1996) [^{11}C]MDL 100907, a radioligand for selective imaging of 5-HT$_{2A}$ receptors with positron emission tomography. Life Sci 58:187–192

Luo H, Hasan A, Sood V, McRee RC, Zeeberg B, Reba RC, McPherson DW, Knapp FF (1996) Evaluation of 1-azabicyclo[2.2.2]oct-3-yl α-fluoroalkyl-α-hydroxy-α-phenylacetates as potential ligands for the study of muscarinic receptor density by positron emission tomography. Nucl Med Biol 23:267–276

Luyt LG, Bigott HM, Welch MJ, Katzenellenbogen JA (2003) 7α- and 17α-substituted estrogens containing tridentate tricarbonyl rhenium/technetium complexes: synthesis of estrogen receptor imaging agents and evaluation using microPET with technetium-94 m. Bioorg Med Chem 11:4977–4989

Mach RH, Huang Y, Buchheimer N, Kuhner R, Wu L, Morton TE, Wang LM, Ehrenkaufer RL, Wallen CA, Wheeler KT (2001) [^{18}F]N-4'-Fluorobenzyl-4-(3–bromophenyl) acetamide for imaging the sigma receptor status of tumors:comparison with [^{18}F]FDG and [^{125}I]IUDR. Nucl Med Biol 28:451–458

Machulla H-J, Heinz A (2005) Radioligands for brain imaging of the κ-opioid system. J Nucl Med 46:386–387

Mankoff DA, Dehdashti F, Shields AF (2000) Characterizing tumors using metabolic imaging: PET imaging of cellular proliferation and steroid receptors. Neoplasia 2:71–88

Marek K, Jennings D, Seibyl J (2003) Imaging the dopamine system to assess disease-modifying drugs: studies comparing dopamine agonists and levodopa. Neurology 61:S43–S48

Martin WR, Eades CG, Thompson JA, Huppler RE, Gilbert PE (1976) The effects of morphine- and nalorphine-like drugs in the nondependent and morphine-dependent chronic spinal dog. J Pharmacol Exp Ther 197:517–532

Matarrese M, Moresco RM, Romeo G, Turolla EA, Simonelli P, Todde S, Belloli S, Carpinelli A, Magni F, Russo F, Galli Kienle M, Fazio F (2002) [^{11}C]RN5: a new agent for the in vivo imaging of myocardial α_1-adrenoceptors. Eur J Pharmacol 453:231–238

Mathias CJ, Hubers D, Low PS, Green MA (2000) Synthesis of [^{99m}Tc]DTPA-folate and its evaluation as a folate–receptor–targeted radiopharmaceutical. Bioconjugate Chem 11:253–257

Mathias CJ, Lewis MR, Reichert DE, Laforest R, Sharp TL, Lewis JS, Yang Z–F, Waters DJ, Snyder PW, Low PS, Welch MJ, Green MA (2003) Preparation of ^{66}Ga- and ^{68}Ga-labeled Ga(III)-deferoxamine-folate as potential folate-receptor-targeted PET radiopharmaceuticals. Nucl Med Biol 30:725–731

Mathis CA, Simpson NR, Mahmood K, Kinahan PE, Mintun MA (1994) [^{11}C]WAY 100635: a radioligand for imaging 5-HT$_{1A}$ receptors with positron emission tomography. Life Sci 55: 403–407

Matsumura K, Uno Y, Scheffel U, Wilson AA, Dannals RF, Wagner HN Jr (1991) In vitro and in vivo characterization of 4-[^{125}I]iododexetimide binding to muscarinic cholinergic receptors in the rat heart. J Nucl Med 32:76–80

Mazière B, Halldin C (2004) PET tracers for brain scanning. In: Ell PJ, Gambhir SS (eds) nuclear medicine in clinical diagnosis and treatment. Churchill Livingstone, Edinburgh, pp 1295–1329

Maziere M, Comar D, Godot JM, Collard P, Cepeda C, Naquet R (1981) In vivo characterization of myocardium muscarinic receptors by positron emission tomography. Life Sci 29:2391–2397

Maziere M, Hantraye P, Prenant C, Sastre J, Comar D (1984) Synthesis of ethyl 8-fluoro-5,6-dihydro-5-[^{11}C]methyl-6-oxo-4H-imidazo [1,5-a] [1,4] benzodiazepine-3-carboxylate (Ro 15-1788-^{11}C): a specific radioligand for the in vivo study of central benzodiazepine receptors by positron emission tomography. Int J Appl Radiat Isot 35:973–976

Mazzi U (2006) Technetium, rhenium and other metals in chemistry and nuclear medicine. SGEditoriali, Padova

McCann UD, Szabo Z, Seckin E, Rosenblatt P, Mathews WB, Ravert HT, Dannals RF, Ricaurte GA (2005) Quantitative PET studies of the serotonin transporter in MDMA Users and controls using [^{11}C]McN5652 and [^{11}C]DASB. Neuropsychopharmacology 30:1741–1750

McLeod DG (1993) Antiandrogenic drugs. Cancer 71:1046–1049

McPherson DW, Greenbaum M, Luo H, Beets AL, Knapp FF (2000) Evaluation of Z-(R,R)-IQNP for the potential imaging of m2 mAChR rich regions of the brain and heart. Life Sci 66:885–896

Merlet P, Delforge J, Syrota A, Angevin E, Maziere B, Crouzel C, Valette H, Loisance D, Castaigne A, Rande JL (1993) Positron emission tomography with ^{11}C CGP-12177 to assess β-adrenergic receptor concentration in idiopathic dilated cardiomyopathy. Circulation 87: 1169–1178

Mertens J, Terriere D, Sipido V, Gommeren W, Janssen PMF, Leysen JE (1994) Radiosynthesis of a new radioiodinated ligand for serotonin-5HT$_2$-receptors, a promising tracer for γ-emission tomography. J Labelled Comp Radiopharm 34:795–806

Mitterhauser M, Wadsak W, Wabnegger L, Mien L–K, Togel S, Langer O, Sieghart W, Viernstein H, Kletter K, Dudczak R (2004) Biological evaluation of 2′-[^{18}F]fluoroflumazenil ([^{18}F]FFMZ), a potential GABA receptor ligand for PET. Nucl Med Biol 31:291–295

Moerlein SM, Perlmutter JS (1992) Binding of 5-(2′-[^{18}F]fluoroethyl)flumazenil to central benzodiazepines receptors measured in living baboon by positron emission tomography. Eur J Pharmacol 218:109–115

Moerlein SM, Parkinson D, Welch MJ (1990) Radiosynthesis of high effective specific-activity [^{123}I]SCH 23982 for dopamine D-1 receptor-based SPECT imaging. Int J Rad Appl Instrum [A] 41:381–385

Moerlein SM, Perlmutter JS, Markham J, Welch MJ (1997) In vivo kinetics of [^{18}F](N-methyl)benperidol: a novel pet tracer for assessment of dopaminergic D$_2$-like receptor binding. J Cereb Blood Flow Metab 17:833–845

Moresco RM, Matarrese M, Soloviev D, Simonelli P, Rigamonti M, Gobbo C, Todde S, Carpinelli A, Galli Kienle M, Fazio F (2000) Synthesis and in vivo evaluation of [^{11}C]ICI 118551 as a putative subtype selective β_2-adrenergic radioligand. Int J Pharm 204:101–109

Mori T, Kasamatsu S, Mosdzianowski C, Welch MJ, Yonekura Y, Fujibayashi Y (2006) Automatic synthesis of 16α-[^{18}F]fluoro-17β-estradiol using a cassette-type [^{18}F]fluorodeoxyglucose synthesizer. Nucl Med Biol 33:281–286

Mortimer JE, Dehdashti F, Siegel BA, Katzenellenbogen JA, Fracasso P, Welch MJ (1996) Positron emission tomography with 2-[^{18}F]fluoro-2-deoxy-D-glucose and 16α-[^{18}F]fluoro-17β-estradiol in breast cancer: correlation with estrogen receptor status and response to systemic therapy. Clin Cancer Res 2:933–939

Mortimer JE, Dehdashti F, Siegel BA, Trinkaus K, Katzenellenbogen JA, Welch MJ (2001) metabolic flare: indicator of hormone responsiveness in advanced breast cancer. J Clin Oncol 19:2797–2803

Mukherjee J, Narayanan TK, Christian BT, Shi B, Dunigan KA, Mantil J (2000) In vitro and in vivo evaluation of the binding of the dopamine D_2 receptor agonist ^{11}C-(R,S)-5-hydroxy-2-(di-n-propylamino)tetralin in rodents and nonhuman primate. Synapse 37:64–70

Mukherjee J, Narayanan TK, Christian BT, Shi B, Yang ZY (2004a) Binding characteristics of high-affinity dopamine D_2/D_3 receptor agonists, ^{11}C-PPHT and ^{11}C-ZYY-339 in rodents and imaging in non-human primates by PET. Synapse 54:83–91

Mukherjee J, Shi B, Christian BT, Chattopadhyay S, Narayanan TK (2004b) ^{11}C-Fallypride: radiosynthesis and preliminary evaluation of a novel dopamine D_2/D_3 receptor PET radiotracer in non-human primate brain. Bioorg Med Chem 12:95–102

Mull ES, Sattigeri VJ, Rodriguez AL, Katzenellenbogen JA (2002) Aryl cyclopentadienyl tricarbonyl rhenium complexes: novel ligands for the estrogen receptor with potential use as estrogen radiopharmaceuticals. Bioorg Med Chem 10:1381–1398

Müller C, Hohn A, Schubiger AP, Schibli R (2006) Preclinical evaluation of novel organometallic ^{99m}Tc-folate and ^{99m}Tc-pteroate radiotracers for folate receptor-positive tumour targeting. Eur J Nucl Med Mol Imaging 33:1007–1016

Murali D, Flores LG, Roberts AD, Nickles RJ, DeJesus OT (2003) Aromatic -amino acid decarboxylase (AAAD) inhibitors as carcinoid tumor-imaging agents: synthesis of ^{18}F-labeled α-fluoromethyl-6-fluoro-m-tyrosine (FM-6-FmT). Appl Radiat Isot 59:237–243

Murphy LC, Watson PH (2006) Is oestrogen receptor-β a predictor of endocrine therapy responsiveness in human breast cancer? Endocr Relat Cancer 13:327–334

Nakatsuka I, Saji H, Shiba K, Shimizu H, Okuno M, Yoshitake A, Yokoyama A (1987) In vitro evaluation of radioiodinated butyrophenones as radiotracer for dopamine receptor study. Life Sci 41:1989–1997

Nicolaas P, Verhoeff LG (1999) Radiotracer imaging of dopaminergic transmission in neuropsychiatric disorders. Psychopharmacology 147:217–249

Nijkamp FP, Henricks PA (1990) Receptors in airway disease. β-adrenoceptors in lung inflammation. Am Rev Respir Dis 141:S145–S150

Nutt DJ, Malizia AL (2001) New insights into the role of the GABA$_A$-benzodiazepine receptor in psychiatric disorder. Br J Psychiatry 179:390–396

Okarvi SM, Jammaz IA (2006) Preparation and in vitro and in vivo evaluation of technetium-99m-labeled folate and methotrexate conjugates as tumor imaging agents. Cancer Biother Radiopharm 21:49–60

Osman S, Lundkvist C, Pike VW, Halldin C, McCarron JA, Swahn C-G, Farde L, Ginovart N, Luthra SK, Gunn RN (1998) characterisation of the appearance of radioactive metabolites in monkey and human plasma from the 5-HT$_{1A}$ receptor radioligand, [carbonyl-^{11}C]WAY-100635–Explanation of high signal contrast in PET and an aid to biomathematical modelling. Nucl Med Biol 25:215–223

Owens MJ (1996/1997) Molecular and cellular mechanisms of antidepressant drugs. Depress Anxiety 4:153–159

Palmer AM, Francis PT, Benton JS, Sims NR, Mann DM, Neary D, Snowden JS, Bowen DM (1987) Presynaptic serotonergic dysfunction in patients with Alzheimer's disease. J Neurochem 48:8–15

Palmieri C, Cheng GJ, Saji S, Zelada–Hedman M, Warri A, Weihua Z, Van Noorden S, Wahlstrom T, Coombes RC, Warner M, Gustafsson JA (2002) Estrogen receptor beta in breast cancer. Endocr Relat Cancer 9:1–13

Panwar P, Shrivastava V, Tandon V, Mishra P, Chuttani K, Sharma RK, Chandra R, Mishra AK (2004) ^{99m}Tc-tetraethylenepentamine-folate — a new ^{99m}Tc-based folate derivative for the detection of folate receptor positive tumors: synthesis and biological evaluation. Cancer Biol Ther 3:995–1001

Parent EE, Dence CS, Sharp TL, Welch MJ, Katzenellenbogen JA (2006a) Synthesis and biological evaluation of a fluorine-18-labeled nonsteroidal androgen receptor antagonist, N-(3-[^{18}F]fluoro-4-nitronaphthyl)-cis-5-norbornene-endo-2,3-dicarboxylic imide. Nucl Med Biol 33:615–624

Parent EE, Jenks C, Sharp T, Welch MJ, Katzenellenbogen JA (2006b) Synthesis and biological evaluation of a nonsteroidal bromine-76-labeled androgen receptor ligand 3-[^{76}Br]bromo-hydroxyflutamide. Nucl Med Biol 33:705–713

Passchier J, van Waarde A (2001) Visualisation of serotonin-1A (5-HT$_{1A}$) receptors in the central nervous system. Eur J Nucl Med 28:119–129

Peremans K, Audenaert K, Hoybergs Y, Otte A, Goethals I, Gielen I, Blankaert P, Vervaet M, Heeringen Cv, Dierckx R (2005) The effect of citalopram hydrobromide on 5-HT$_{2A}$ receptors in the impulsive-aggressive dog, as measured with ^{123}I-5-I-R91150 SPECT. Eur J Nucl Med Mol Imaging 32:708–716

Piccini P, Whone A (2004) Functional brain imaging in the differential diagnosis of Parkinson's disease. Lancet Neurol 3:284–290

Pike VW, McCarron JA, Lammertsma AA, Osman S, Hume SP, Sargent PA, Bench CJ, Cliffe IA, Fletcher A, Grasby PM (1996) Exquisite delineation of 5-HT$_{1A}$ receptors in human brain with PET and [carbonyl-^{11}C] WAY-100635. Eur J Pharmacol 301:R5–R7

Pike VW, Law MP, Osman S, Davenport RJ, Rimoldi O, Giardina D, Camici PG (2000) Selection, design and evaluation of new radioligands for PET studies of cardiac adrenoceptors. Pharm Acta Helv 74:191–200

Pleis JR, Lethbridge CM (2006) Summary health statistics for U.S. adults: National Health Interview Survey, 2005. Vital Health Stat 10:1–153

Plisson C, McConathy J, Martarello L, Malveaux EJ, Camp VM, Williams L, Votaw JR, Goodman MM (2004) Synthesis, radiosynthesis, and biological evaluation of carbon-11 and iodine-123 labeled 2-carbomethoxy-3-[4′-((Z)-2-haloethenyl)phenyl]tropanes: candidate radioligands for in vivo imaging of the serotonin transporter. J Med Chem 47:1122–1135

Pomper MG, Katzenellenbogen JA, Welch MJ, Brodack JW, Mathias CJ (1988) 21-[^{18}F]fluoro-16α-ethyl-19-norprogesterone: synthesis and target tissue selective uptake of a progestin receptor based radiotracer for positron emission tomography. J Med Chem 31:1360–1363

Qing F, Rahman SU, Rhodes CG, Hayes MJ, Sriskandan S, Ind PW, Jones T, Hughes JM (1997) Pulmonary and cardiac β-adrenoceptor density in vivo in asthmatic subjects. Am J Respir Crit Care Med 155:1130–1134

Quinlivan M, Mattner F, Papazian V, Zhou J, Katsifis A, Emond P, Chalon S, Kozikowski A, Guilloteau D, Kassiou M (2003) Synthesis and evaluation of iodine-123 labelled tricyclic tropanes as radioligands for the serotonin transporter. Nucl Med Biol 30:741–746

Quirion R, Bowen WD, Itzhak Y, Junien JL, Musachio J, Rothman RB, Tsung-Ping S, Tam SW, Taylor DP (1992) A proposal for the classification of sigma binding sites. Trends Pharmacol Sci 13:85–86

Ravert HT, Scheffel U, Mathews WB, Musachio JL, Dannals RF (2002) [^{11}C]–GR89696, a potent kappa opiate receptor radioligand; in vivo binding of the R and S enantiomers. Nucl Med Biol 29:47–53

Reddy JA, Xu LC, Parker N, Vetzel M, Leamon CP (2004) Preclinical evaluation of ^{99m}Tc-EC20 for imaging folate receptor-positive tumors. J Nucl Med 45:857–866

Reddy JA, Allagadda VM, Leamon CP (2005) Targeting therapeutic and imaging agents to folate receptor positive tumors. Curr Pharm Biotechnol 6:131–150

Rijks LJ, Boer GJ, Endert E, de Bruin K, van den Bos JC, van Doremalen PA, Schoonen WG, Janssen AG, van Royen EA (1996) The stereoisomers of 17α-[^{123}I]iodovinyloestradiol and its 11α-methoxy derivative evaluated for their oestrogen receptor binding in human MCF-7 cells and rat uterus, and their distribution in immature rats. Eur J Nucl Med Mol Imaging 23:295–307

Rijks LJM, van den Bos JC, van Doremalen PAPM, Boer GJ, de Bruin K, Janssen AGM, van Royen EA (1998) New iodinated progestins as potential ligands for progesterone receptor imaging in breast cancer. Part 2: In vivo pharmacological characterization. Nucl Med Biol 25:791–798

Rossin R, Pan D, Qi K, Turner JL, Sun X, Wooley KL, Welch MJ (2005) ^{64}Cu-labeled folate-conjugated shell cross-linked nanoparticles for tumor imaging and radiotherapy: synthesis, radiolabeling, and biologic evaluation. J Nucl Med 46:1210–1218

Rowland DJ, Tu Z, Xu J, Ponde D, Mach RH, Welch MJ (2006) Synthesis and in vivo evaluation of 2 high-affinity ^{76}Br-labeled σ₂-receptor ligands. J Nucl Med 47:1041–1048

Ryzhikov NN, Seneca N, Krasikova RN, Gomzina NA, Shchukin E, Fedorova OS, Vassiliev DA, Gulyas B, Hall H, Savic I, Halldin C (2005) Preparation of highly specific radioactivity [^{18}F]flumazenil and its evaluation in cynomolgus monkey by positron emission tomography. Nucl Med Biol 32:109–116

Saigal N, Pichika R, Easwaramoorthy B, Collins D, Christian BT, Shi B, Narayanan TK, Potkin SG, Mukherjee J (2006) Synthesis and biologic evaluation of a novel serotonin 5-HT$_{1A}$ receptor radioligand, ^{18}F-labeled mefway, in rodents and imaging by PET in a nonhuman primate. J Nucl Med 47:1697–1706

Samnick S, Remy N, Ametamey S, Bader JB, Brandau W, Kirsch C-M (1998) ^{123}I-MSP and F[^{11}C]MSP: new selective 5-HT$_{2A}$ receptor radiopharmaceuticals for in vivo studies of neuronal 5-HT$_2$ serotonin receptors. Synthesis, in vitro binding study with unlabelled analogues and preliminary in vivo evaluation in mice. Life Sci 63:2001–2013

Sanchez-Pernaute R, Brownell AL, Isacson O (2002) functional imaging of the dopamine system: in vivo evaluation of dopamine deficiency and restoration. Neurotoxicology 23:469–478

Santos AF, Huang H, Tindall DJ (2004) The androgen receptor: a potential target for therapy of prostate cancer. Steroids 69:79–85

Schafers MA, Wichter T, Schafers KP, Rahman S, Rhodes CG, Lammertsma AA, Lerch H, Knickmeier M, Hermansen F, Schober O, Camici PG, Breithardt G (2001) Pulmonary β-adrenoceptor density in arrhythmogenic right ventricular cardiomyopathy and idiopathic tachycardia. Basic Res Cardiol 96:91–97

Schins A, Van Kroonenburgh M, Van Laere K, D'Haenen H, Lousberg R, Crijns H, Eersels J, Honig A (2005) Increased cerebral serotonin-2A receptor binding in depressed patients with myocardial infarction. Psychiatry Res 139:155–163

Schirrmacher E, Schirrmacher R, Thews O, Dillenburg W, Helisch A, Wessler I, Buhl R, Hohnemann S, Buchholz H–G, Bartenstein P, Machulla H-J, Rosch F (2003) Synthesis and preliminary evaluation of (R,R)(S,S) 5-(2-(2-[4-(2-[^{18}F]fluoroethoxy)phenyl]-1-methylethylamino)-1-hydroxyethyl)-benzene-1,3-diol ([^{18}F]FEFE) for the in vivo visualisation and quantification of the β₂-adrenergic receptor status in lung. Bioorg Med Chem Lett 13:2687–2692

Seimbille Y, Rousseau J, Benard F, Morin C, Ali H, Avvakumov G, Hammond GL, van Lier JE (2002) ^{18}F-labeled difluoroestradiols: preparation and preclinical evaluation as estrogen receptor-binding radiopharmaceuticals. Steroids 67:765–775

Seimbille Y, Benard F, Rousseau J, Pepin E, Aliaga A, Tessier G, van Lier JE (2004) Impact on estrogen receptor binding and target tissue uptake of [^{18}F]fluorine substitution at the 16α-position of fulvestrant (faslodex; ICI 182,780). Nucl Med Biol 31:691–698

Seo JW, Comninos JS, Chi DY, Kim DW, Carlson KE, Katzenellenbogen JA (2006) Fluorine-substituted cyclofenil derivatives as estrogen receptor ligands: synthesis and structure-affinity relationship study of potential positron emission tomography agents for imaging estrogen receptors in breast cancer. J Med Chem 49:2496–2511

Shiue CY, Welch MJ (2004) Update on PET radiopharmaceuticals: life beyond fluorodeoxyglucose. Radiol Clin North Am 42:1033–1053

Shiue CY, Bai LQ, Teng RR, Arnett CD, Dewey SL, Wolf AP, McPherson DW, Fowler JS, Logan J, Holland MJ (1991) A comparison of the brain uptake of N-(cyclopropyl[^{11}C]methyl)norbuprenorphine ([^{11}C]buprenorphine) and N-(cyclopropyl[^{11}C]-methyl)nordiprenorphine ([^{11}C]diprenorphine) in baboon using PET. Int J Rad Appl Instrum B 18:281–288

Shiue CY, Shiue GG, Zhang SX, Wilder S, Greenberg JH, Benard F, Wortman JA, Alavi AA (1997) N-(N-Benzylpiperidin-4-yl)-2-[^{18}F]fluorobenzamide: a potential ligand for PET imaging of σ receptors. Nucl Med Biol 24:671–676

Shiue CY, Pleus RC, Shiue GG, Rysavy JA, Sunderland JJ, Cornish KG, Young SD, Bylund DB (1998) Synthesis and biological evaluation of [^{11}C]MK-912 as an α_2-adrenergic receptor radioligand for PET studies. Nucl Med Biol 25:127–133

Sibley DR, Monsma JFJ (1992) Molecular biology of dopamine receptors. Trends Pharmacol Sci 13:61–69

Sibley DR, De Lean A, Creese I (1982) Anterior pituitary dopamine receptors. Demonstration of interconvertible high and low affinity states of the D-2 dopamine receptor. J Biol Chem 257:6351–6361

Siegel BA, Dehdashti F, Mutch DG, Podoloff DA, Wendt R, Sutton GP, Burt RW, Ellis PR, Mathias CJ, Green MA, Gershenson DM (2003) Evaluation of ^{111}In-DTPA-folate as a receptor-targeted diagnostic agent for ovarian cancer: initial clinical results. J Nucl Med 44:700–707

Skaddan MB, Wust FR, Jonson S, Syhre R, Welch MJ, Spies H, Katzenellenbogen JA (2000) Radiochemical synthesis and tissue distribution of Tc-99m-labeled 7α-substituted estradiol complexes. Nucl Med Biol 27:269–278

Small EJ, Halabi S, Dawson NA, Stadler WM, Rini BI, Picus J, Gable P, Torti FM, Kaplan E, Vogelzang NJ (2004) antiandrogen withdrawal alone or in combination with ketoconazole in androgen-independent prostate cancer patients:a phase iii trial (CALGB 9583). J Clin Oncol 22:1025–1033

Smith JS, Zubieta JK, Price JC, Flesher JE, Madar I, Lever JR, Kinter CM, Dannals RF, Frost JJ (1999) Quantification of δ-opioid receptors in human brain with N1'-([^{11}C]Methyl) naltrindole and positron emission tomography. J Cereb Blood Flow Metab 19:956–966

Sobrio F, Amokhtari M, Gourand F, Dhilly M, Dauphin F, Barre L (2000) Radiosynthesis of [^{18}F]Lu29-024: a potential PET ligand for brain imaging of the serotonergic 5-HT$_2$ receptor. Bioorg Med Chem 8:2511–2518

Soloviev DV, Matarrese M, Moresco RM, Todde S, Bonasera TA, Sudati F, Simonelli P, Magni F, Colombo D, Carpinelli A, Galli Kienle M, Fazio F (2001) Asymmetric synthesis and preliminary evaluation of (R)- and (S)-[^{11}C]bisoprolol, a putative β_1-selective adrenoceptor radioligand. Neurochem Int 38:169–180

Sprenger T, Berthele A, Platzer S, Boecker H, Tolle TR (2005) What to learn from in vivo opioidergic brain imaging? Eur J Pain 9:117–121

Stamatakis EA, Hetherington MM (2003) Neuroimaging in eating disorders. Nutr Neurosci 6: 325–334

Starke K (1981) α-Adrenoceptor subclassification. Rev Physiol Biochem Pharmacol 88: 199–236

Stockmeier CA (2003) Involvement of serotonin in depression: evidence from postmortem and imaging studies of serotonin receptors and the serotonin transporter. J Psychiatr Res 37: 357–373

Sucharov CC (2007) β-adrenergic pathways in human heart failure. Expert Rev Cardiovasc Ther 5:119–124

Suehiro M, Dannals RF, Scheffel U, Stathis M, Wilson AA, Ravert HT, Villemagne VL, Sanchez-Roa PM, Wagner HN Jr, (1990) In vivo labeling of the dopamine D$_2$ receptor with N-^{11}C-methyl-benperidol. J Nucl Med 31:2015–2021

Sun C, Sze R, Zhang M (2006) Folic acid-PEG conjugated superparamagnetic nanoparticles for targeted cellular uptake and detection by MRI. J Biomed Mater Res A 78:550–557

Takahashi N, Yang DJ, Kohanim S, Oh CS, Yu DF, Azhdarinia A, Kurihara H, Zhang X, Chang JY, Edmund KE (2008) Targeted functional imaging of estrogen receptors with ^{99m}Tc-GAP-EDL. Eur J Nucl Med Mol Imaging (in press)

Takamatsu S, Furukawa T, Mori T, Yonekura Y, Fujibayashi Y (2005) Noninvasive imaging of transplanted living functional cells transfected with a reporter estrogen receptor gene. Nucl Med Biol 32:821–829

Talbot PS, Laruelle M (2002) The role of in vivo molecular imaging with PET and SPECT in the elucidation of psychiatric drug action and new drug development. Eur Neuropsychopharmacol 12:503–511

Talbot PS, Narendran R, Butelman ER, Huang Y, Ngo K, Slifstein M, Martinez D, Laruelle M, Hwang DR (2005) ^{11}C-GR103545, a radiotracer for imaging κ-opioid receptors in vivo with PET: synthesis and evaluation in baboons. J Nucl Med 46:484–494

Tan PZ, Baldwin RM, Van Dyck CH, Al-Tikriti M, Roth B, Khan N, Charney DS, Innis RB (1999) Characterization of radioactive metabolites of 5-HT$_{2A}$ receptor PET ligand [^{18}F]altanserin in human and rodent. Nucl Med Biol 26:601–608

Tewson TJ, Stekhova S, Kinsey B, Chen L, Wiens L, Barber R (1999) Synthesis and biodistribution of R- and S-isomers of [^{18}F]-fluoropropranolol, a lipophilic ligand for the β-adrenergic receptor. Nucl Med Biol 26:891–896

Tipre DN, Zoghbi SS, Liow JS, Green MV, Seidel J, Ichise M, Innis RB, Pike VW (2006) PET Imaging of brain 5-HT$_{1A}$ receptors in rat in vivo with ^{18}F-FCWAY and improvement by successful inhibition of radioligand defluorination with miconazole. J Nucl Med 47:345–353

Trump DP, Mathias CJ, Yang Z, Low PS, Marmion M, Green MA (2002) Synthesis and evaluation of ^{99m}Tc(CO)$_3$-DTPA-folate as a folate-receptor-targeted radiopharmaceutical. Nucl Med Biol 29:569–573

Tsoukalas C, Pirmettis I, Patsis G, Pelecanou M, Bodo K, Raptopoulou CP, Terzis A, Papadopoulos M, Chiotellis E (2003) Novel oxorhenium and oxotechnetium MO(NS)(S)$_2$ complexes in the development of 5-HT$_{1A}$ receptor imaging agents. J Inorg Biochem 93: 213–220

Tu Z, Dence CS, Ponde DE, Jones L, Wheeler KT, Welch MJ, Mach RH (2005) Carbon-11 labeled σ$_2$ receptor ligands for imaging breast cancer. Nucl Med Biol 32:423–430

Turner MR, Cagnin A, Turkheimer FE, Miller CCJ, Shaw CE, Brooks DJ, Leigh PN, Banati RB (2004) Evidence of widespread cerebral microglial activation in amyotrophic lateral sclerosis: an [^{11}C](R)-PK11195 positron emission tomography study. Neurobiol Dis 15:601–609

Tyacke RJ, Robinson ESJ, Schnabel R, Lewis JW, Husbands SM, Nutt DJ, Hudson AL (2002) N1′-fluoroethyl-naltrindole (BU97001) and N1′-fluoroethyl-(14-formylamino)-naltrindole (BU97018) potential δ-opioid receptor PET ligands. Nucl Med Biol 29:455–462

Ueki J, Rhodes CJ, Hughes JM, De–Silva R, Lefroy DC, Ind PW, Qing F, Brady F, Luthra SK, Steel CJ (1993) In vivo quantification of pulmonary β-adrenoceptor density in humans with (S)-[^{11}C]CGP–12177 and PET. J Appl Physiol 75:559–565

Valette H, Dolle F, Guenther I, Demphel S, Rasetti C, Hinnen F, Fuseau C, Crouzel C (1999) Preliminary evaluation of 2-[4-[3-(tert-Butylamino)-2-hydroxypropoxy]phenyl]-3-methyl-6-methoxy-4(3H)-quinazolinone ([+/−]HX-CH 44) as a selective β$_1$-adrenoceptor ligand for PET. Nucl Med Biol 26:105–109

Valk PE, Bailey DL, Townsend DW, Maisey MN (2003) Positron emission tomography: basic science and clinical practice. Springer, London

van den Bos JC, Rijks LJM, van Doremalen PAPM, de Bruin K, Janssen AGM, van Royen EA (1998) New iodinated progestins as potential ligands for progesterone receptor imaging in breast cancer. Part 1: synthesis and in vitro pharmacological characterization. Nucl Med Biol 25:781–789

Van Den Bossche B, Van de Wiele C (2004) receptor imaging in oncology by means of nuclear medicine: current status. J Clin Oncol 22:3593–3607

Van der Mey M, Windhorst AD, Klok RP, Herscheid JDM, Kennis LE, Bischoff F, Bakker M, Langlois X, Heylen L, Jurzak M, Leysen JE (2006) Synthesis and biodistribution of

[^{11}C]R107474, a new radiolabeled α_2-adrenoceptor antagonist. Bioorg Med Chem 14:4526–4534

van Waarde A, Visser TJ, Elsinga PH, de Jong BM, van der Mark TW, Kraan J, Ensing K, Pruim J, Willemsen ATM, Brodde O-E, Visser GM, Paans AMJ, Vaalburg W (1997) Imaging β-adrenoceptors in the human brain with (S)-1′-[^{18}F]fluorocarazolol. J Nucl Med 38:934–939

van Waarde A, Elsinga PH, Doze P, Heldoorn M, Jaeggi KA, Vaalburg W (1998) A novel β-adrenoceptor ligand for positron emission tomography: evaluation in experimental animals. Eur J Pharmacol 343:289–296

van Waarde A, Buursma AR, Hospers GAP, Kawamura K, Kobayashi T, Ishii K, Oda K, Ishiwata K, Vaalburg W, Elsinga PH (2004) Tumor imaging with 2 σ-receptor ligands, ^{18}F-FE-SA5845 and ^{11}C-SA4503: a feasibility study. J Nucl Med 45:1939–1945

van Waarde A, Maas B, Doze P, Slart RH, Frijlink HW, Vaalburg W, Elsinga PH (2005) positron emission tomography studies of human airways using an inhaled β-adrenoceptor antagonist, S-^{11}C-CGP 12388. Chest 128:3020–3027

van Waarde A, Been LB, Ishiwata K, Dierckx RA, Elsinga PH (2006) early response of σ-receptor ligands and metabolic PET tracers to 3 forms of chemotherapy: an in vitro study in glioma cells. J Nucl Med 47:1538–1545

VanBrocklin HF, Blagoev M, Hoepping A, O'Neil JP, Klose M, Schubiger PA, Ametamey S (2004) A new precursor for the preparation of 6-[^{18}F]fluoro-m-tyrosine ([^{18}F]FMT): efficient synthesis and comparison of radiolabeling. Appl Radiat Isot 61:1289–1294

Vandecapelle M, De Vos F, Vermeirsch H, De Ley G, Audenaert K, Leysen D, Dierckx RA, Slegers G (2001) In vivo evaluation of 4-[^{123}I]iodo-N-{2-[4-(6-trifluoromethyl-2-pyridinyl)-1-piperazinyl]ethyl}benzamide, a potential SPECT radioligand for the 5-HT$_{1A}$ receptor. Nucl Med Biol 28:639–643

Verhagen A, Luurtsema G, Pesser JW, de Groot TJ, Wouda S, Oosterhuis JW, Vaalburg W (1991) Preclinical evaluation of a positron emitting progestin ([^{18}F]fluoro-16α-methyl-19-norprogesterone) for imaging progesterone receptor positive tumours with positron emission tomography. Cancer Lett 59:125–132

Verhagen A, Studeny M, Luurtsema G, Visser GM, De Goeij CCJ, Sluyser M, Nieweg OE, van der Ploeg E, Go KG, Vaalburg W (1994) Metabolism of a [^{18}F]fluorine labeled progestin (21-[^{18}F]fluoro-16α-ethyl-19-norprogesterone) in humans: a clue for future investigations. Nucl Med Biol 21:941–952

Versijpt J, Van Laere KJ, Dumont F, Decoo D, Vandecapelle M, Santens P, Goethals I, Audenaert K, Slegers G, Dierckx RA, Korf J (2003a) Imaging of the 5-HT$_{2A}$ system: age-, gender-, and Alzheimer's disease-related findings. Neurobiol Aging 24:553–561

Versijpt JJ, Dumont F, van Laere KJ, Decoo D, Santens P, Audenaert K, Achten E, Slegers G, Dierckx RA, Korf J (2003b) Assessment of neuroinflammation and microglial activation in Alzheimer's disease with radiolabelled PK11195 and single photon emission computed tomography. Eur Neurol 50:39–47

Vilner BJ, John CS, Bowen WD (1995) σ$_1$ and σ$_2$ receptors are expressed in a wide variety of human and rodent tumor cell lines. Cancer Res 55:408–413

Visser TJ, van Waarde A, Jansen TJH, Visser GM, van der Mark TW, Kraan J, Ensing K, Vaalburg W (1997a) Stereoselective synthesis and biodistribution of potent [^{11}C]-labeled antagonists for positron emission tomography imaging of muscarinic receptors in the airways. J Med Chem 40:117–124

Visser TJ, van Waarde A, van der Mark TW, Kraan J, Elsinga PH, Pruim J, Ensing K, Jansen T, Willemsen ATM, Franssen EJF, Visser GM, Paans AMJ, Vaalburg W (1997b) Characterization of pulmonary and myocardial β–adrenoceptors with S-1′-[fluorine-18]fluorocarazolol. J Nucl Med 38:169–174

Visser TJ, van Waarde A, Doze P, Elsinga PH, van der Mark TW, Kraan J, Ensing K, Vaalburg W (1998) Characterisation of β$_2$–adrenoceptors, using the agonist [^{11}C]formoterol and positron emission tomography. Eur J Pharmacol 361:35–41

Visser TJ, van Waarde A, van der Mark TW, Kraan J, Ensing K, Willemsen ATM, Elsinga PH, Vaalburg W (1999) Detection of muscarinic receptors in the human lung using PET. J Nucl Med 40:1270–1276

Wagner HN, Jr., Burns HD, Dannals RF, Wong DF, Langstrom B, Duelfer T, Frost JJ, Ravert HT, Links JM, Rosenbloom SB, Lukas SE, Kramer AV, Kuhar MJ (1983) Imaging dopamine receptors in the human brain by positron tomography. Science 221:1264–1266

Wagner S, Kopka K, Law MP, Riemann B, Pike VW, Schober O, Schafers M (2004) Synthesis and first in vivo evaluation of new selective high affinity β_1-adrenoceptor radioligands for SPECT based on ICI 89,406. Bioorg Med Chem 12:4117–4132

Wang S, Lee RJ, Mathias CJ, Green MA, Low PS (1996) Synthesis, purification, and tumor cell uptake of ^{67}Ga-deferoxamine-folate, a potential radiopharmaceutical for tumor imaging. Bioconjugate Chem 7:56–62

Wang S, Luo J, Lantrip DA, Waters DJ, Mathias CJ, Green MA, Fuchs PL, Low PS (1997) Design and synthesis of [^{111}In]DTPA-folate for use as a tumor-targeted radiopharmaceutical. Bioconjugate Chem 8:673–679

Waterhouse RN, Chapman J, Izard B, Donald A, Belbin K, O'Brien JC, Collier TL (1997) Examination of four ^{123}I-labeled piperidine-based sigma receptor ligands as potential melanoma imaging agents: initial studies in mouse tumor models. Nucl Med Biol 24:587–593

Waterhouse RN, Stabin MG, Page JG (2003) Preclinical acute toxicity studies and rodent-based dosimetry estimates of the novel σ_1 receptor radiotracer [^{18}F]FPS. Nucl Med Biol 30:555–563

Wedeking PW, Wager RE, Arunachalam T, Ramalingam K, Linder KE, Ranganathan RS, Nunn AD, Raju N, Tweedle MF (2002) Metal complexes derivatized with folate for use in diagnostic and therapeutic application. US Patent 6221334

Welch MJ, Redvanly CS (2003) Handbook of radiopharmaceuticals: radiochemistry and applications. Wiley, Chichester

Weng YH, Yen TC, Chen MC, Kao PF, Tzen KY, Chen RS, Wey SP, Ting G, Lu CS (2004) sensitivity and specificity of ^{99m}Tc-TRODAT-1 SPECT imaging in differentiating patients with idiopathic Parkinson's disease from healthy subjects. J Nucl Med 45:393–401

Westkaemper RB, Glennon RA (2002) Application of ligand SAR, receptor modeling and receptor mutagenesis to the discovery and development of a new class of 5-HT$_{2A}$ ligands. Curr Top Med Chem 2:575–598

Wheeler KT, Wang LM, Wallen CA, Childers SR, Cline JM, Keng PC, Mach RH (2000) Sigma-2 receptors as a biomarker of proliferation in solid tumors. Br J Cancer 82:1223–1232

Wichter T, Schafers M, Rhodes CG, Borggrefe M, Lerch H, Lammertsma AA, Hermansen F, Schober O, Breithardt G, Camici PG (2000) Abnormalities of cardiac sympathetic innervation in arrhythmogenic right ventricular cardiomyopathy: quantitative assessment of presynaptic norepinephrine reuptake and postsynaptic β-adrenergic receptor density with positron emission tomography. Circulation 101:1552–1558

Wilson AA, McCormick P, Kapur S, Willeit M, Garcia A, Hussey D, Houle S, Seeman P, Ginovart N (2005) Radiosynthesis and evaluation of [^{11}C]-(+)-4–propyl-3,4,4a,5,6,10b-hexahydro-2h-naphtho[1,2-b][1,4]oxazin-9-ol as a potential radiotracer for in vivo imaging of the dopamine D$_2$ high-affinity state with positron emission tomography. J Med Chem 48:4153–4160

Wong DF, Brasic JR (2001) In vivo imaging in neurotransmitter systems in neuropsychiatry. Clin Neurosc Res 1:35–45

Wong DF, Yung B, Dannals RF, Shaya EK, Ravert HT, Chen CA, Chan B, Folio T, Scheffel U, Ricaurte GA, Neumeyer JL, Wagner HN Jr, Michael JK (1993) In vivo imaging of baboon and human dopamine transporters by positron emission tomography using [^{11}C]WIN 35,428. Synapse 15:130–142

Wu WL, Burnett DA, Spring R, Greenlee WJ, Smith M, Favreau L, Fawzi A, Zhang H, Lachowicz JE (2005) Dopamine D$_1$/D$_5$ receptor antagonists with improved pharmacokinetics: design, synthesis, and biological evaluation of phenol bioisosteric analogues of benzazepine D$_1$/D$_5$ antagonists. J Med Chem 48:680–693

Yamada S, Ishima T, Tomita T, Hayashi M, Okada T, Hayashi E (1984) Alterations in cardiac α and β adrenoceptors during the development of spontaneous hypertension. J Pharmacol Exp Ther 228:454–460

Yamada S, Ohkura T, Uchida S, Inabe K, Iwatani Y, Kimura R, Hoshino T, Kaburagi T (1996) A sustained increase in β-adrenoceptors during long-term therapy with metoprolol and bisoprolol in patients with heart failure from idiopathic dilated cardiomyopathy. Life Sci 58:1737–1744

Yamaguchi I, Kopin IJ (1980) Differential inhibition of α_1 and α_2 adrenoceptor-mediated pressor responses in pithed rats. J Pharmacol Exp Ther 214:275–281

Yang ZY, Perry B, Mukherjee J (1996) Fluorinated benzazepines: 1. Synthesis, radiosynthesis and biological evaluation of a series of substituted benzazepines as potential radiotracers for positron emission tomographic studies of dopamine D-1 receptors. Nucl Med Biol 23:793–805

Yoo J, Dence CS, Sharp TL, Katzenellenbogen JA, Welch MJ (2005) Synthesis of an estrogen receptor-selective radioligand: 5-[^{18}F]fluoro-(2R*,3S*)-2,3-bis(4-hydroxyphenyl)pentanenitrile and comparison of in vivo distribution with 16-[^{18}F]fluoro-17-estradiol. J Med Chem 48:6366–6378

Yoshida Y, Kurokawa T, Sawamura Y, Shinagawa A, Okazawa H, Fujibayashi Y, Kotsuji F (2007) The positron emission tomography with F18 17β-estradiol has the potential to benefit diagnosis and treatment of endometrial cancer. Gynecol Oncol 104:764-766

Zanzonico PB, Finn R, Pentlow KS, Erdi Y, Beattie B, Akhurst T, Squire O, Morris M, Scher H, McCarthy T, Welch M, Larson SM, Humm JL (2004) PET-based radiation dosimetry in man of ^{18}F-fluorodihydrotestosterone, a new radiotracer for imaging prostate cancer. J Nucl Med 45:1966–1971

Zessin J, Deuther-Conrad W, Kretzschmar M, Wust F, Pawelke B, Brust P, Steinbach J, Bergmann R (2006) [^{11}C]SMe-ADAM, an imaging agent for the brain serotonin transporter: synthesis, pharmacological characterization and microPET studies in rats. Nucl Med Biol 33:53–63

Zhang MR, Kida T, Noguchi J, Furutsuka K, Maeda J, Suhara T, Suzuki K (2003a) [^{11}C]DAA1106: radiosynthesis and in vivo binding to peripheral benzodiazepine receptors in mouse brain. Nucl Med Biol 30:513–519

Zhang MR, Maeda J, Furutsuka K, Yoshida Y, Ogawa M, Suhara T, Suzuki K (2003b) [^{18}F]FMDAA1106 and [^{18}F]FEDAA1106: two positron-emitter labeled ligands for peripheral benzodiazepine receptor (PBR). Bioorg Med Chem Lett 13:201–204

Zhu Z, Guo N, Narendran R, Erritzoe D, Ekelund J, Hwang DR, Bae SA, Laruelle M, Huang Y (2004) The new PET imaging agent [11C]AFE is a selective serotonin transporter ligand with fast brain uptake kinetics. Nucl Med Biol 31:983–994

Zisterer DM, Williams DC (1997) Peripheral-type benzodiazepine receptors. Gen Pharmacol 29:305–314

Zubieta JK, Gorelick DA, Stauffer R, Ravert HT, Dannals RF, Frost JJ (1996) Increased mu opioid receptor binding detected by PET in cocaine-dependent men is associated with cocaine craving. Nat Med 2:1225–1229

Zubieta JK, Smith YR, Bueller JA, Xu Y, Kilbourn MR, Jewett DM, Meyer CR, Koeppe RA, Stohler CS (2001) Regional mu opioid receptor regulation of sensory and affective dimensions of pain. Science 293:311–315

Enzymes/Transporters

Regine Garcia Boy, Eva-Maria Knapp, Michael Eisenhut, Uwe Haberkorn, and Walter Mier(✉)

Abstract Tracers that specifically target tumours are highly warranted for diagnosis and to monitor cancer chemotherapy response. However, as cancer cells arise from normal cells they do not substantially differ from the normal cells and therefore tumour specific targets are rare. Fortunately, the process of malignant transformation is associated with the up- or down-regulation of enzymes and transporters that play a crucial role in tumour growth. Consequently diagnostic imaging procedures have attained their major success with tracers that target enzymes and transporters that are over-expressed in tumours. The glucose transporters, the multi drug resistance transporters (MDRPs), several kinases and the family of cathepsins are prominent examples for enzymes and receptors that can be targeted for molecular imaging.

Walter Mier

Universitätsklinikum Heidelberg, Abteilung für Nuklearmedizin, Im Neuenheimer Feld 400, 69120 Heidelberg

walter.mier@med.uni-heidelberg.de

W. Semmler and M. Schwaiger (eds.), *Molecular Imaging II.*
Handbook of Experimental Pharmacology 185/II.
© Springer-Verlag Berlin Heidelberg 2008

1 Introduction

Traditionally, diagnostic imaging was restricted to the visualisation of the final morphological changes of the diseased tissue/organ. Modern molecular imaging techniques allow the visualisation of early stages of diseases and therefore enable better therapy.

By visualising changes of crucial structures, predictions about the health status of a cell can be made long before macroscopically or microscopically visible changes in cell morphology occur. Imaging also plays an important role in pharmacotherapy, as the effects caused by the application of drugs can be closely monitored.

Detecting a small number of degenerated cells surrounded by healthy tissue is a major challenge, but the first step in identifying pathological changes. Ideally, the diagnostic methods should be able to detect the one mutated cell with specific changes and the ability to potentially, at a much later stage, develop into a malignant tumour.

In general, there is no expectation that tumour specificity exists. The biosynthesis of enzymes and transporters in the tumour cell is based on essentially the same DNA as in the normal cell. Nevertheless, the DNA expression in tumour cells often differs from that in a healthy cell; the expression of structures which play a crucial role in tumour growth can be either up-regulated or down-regulated. Examples for these processes are the up-regulation of enzymes in DNA synthesis, or the down-regulation of apoptosis induction, such as the expression of the p53 protein.

The challenge to develop specific tracers thus results not only in improving labelling techniques and their specificity but also in specifically delivering the labelled compound to the desired target.

Transporters and enzymes are major targets for the specific targeting of transformed tissue, be it a tumour or other pathologic condition. Both transporters and enzymes lead to a strong amplification of the tracer accumulation and are therefore potentially suited for imaging modalities that suffer from a low sensitivity, such as optical in-vivo imaging. Table 1 provides a summary of the most common transporters and enzymes for molecular imaging.

2 Enzymes

Enzymatic reactions are often visualised by applying a tagged substrate and monitoring the formation of a detectable product. To discriminate between unprocessed substrate and product, it is favourable that only one of them can be detected under the experimental conditions. The advantage when using enzymatic reactions as labelling tools is that the enzyme is regenerated after catalysing the fluorescence-forming reaction and, thus, a strong signal amplification takes place. Consequently, small differences in enzyme concentration will result in considerably more distinguishable differences in signal response. The different possibilities of exploiting enzymatic activity for molecular imaging are illustrated in Fig. 1a-c.

Table 1 Summary of enzymes and transporters and the different substrates used for their respective visualisation

Transporter	Substrate/visualisation with	Reference
Glucose	^{18}F-FDG	[1]
Amino acids	^{18}F-FET, ^{11}C-methionine	[2]
Organic anion transport (OATP)	Bile acids, radiolabelled or fluorescent	[3]
Nucleoside	FLT, fluorescent nucleoside analogues	[4]
Monocarboxylic Acid	^{14}C-acetate	[5]
Na$^+$/I$^-$ symporter	^{123}I-iodide (SPECT), ^{124}I-iodide (PET)	[6]
MDR transporters	Vinblastin, cytostatic drugs, verapamil, fluorescein-MTX	[7]
Sodium-neurotransmitter symporter (= sodium monoamine transporter)	Dopamine transporter: ^{99m}Tc-labeled tropane derivatives, ^{11}C-CFT, ^{11}C-nomifensine; Serotonine transporter: [^{11}C]RTI-357	[8]
Reduced folate/thiamine transporter	Fluorescein-MTX (flow cytometry)	[9]
Steroids/ bile acids	Radiolabelled bile acids	[10]

Enzyme	Substrate	Reference
Kinases	^{3}H-thymidine, ^{18}F-FLT	[11]
Caspases	DEVD-peptides (caspase 3)	[12]
Cathepsins	Quenched fluorophors via NIRF	[13]
MMPs	Qadiolabelled peptide inhibitors	[14]
β-Galactosidase/ hexokinase	^{18}F-FDG	[1]
Esterases	^{99m}Tc-Neurolite	[15]

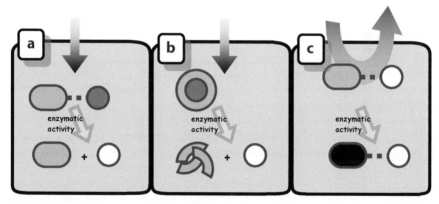

Fig. 1a-c General modes of action of enzyme activated tracers. **a** Probes for optical imaging; **b** MRT contrast agents; **c** radiotracers. In **a**, the enzymatic activity releases a fluorescent metabolite (*white circle*). In **b**, the enzymatic activity unwraps a paramagnetic ion (*white circle*). In contrast, the radioactive decay cannot be modulated by changing the chemical environment of the radioisotope (*white circle*); trapping is achieved by enzymatic conversion of a tracer penetrating the cell membrane in either direction into an non-penetrating form

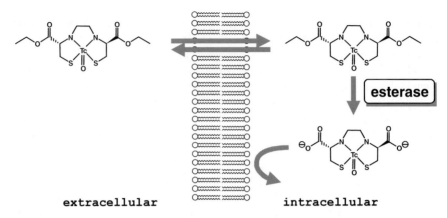

Fig. 2 Enzyme catalysed intracellular trapping of the brain perfusion agent Neurolite

An illustrative example for a tracer that is trapped as a consequence of enzyme activity is Neurolite [L,L-ethylcysteinate labelled with technetium-99 m (^{99m}Tc)]. This SECT tracer is used for the investigation of perturbations of cerebral perfusion that cause a functional impairment in the CNS (Walovitch et al. 1989; Saha et al. 1994). The lipophilic complex can readily penetrate the blood brain barrier and can therefore be used to monitor the perfusion and regional cerebral blood flow (CBF). Trapping is achieved by the esterase-catalysed intracellular cleavage of the ethyl ester bonds (Jacquier-Sarlin et al. 1996). This cleavage leads to the release of a carboxylate product, which is a polar metabolite that is unable to disappear from the site of accumulation (shown in Fig. 2).

2.1 Kinases

Proliferation is an important marker to describe the pathological status of a cell. Often, the first reaction to an external influence results in changes in cell proliferation; the cell goes through either a faster or slower cell cycle.

In order to proliferate faster, the cell needs a supply of nitrogen and carbon building blocks (= nucleosides) and energy. This is why tumour cells in many cases show an up-regulation of both ribonucleotide-synthesizing enzymes and glucose transporters, as well as proteolytic enzymes to recycle other proteins.

The "gold standard" for studying tumour cell proliferation is radiolabelled ^{3}H-thymidine, which has been used for more than 40 years. Many efforts have been made to further develop thymidine-derived tracers containing either gamma or positron-emitting radionuclides, which can be used for SPECT or PET scans. One of the most valuable developments in the latter field is the ^{18}F-fluorothymidine (FLT).

Unlabelled FLT had been known for more than a decade for its antiviral properties, which made it a promising compound for HIV treatment (Matthes et al. 1988). By labelling this substance with the positron emitting ^{18}F, another application emerged: FLT can now be used as a reliable and easily detectable proliferation marker in a way comparable with both that of ^{3}H-thymidine and 2-[^{18}F]fluoro-2-deoxy-β-D-glucose (FDG).

Although labelled FLT is yet to be thoroughly investigated and compared with other PET active tracers, several advantages over ^{3}H-thymidine and FDG cannot be disregarded. Opposite to ^{3}H-thymidine, its detection does not solely depend on cell proliferation or incorporation into DNA and thus thymidine kinase activity. Also, cell-cycle-arrested cells and thymidine-kinase-deficient mutants are able to take up FLT.

Another advantage of FLT is the fact that it can be used as a diagnostic marker in tissues with a high glucose uptake background, such as brain tissue, where the use of FDG is limited by the distinguishability between glucose transporter overexpressing cells and healthy cells (Rasey et al. 2002; Haberkorn et al. 1997, 2001).

2.2 β-Galactosidase

β-Galactosidase, or the gene encoding it, *lacZ*, is frequently used as a tool to identify a successful plasmid transfection. Thus, the imaging of β-galactosidase is a helpful tool in molecular biology and genetics. When living organisms undergo optical imaging, the fact that they are rarely transparent to the light used for visualisation often represents a limiting factor during detection. Thus, alternative detection methods, such as magnetic resonance imaging (MRI) are a helpful tool. In order to visualise galactosidase imaging, a galactose-coupled gadolinium chelator has been synthesised by Louie et al. (2000). This chelator occupies seven of the nine Gd coordination sites, the two remaining are taken by a galactose residue. Galactosidase cleaves the sugar moiety causing the complex to irreversibly shift into its active (= detectable) state, as shown in Fig. 3.

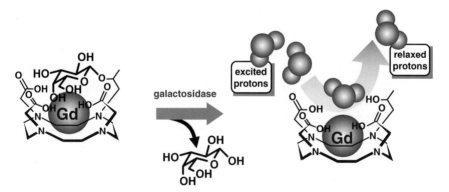

Fig. 3 Mode of action of a galactose-coupled Gd-chelator used to visualise galactosidase activity. After cleavage of the galactose moiety, the chelator does no longer occupy all of the Gd complex valencies. The valencies become accessible to water that is relaxed and can be detected by MRI

2.3 Proteases/ Proteolytic enzymes

The recycling of building blocks, such as amino acids, plays an important role during the cell cycle. Proteases digest proteins into peptides and single amino acids, so they can be reused. Due to their increased metabolic rate, tumour tissues often show increased protease levels.

In the following paragraphs, two kinds of proteases, the cathepsin family and the matrix metalloproteinases (MMPs), as well as the possibilities to visualise them will be discussed.

2.4 Cathepsins

Cathepsins are lysosomal cysteine proteases which have been associated with tumour progression as well as metastasis formation. Cathepsin imaging can be done with the help of near-infrared fluorescence (NIRF), using a probe consisting of alternating fluorophors and quenchers as illustrated in Fig. 4. The light released by the fluorophors is immediately absorbed by adjacent groups. After cleavage the emitted light can be detected using the appropriate instrumentation (Redwood et al. 1992; Navab et al. 1997; Coulibaly et al. 1999; Bremer et al. 2001).

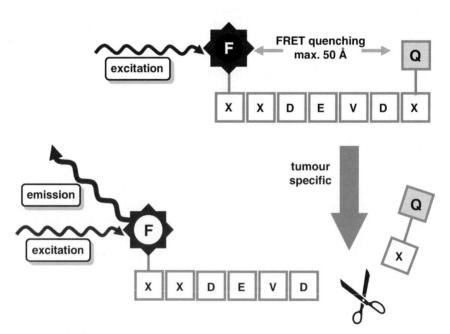

Fig. 4 Tracer molecule consisting of a fluorophor (F) and a quencher (Q) in close proximity. After cleavage by a tumour-specific protease, the fluorescent substrate is separated from the quencher and, after excitation, emits detectable light

2.5 Cystein Aspartate-specific Proteases (Caspases)

The caspase enzyme family consists of at least 14 known members (Hu et al. 1998). While all play a significant role in the induction of apoptosis, some also have been shown to take part in pro-inflammatory processes (Miura et al. 1993). As caspase activation is irreversible and one of the earliest markers in the apoptotic process, it represents a valuable diagnostic target. By linking rhodamine to a caspase-specific substrate, e.g. a peptide with the recognition sequence DEVD, a non-fluorescent compound is generated, which can enter living cells. After cleavage, the intracellular fluorescent rhodamine can be detected after laser excitation (Hug et al. 1999).

2.6 MMPs

As their name suggests, MMPs are expressed on the cell surface. The MMP family consists of multiple members (MMP1-25) with diverse structures and functions. Their main function is to digest protein-associated constructs connecting the matrices of adjacent cells. Thus, MMPs play a crucial role in cell-cell interaction, the basis of membrane degradation and cell migration, as well as tumour metastasis formation, apoptosis and angiogenesis.

Great efforts have been made to develop specific imaging strategies for MMP-2 and MMP-9, found in tissues of aggressively metastasising tumours. To a small peptide inhibitor containing ten amino acids, a D-Tyr was added which could then be radiolabelled using the Iodogene method and functioned both as a potent inhibitor and as an imaging tool (Kuhnast et al. 2004). Other MMP-inhibiting peptides containing ^{64}Cu-DOTA, or functional groups labelled with ^{11}C or ^{18}F have also been described (Li et al. 2002; Furumoto et al. 2003).

3 Transporters

The intracellular and extracellular concentrations of nutrients and electrolytes play a critical role in cell physiology. Not only does the osmotic pressure highly depend on the compounds present but also the cell's ability to proliferate is directly related to a sufficient supply of building blocks.

Molecules can enter the cell using three different paths: passive diffusion, facilitated diffusion through channels and active transport.

Lipophilic substances can enter the cell by passive diffusion through the phospholipids bilayer along a concentration gradient, while more hydrophilic, especially charged, molecules likewise use facilitated diffusion via ion channels.

Compounds that the cell requires in high concentration have to be transported against their concentration gradient. This transport is provided by very selective ATP consuming ion pumps. Frequently, these pumps function like revolving doors

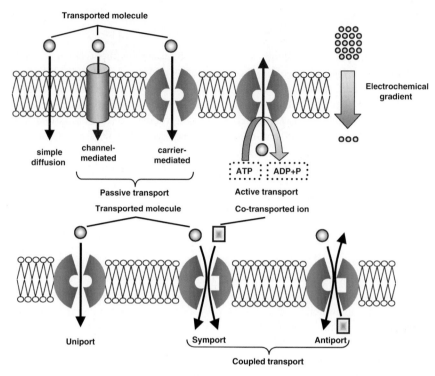

Fig. 5 Different carrier-mediated routes of the transportation for ions and molecules through the lipid bilayer membrane. The *lower figure* shows the three types of facilitated transport through a membrane, all of which require an electrochemical gradient

transporting more than one compound at once, either from the same side or from different sides of the cell membrane. Examples are the myocardial Na^+/K^+-ATPase (exchange of sodium and potassium, both against a concentration gradient) and the ubiquitously expressed sodium glucose co-transporters (transport of sodium along and of glucose against a concentration gradient).

The different transport mechanisms can be seen in Fig. 5.

3.1 FDG

The above-mentioned glucose transporters have been found to be frequently over-expressed in rapidly proliferating tissue, e.g. tumour tissue (Yamamoto et al. 1990). Based on the increased proliferation rate and thus increased metabolic rate, the degenerated cell compensates the increased glycolytic metabolism and thus the resulting energy shortage by over-expressing glucose transporters in the cell membrane. An increased number of glucose transporters in the cell membrane can be detected with the help of the PET-active compound FDG (Som et al. 1980).

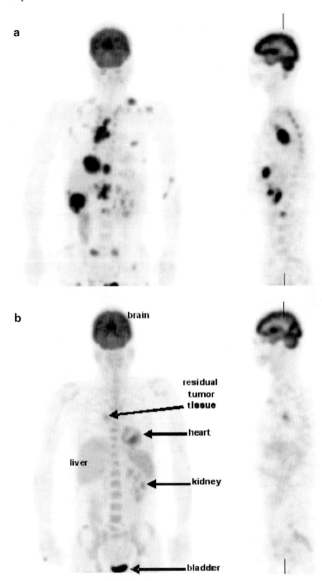

Fig. 6 Projection and sagittal view of an ^{18}F-FDG PET scan of a SCLC patient prior **a** and after **b** chemotherapy. Whereas the scan after chemotherapy shows almost the normal distribution of ^{18}F-FDG, multiple metastases are detected in **a**

Without a doubt, FDG is the most useful and the most frequently used PET radiopharmaceutical. *See* Fig. 6, for example.

Once it has entered the cell, FDG is subject to the energy-producing glucose metabolism. FDG is phosphorylated by the enzyme hexokinase, but in the consecutive step, the fluoro-substituent prevents the phosphorylated intermediate from being

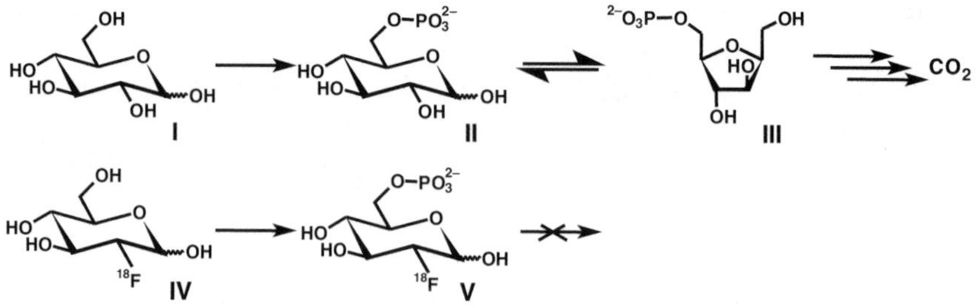

Fig. 7 Summary of glucose metabolism (I-III) and metabolism of FDG (IV-V) inside a cell. Glucose (I) enters a cell via glucose transporters and is quickly phosphorylated by hexokinase, yielding glucose-6-phosphate (II). Glucose-6-phosphate is processed by glucose isomerase, which consecutively enters further metabolism, yielding CO_2 in the end. In contrast, metabolism of FDG (IV) ends after phosphorylation (V), as phosphorylated FDG is not a substrate for glucose isomerase

recognised and further processed by the enzyme phosphohexose isomerase. Furthermore, the addition of a negatively charged phosphate residue keeps FDG-P from leaving the cell again. The molecule is thus metabolically trapped inside the cell and can easily be detected using PET scans (Fig. 7) (Suolinna et al. 1986).

The intracellular FDG concentration can directly be correlated with the expression of glucose transporters on the cell membrane.

3.2 Multidrug-resistance Proteins (MDRs)

Not every compound that enters a cell also reaches its final target. To protect the cell from xenobiotics, so-called multidrug-resistance transmembrane P-glycoproteins, or MDR proteins, non-specifically transport compounds to the extracellular space so they can be excreted. When exposed to a substance over a longer period of time, e.g. cytostatics in the case of tumour cells, susceptible cells can develop a resistance. An over-expression of MDR proteins is often the cause of tumours becoming refractory after some cycles of chemotherapy. There are two ways to overcome the resistance: increase the dosage – this will result in a temporary sensitivity, which may decrease with the course of time – or switch to another compound or a combination of several substances.

Radiolabelled MDR modulators, like verapamil, or cytostatic agents, like daunorubicin and colchicin, can be used to monitor the function of the drug efflux pump in vivo (Hendrikse et al. 1999).

3.3 Na$^+$/I$^-$ Symporter

Iodide ions are important for the biosynthesis of thyroid hormones. They are shuttled into the cell by active transport through the sodium iodide symporter (NIS). Iodide is then oxidized by the iodoperoxidase and incorporated into the thyroid hormone precursors. As iodide is the key for this biosynthesis, the iodine concentration in the thyroid gland is a manifold of that in other parts of the body.

Most thyroid cancers keep their ability to take up iodide via the NIS. Radiolabelled iodine, ^{131}I, ^{125}I, ^{124}I and ^{123}I, can thus be used both as a diagnostic tool after surgical removal of the thyroid gland as well as a therapeutic to specifically target the thyroid gland (Sherman 2002).

3.4 Amino Acid Transporters

Similar to glucose, amino acids represent important building blocks the cell requires to proliferate. They are not only essential constituents of proteins, but also important precursors in the biosynthesis of neurotransmitters and hormones (Del Sol et al. 2001). The increased metabolism and proliferation rate of tumour cells correlates with an increased need for amino acids, and often an increased expression of amino acid transporters. Imaging of these transporters can give valuable hints concerning the degree of malignant transformation of a tissue.

Amino acids can enter the cell using different transport systems, the most frequently expressed being the so-called L transport system and the A transport system. In the L transport system, larger amino acids are carried through the membranes in a 1:1 antiport system: For every amino acid entering the cell, one amino acid is transported out. This means, that in order to increase the amount of amino acids inside a cell, another transport system must exist, the so-called A transport system. In this sodium-dependent system, a symport of sodium ions and amino acid molecules takes place. Other amino acid carriers are the CATs (cationic amino acid transporters) (MacLeod et al. 1994) for the transport of cationic and dipolar amino acids, as well as the proton dependent amino acid and peptide transporters (PEPT and PAT, respectively).

To visualise amino acid transporters, radiolabelled amino acids are used most frequently, such as [^{11}C-methyl]-L-methionine (MET), 3-[^{123}I]iodo-α-methyl-L-tyrosine (IMT), and O-(2-[^{18}F]fluoroethyl)-L-tyrosine (FET) (Wester et al. 1999; Jager et al. 2001). Unlike the glucose-based tracer FDG, labelled amino acids show a low uptake into inflammatory tissue and are thus valuable tracers in cancer diagnostics (Kaim et al. 2002). In addition, these molecules show a high stability, low metabolism, and both the parent compounds and their metabolites are rapidly excreted by the kidneys (Pauleit et al. 2003).

References

Bremer C, Tung CH, Weissleder R (2001) In vivo molecular target assessment of matrix metalloproteinase inhibition. Nat Med 7(6):743–748

Coulibaly S et al (1999) Modulation of invasive properties of murine squamous carcinoma cells by heterologous expression of cathepsin B and cystatin C. Int J Cancer 83(4):526–531

Del Sole A et al (2001) Anatomical and biochemical investigation of primary brain tumours. Eur J Nucl Med 28(12):1851–1872

Dienel GA et al (2001) Preferential labeling of glial and meningial brain tumors with [2-(14)C] acetate. J Nucl Med 42(8):1243–1250

Furumoto S et al (2003) Tumor detection using 18F-labeled matrix metalloproteinase-2 inhibitor. Nucl Med Biol 30(2):119–125

Gutmann H et al (2000) P-glycoprotein- and mrp2-mediated octreotide transport in renal proximal tubule. Br J Pharmacol 129(2):251–256

Haberkorn U (1997) PET 2-fluoro-2-deoxyglucose uptake in rat prostate adenocarcinoma during chemotherapy with gemcitabine. J Nucl Med 38(8):1215–1221

Haberkorn U (2001) Apoptosis and changes in glucose transport early after treatment of Morris hepatoma with gemcitabine Eur J Nucl Med 28(4):418–425

Hartmann H (1988) Enhanced in vitro inhibition of HIV-1 replication by 3′-fluoro-3′-deoxythymidine compared to several other nucleoside analogs. AIDS Res Hum Retroviruses 4(6):457–466

Hendrikse NH (1999) Visualization of multidrug resistance in vivo. Eur J Nucl Med 26(3):283–293

Hu S (1998) Caspase-14 is a novel developmentally regulated protease. J Biol Chem 273(45):29648–29653

Hug H (1999) Rhodamine 110-linked amino acids and peptides as substrates to measure caspase activity upon apoptosis induction in intact cells. Biochemistry 38(42):13906–13911

Mills CO (1997) Cholyllysyl fluroscein and related lysyl fluorescein conjugated bile acid analogues Yale J Biol Med 70(4):447–457

Jacquier-Sarlin MR, Polla BS, Slosman DO (1996) Cellular basis of ECD brain retention. J Nucl Med 37(10):1694–1697

Kuhnast B (2004) Targeting of gelatinase activity with a radiolabeled cyclic HWGF peptide. Nucl Med Biol 31(3):337–444

Jager PL (2001) Radiolabeled amino acids: basic aspects and clinical applications in oncology. J Nucl Med 42(3):432–445

Kaim AH (2002) (18)F-FDG and (18)F-FET uptake in experimental soft tissue infection. Eur J Nucl Med Mol Imaging 29(5):648–654

Li WP (2002) DOTA-D-Tyr(1)-octreotate: a somatostatin analogue for labeling with metal and halogen radionuclides for cancer imaging and therapy. Bioconjug Chem 13(4):721–728

Louie AY (2000) In vivo visualization of gene expression using magnetic resonance imaging. Nat Biotechnol 18(3):321–325

MacLeod CL, Finley KD, Kakuda DK (1994) y(+)-type cationic amino acid transport: expression and regulation of the mCAT genes. J Exp Biol 196:109–121

Matthes E, Lehmann C, Scholz D, Rosenthal HA, Langen P (1988) Phosphorylation, anti-HIV activity and cytotoxicity of 3'-fluorothymidine. Biochem Biophys Res Commun. Jun 16; 153(2):825–31. PMID: 3164184 [PubMed - indexed for MEDLINE]

Miura M (1993) Induction of apoptosis in fibroblasts by IL-1 beta-converting enzyme, a mammalian homolog of the C elegans cell death gene ced-3. Cell 75(4):653–660

Navab R, Mort JS, Brodt P (1997) Inhibition of carcinoma cell invasion and liver metastases formation by the cysteine proteinase inhibitor E-64. Clin Exp Metastasis 15(2):121–129

Pauleit D (2003) Whole-body distribution and dosimetry of O-(2-[18F]fluoroethyl)-L-tyrosine. Eur J Nucl Med Mol Imaging 30(4):519–524

Rasey JS (2002) Validation of FLT uptake as a measure of thymidine kinase-1 activity in A549 carcinoma cells. J Nucl Med 43(9):1210–1217

Redwood SM (1992) Abrogation of the invasion of human bladder tumor cells by using protease inhibitor(s). Cancer 69(5):1212–1219

Saha GB, MacIntyre WJ, Go RT (1994) Radiopharmaceuticals for brain imaging.Semin Nucl Med 24(4):324–493

Schuhmann-Giampieri G (1993) Nonlinear pharmacokinetic modeling of a gadolinium chelate used as a liver-specific contrast agent for magnetic resonance imaging. Arzneimittelforschung 43(9):1020–1024

Sherman SI (2002) Optimizing the outcomes of adjuvant radioiodine therapy in differentiated thyroid carcinoma. J Clin Endocrinol Metab 87(9):4059–4062

Shields AF (1998) Imaging proliferation in vivo with [F-18]FLT and positron emission tomography. Nat Med 4(11):1334–1336

Som P (1980) A fluorinated glucose analog, 2-fluoro-2-deoxy-D-glucose (F-18): nontoxic tracer for rapid tumor detection. J Nucl Med 21(7):670–675

Suolinna EM (1986) Metabolism of 2-[18F]fluoro-2-deoxyglucose in tumor-bearing rats: chromatographic and enzymatic studies. Int J Rad Appl Instrum B 13(5):577–581

Tung CH (1999) Preparation of a cathepsin D sensitive near-infrared fluorescence probe for imaging. Bioconjug Chem 10(5):892–896

Volkow ND et al (1996) PET evaluation of the dopamine system of the human brain. J Nucl Med 37(7):1242–1256

Walovitch RC (1989) Characterization of technetium-99m-L, L-ECD for brain perfusion imaging, Part 1: Pharmacology of technetium-99 m ECD in nonhuman primates. J Nucl Med 30(11):1892–1901

Wester HJ (1999) Synthesis and radiopharmacology of O-(2-[18F]fluoroethyl)-L-tyrosine for tumor imaging. J Nucl Med 40(1):205–212

Pope LE et al (1989) Visualization of membrane-associated folate transport proteins. Adv Enzyme Regul 28:3–11

Yamamoto T et al (1990) Over-expression of facilitative glucose transporter genes in human cancer. Biochem Biophys Res Commun 170(1):223–230

Phage Peptide Display

Jessica Newton and Susan L. Deutscher(✉)

Abstract Molecular imaging is at the forefront in the advancement of in-vivo diagnosis and monitoring of cancer. New peptide-based molecular probes to facilitate cancer detection are rapidly evolving. Peptide-based molecular probes that target apoptosis, angiogenesis, cell signaling and cell adhesion events are in place. Bacteriophage (phage) display technology, a molecular genetic approach to ligand discovery, is commonly employed to identify peptides as tumor-targeting molecules. The peptide itself may perhaps have functional properties that diminish tumor growth or metastasis. More often, a selected peptide is chemically synthesized, coupled to a radiotracer or fluorescent probe, and utilized in the development of new noninvasive molecular imaging probes. A myriad of peptides that bind cancer cells and cancer-associated antigens have been reported from phage library selections. Phage selections have also been performed in live animals to obtain peptides with optimal stability and targeting properties in vivo. To this point, few in-vitro, in-situ, or in-vivo selected peptides have shown success in the molecular imaging of cancer, the notable exception being vascular targeting peptides identified via in-vivo selections. The success of vasculature targeting peptides, such as those with an RGD motif that bind $\alpha_v\beta_3$ integrin, may be due to the abundance and expression patterns of

Susan L. Deutscher
Department of Biochemistry, M743 Medical Sciences Bldg., University of Missouri, Columbia, MO 65212
deutschers@missouri.edu

W. Semmler and M. Schwaiger (eds.), *Molecular Imaging II.*
Handbook of Experimental Pharmacology 185/II.
© Springer-Verlag Berlin Heidelberg 2008

integrins in tumors and supporting vasculature. The discovery of molecular probes that bind tumor-specific antigens has lagged considerably. One promising means to expedite discovery is through the implementation of selected phage themselves as tumor-imaging agents in animals.

1 Cancer Biomarkers and Phage Display

New approaches are emerging to better diagnose and treat cancer. Molecular imaging, combining novel molecular probes and imaging technologies, has facilitated the in-vivo visualization of processes involved in tumorigenesis and has obvious clinical applications. However, for this approach to work, biomarkers or antigens specifically expressed on tumor cells or necessary for the sustaining of tumor cell growth must be exploited. Identification of new tumor-associated targets has been facilitated by the conclusion of the human genome project and a better understanding of the process of tumorigenesis and metastasis (Kim and Wang 2003; Waltz 2006).

Combinatorial chemistry and phage display provides an opportunity to identify new tumor targeting agents. The development of cancer imaging or therapeutic compounds has customarily relied on isolation of products from natural extracts, or from screening compound databases or structure-based rational drug design. These approaches are laborious and do not take advantage of modern robotics and molecular biology advances. Recent efforts have focused on the use of combinatorial technologies for the preparation and screening of chemically synthetic or genetically encoded libraries as sources for new cancer targeting agents. Chemical synthetic combinatorial libraries consisting of millions of peptides, employed since the late 1980s, have been extensively described (Houghten et al. 1991; Marik and

Fig. 1 Affinity selection of a phage display library. A phage display library is selected against a desired target (purified antigen, cell line, live organism) to find the fittest subpopulation, which is then amplified and reselected again. This process is termed affinity selection and is repeated four to five times, resulting in an enriched population theoretically containing phage clones with high affinity for the presented target. There are numerous forms of affinity selection. Smith and Petrenko described in detail affinity selection and enrichment. In-vitro affinity selection can be used to select phage clones that bind to a purified target (protein, nucleic acid, carbohydrate, etc) (Kumada et al. 2005) or a cultured cell (Giordano et al. 2001). In-situ and ex-vivo affinity selection has been used to select for phage clones that bind to specific tissues (Shukla and Krag 2005; Maruta et al. 2003), while in-vivo affinity selection allows for the selection of phage clones with specific pharmacokinetic properties (Pasqualini and Ruoslahti 1996; Newton et al. 2006). High throughput screening through the use of robotics enables rapid handling of large and complex phage library populations, thus allowing for unprecedented monitoring and screening of the affinity selection process (Walter et al. 2001; Crameri and Kodzius 2001). Analysis of the resulting affinity selected phage clones is necessary and can be accomplished through the study of synthetic peptide (Samoylov et al. 2002; Fleming et al. 2005; Voss et al. 2002); Nowak et al. 2006) or phage particle (Jaye et al. 2004; Landon et al. 2004a; Kelly et al. 2006a; Chen et al. 2004; Newton et al. 2006)

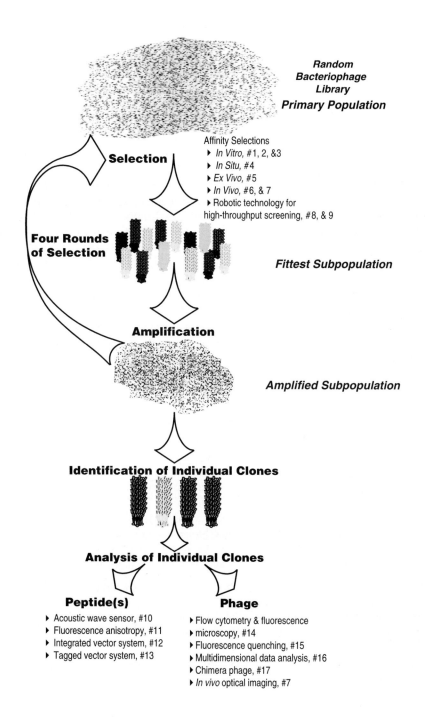

Random
Bacteriophage
Library
Primary Population

Selection

Affinity Selections
- ▸ *In Vitro,* #1, 2, &3
- ▸ *In Situ,* #4
- ▸ *Ex Vivo,* #5
- ▸ *In Vivo,* #6, & 7
- ▸ Robotic technology for
high-throughput screening, #8, & 9

**Four Rounds
of Selection**

Fittest Subpopulation

Amplification

Amplified Subpopulation

Identification of Individual Clones

Analysis of Individual Clones

Peptide(s)
- ▸ Acoustic wave sensor, #10
- ▸ Fluorescence anisotropy, #11
- ▸ Integrated vector system, #12
- ▸ Tagged vector system, #13

Phage
- ▸ Flow cytometry & fluorescence
- ▸ microscopy, #14
- ▸ Fluorescence quenching, #15
- ▸ Multidimensional data analysis, #16
- ▸ Chimera phage, #17
- ▸ *In vivo* optical imaging, #7

Lam 2005). In 1985, George P. Smith demonstrated that a foreign peptide sequence could be fused to coat protein III or VIII of filamentous phage (a bacterial virus) and displayed on the surface of the phage (Smith 1985). The expression of foreign sequences on phage is not restricted to small peptides, as antibody fragments, receptors and enzymes have also been displayed (Atwell and Wells 1999; Barbas et al. 1991). For the development of cancer diagnostics, including imaging, there are incentives to use genetically encoded combinatorial libraries. The genetic encoding of a library allows the resynthesis and rescreening of molecules with a desired binding activity. The resulting amplification of interacting molecules in subsequent rounds of "affinity selection" can yield very rare, specific binders from an enormous collection of molecules.

Typically, phage libraries are generated to encode small foreign peptides, which can range in size from 6 to 45 amino acids, while retaining large diversity. Peptide libraries may be displayed as linear or cysteine-constrained sequences. To accomplish a survey or affinity selection, the library is passed over the desired target; binding clones are captured, while nonbinding clones are washed away (Fig. 1). The captured phage retain infectivity and can therefore be propagated and cloned by infecting fresh bacterial host cells. Traditionally, the process of affinity selection is an iterative process of several rounds of selection, elution, and amplification of phage (Fig. 1). However, affinity selections can be tedious and time-consuming, often requiring weeks to months to obtain sequence data on displayed peptides that are candidate "winners". Recently, new developments in high throughput methods have allowed for the screening and characterization of large numbers of phage clones simultaneously. Most procedures are performed in multiwell plates and involve fluorometric and/or spectrophotometric data measurements (Crameri and Kodzius 2001; Jaye et al. 2003; Kelly et al. 2006a; Landon et al. 2004a; Rahim et al. 2003; Walter et al. 2001). This format is easily automatable and the addition of robotic technology enables the rapid handling of large and complex phage library populations, thus allowing for unprecedented monitoring and screening of the affinity selection process (Crameri and Kodzius 2001; Walter et al. 2001). Other advancements include faster more stringent selection and washing conditions (Giordano et al. 2001; Kumada et al. 2005), improved DNA sequencing (Jaye et al. 2003; Rahim et al. 2003) for quick identification of selected clones, the use of labeled or modified phage (Chen et al. 2004; Jaye et al. 2004; Newton et al. 2006), and implementation of multidimensional data analysis (Kelly et al. 2006a). The ability to analyze the selected phage themselves both during early and final rounds of selection has an advantage over the screening of synthetic peptides. Phage particles can have 300–600 covalently attached fluorochrome molecules per phage particle (Jaye et al. 2004; Newton et al. 2006), resulting in signal amplification. Also, synthetic versions of a selected peptide do not always possess identical binding characteristics as its phage displayed counterpart. Thus, direct detection of labeled phage conjugates provides a greater level of convenience and the potential to detect phage with low target avidity or low target density.

2 Tumor-targeting Peptides from Phage Display

Monoclonal antibodies (MAbs), and recombinant antibody fragments selected from phage display libraries have had the most success in cancer imaging and therapeutic applications (Goldenberg 2002; Meredith et al. 1994; Popkov et al. 2004). The power of combinatorial chemistry and phage display is exemplified by studies with anti-ErbB-2 antibodies. The efficacy of the originally FDA- approved MAb HerceptinTM (anti-Her2/neu), has been greatly improved through phage display and molecular engineering approaches to create antibody fragments with better tumor targeting, faster clearance, and reduced side-effects (Goldenberg 1999; Orlova et al. 2006). Peptides comprise only a small percentage of cancer imaging or therapeutic agents but may offer advantages over antibodies for in-vivo applications because of rapid blood clearance, increased diffusion, nonimmunogenicity, and straightforward synthesis (Behr et al. 2001; Heppeler et al. 2000). As far as cancer, regulatory peptides that bind receptors overexpressed on tumors have been robustly pursued in imaging and therapy studies. However, only a handful of peptides that target a few receptors have shown success, including somatostatin (Bakker et al. 1991), bombesin/gastrin-releasing peptide (GRP) (Van de Wiele et al. 2001), vasoactive intestinal peptide (VIP) (Virgolini 1997), and α-melanocyte-stimulating hormone (α-MSH) derivatives (Chen et al. 2000).

2.1 Targeting Peptides to Known Antigens or Biomarkers

Phage display has contributed peptides that target numerous receptors, enzymes, ligands, and carbohydrates that are involved in tumor development, growth, and metastasis (Table 1). Some of these peptides have clear prospective anti-cancer applications. For example, numerous laboratories have isolated peptides from phage display libraries that bind the ErbB-2 receptor (Houimel et al. 2001; Karasseva et al. 2002; Stortelers et al. 2002; Urbanelli et al. 2001). One such peptide, KCCYSL bound to ErbB-2 with a Kd of 1 μM, but the four-copy multiple antigen peptide (MAP) constructs displayed a 100-fold increased affinity for ErbB-2 receptor-expressing cell lines (Karasseva et al. 2002). Peptides that bind angiogenesis factors have been reported. Many peptides which block the growth factor-receptor interactions have been isolated, including ephrin-A-2 (Koolpe et al. 2002), fibroblast growth factor (FGF) (Fan et al. 2002; Maruta et al. 2002), insulin-like growth factor (IGF) (Skelton et al. 2001), transforming growth factor-β (TGFβ) (Michon et al. 2002), and vascular endothelial growth factor (VEGF) (Binetruy-Tournaire et al. 2000; Hetian et al. 2002). The efficacy of phage display-derived peptides to inhibit urokinase plasminogen activator (uPA) receptor-mediated, metastasis-related tissue remodeling was demonstrated when peptides, which were selected for binding uPA receptor (Goodson et al. 1994; Ke et al. 1997; Yang and Craik 1998), were able to block tumor cell extravasation (Ploug et al. 2001). Phage display selections have been utilized to target proteases and determine substrate specificity of numerous

Table 1 Tumor-targeting and tumorigenesis-inhibiting peptides derived by using phage display

Target	Sequence	Reference
Protein/Receptor Target		
ErbB-2	MARSGL, MARAKE, MSRTMS; KCCYSL; WRR, WKR, WVR, WVK, WIK, WTR, WVL, WLL, WRT, WRG, WVS, WVA; MYWGDSHWLQYWYE	(Houimel et al. 2001; Karasseva et al. 2002; Kumar and Deutscher; Stortelers et al. 2002; Urbanelli et al. 2001)
Ephrin receptor (EphA2 and EphB)	MQLPLAT, EWLS, SNEW, TNYL	(Koolpe et al. 2005; Koolpe et al. 2002)
Glucose-regulated protein 78	WIFPWIQL, WDLAWMFRLPVG; CTVALPGGYVRVC	(Arap et al. 2004; Kim et al. 2006)
HSP90	CVPELGHEC	(Vidal et al. 2004)
Interleukin-11 Receptor α	CGRRAGGSC	(Zurita et al. 2004)
PSA	CVAYCIEHHCWTC, CVFAHNYDYLVC, CVFTSNYAFC	(Pakkala et al. 2004)
Angiogenesis		
VCAM-1	VHSPNKK	(Kelly et al. 2006b)
Endothelium/$\alpha v\beta_3$/$\alpha 5\beta_1$ integrin	CDCRGDCFC, CRGDGWC, XRGDX[a]	(Arap et al. 1998; Cai et al. 2006; Chen et al. 2005b; Cheng et al. 2005; Haubner and Wester 2004; Kwon et al. 2005; Su et al. 2002; Wang et al. 2004; Ye et al. 2006)
MMP-2/MMP-9	PXX↓(Ser/Thr); CTTHWGFTLC; SGKGPRQITAL	(Chen et al. 2005a; Kridel et al. 2001; Kuhnast et al. 2004)
MMP-11	A(A/Q)(N/A)↓(L/Y)(T/V/M/R)(R/K)	(Pan et al. 2003)
FGF receptor	VYMSPF; MQLPLAT	(Fan et al. 2002; Maruta et al. 2002)
VEGF receptor	ATWLPPR; HTMYYHHYQHHL	(Binetruy-Tournaire et al. 2000; Hetian et al. 2002)
IGF-1	SEVGCRAGPLQWLCEKYFG	(Skelton et al. 2001)
TGF-β receptor	CGLLPVGRPDRNVWRWLC, CKGQCDRFKGLPEWC	(Michon et al. 2002)
uPA	SGRSA; WGFP; LWXXAr(Ar=Y,W,F,H), XFXXYLW	(Goodson et al. 1994; Ke et al. 1997; Ploug et al. 2001; Yang and Craik 1998)
uPAR	AEPMPHSLNFSQYLWYT	(Fong et al. 2002)
Carbohydrate/Lectins		
TFA	WAY(W/F)SP	(Peletskaya et al. 1996; Peletskaya et al. 1997)
E-selectin	IELLQAR; DITWDQLWDLMK	(Fukuda et al. 2000; Funovics et al. 2005; Martens et al. 1995)
Galectin-3	AYTKCSRQWRTCMTTH, PQNSKIPGPTFLDPH, SMEPALPDWWWKMFK, ANTPCGPYTHDCPVKR	(Kumar and Deutscher; Zou et al. 2005)

(continued)

Table 1 (continued)

Cultured Cell Surface Targets		
Hepatocarcinoma	TACHQHVRMVRP	(Du et al. 2006)
Neuroblastoma, Breast	VPWMEPAYQRFL	(Askoxylakis et al. 2006; Askoxylakis et al. 2005)
Prostate Carcinoma	DPRATPGS; FRPNRAQDYNTN	(Romanov et al. 2001; Zitzmann et al. 2005)
HUVEC/Gastric Cancer	CTKNSYLMC	(Liang et al. 2006)
Cervical Carcinoma	C(R/Q)L/RT(G/N)XXG(A/V)GC	(Robinson et al. 2005)
Colorectal HT29	CPIEDRPMC; HEWSYLAPYPWF	(Kelly et al. 2004; Kelly and Jones 2003; Rasmussen et al. 2002)
Glioma	MCPKHPLGC	(Spear et al. 2001)
B Cell Lymphoma	RMWPSSTVNLSAGRR; SAKTAVSQRVWLPSHRGGEP, KSREHVNNSACPSKRITAAL	(Ding et al. 2006; McGuire et al. 2006)
NCI-60 Binding Peptides	EGFR: RVS, AGS, AGL, GVR, GGR, GGL, GSV, GVS	(Kolonin et al. 2006)
In vivo Selected		
Prostate Carcinoma	GTRQGHTMRLGVSDG, IAGLATPGWSHWLAL	(Newton et al. 2006)
Tramp Prostate	SMSIARL	(Arap et al. 2002a)
Thyroid Carcinoma	HTFEPGV	(Bockmann et al. 2005)
Rat Tracheal Tumor	NRSLKRISNKRIRRK, LRIKRKRRKRKKTRK	(Kennel et al. 2000)
Organ-Specific Motifs	Bone marrow: GGG, GFS, LWS; Fat: EGG, LLV, LSP; Muscle: LVS; Prostate: AGG; Skin: GRR, GGH, GTV	(Arap et al. 2002b)

Sequences successfully used in imaging [a] RGD containing and RGD variants

metalloproteases, including MMP-2, MMP-9, and MMP-11 (Kridel et al. 2001; Pan et al. 2003). The substrates and peptide inhibitors are being used to develop molecular probes to image and inhibit tissue remodeling associated with tumor cell invasion (Kuhnast et al. 2004).

Peptides specific for tumor-associated carbohydrates and interacting lectins have also been isolated from phage display libraries (Peletskaya et al. 1997). Peptides that bind the disaccharide tumor marker TFA inhibit both homotypic human breast cancer cell aggregation as well as heterotypic aggregation between cancer cells and the endothelium (Glinsky et al. 2000, 2001). They also inhibit the interaction of TFA with its ligand gal-3, suggesting both targets may be exploited in developing new molecular probes of carcinogenesis (Zou et al. 2005).

2.2 Integrin and Other Vasculature-targeting Peptides

One of the best examples of the power of phage display is in its application to vascular biology, from which new peptide-based cancer diagnostic and therapeutics have emerged. In 1996, Rouslahti and Pasqualini reported a breakthrough in phage display technology by performing their selections in living animals to obtain endothelium-targeting peptides (Arap et al. 1998; Pasqualini and Ruoslahti 1996). Peptides were selected that targeted the vasculature of various organs, including brain, kidney, lung, skin, pancreas, intestine, uterus and prostate. In particular, peptides containing an ArgGlyAsp (RGD) motif dominated the selections and were shown to target organ and tumor vasculature via the integrin $\alpha_v\beta_3$. Integrins are transmembrane heterodimeric cell-surface receptors expressed in a variety of cancer cells and endothelial cells and mediate adhesion to vitronectin, fibrinogen, laminin, etc., through the RGD motif (Pasqualini and Ruoslahti 1996; van der Flier and Sonnenberg 2001). Screening results indicated that different integrins exhibit subtly different peptide-binding specificities (van der Flier and Sonnenberg 2001). For example, peptides that bind $\alpha_5\beta_1$ integrin favored the CRGDGWC sequence, while those selected for $\alpha_v\beta_5$ integrin preferred the CDCRGDCFC (RGD-4C) sequence, suggesting that integrins interact preferentially to different ECM proteins (Kolonin et al. 2001). Numerous other vascular-targeting peptides have been identified by in-vivo selection in mice (Koivunen et al. 1999). Pasqualini's group went on to select a disulfide-constrained random phage library in a brain-dead human, and thousands of peptide motifs were identified (Table 1). Analysis of the selected motifs revealed that the distribution of the peptides was nonrandom and has allowed for mapping of the human vasculature (Arap et al. 2002b). Importantly, many of the peptides selected have been used for the subsequent identification of the corresponding cell-surface target (Zurita et al. 2004). In addition, discovery of these new vascular addresses has facilitated tissue-specific targeting of normal vasculature and angiogenesis-related targeting of tumor blood vessels. Recently, the National Cancer Institute panel of human cancer cell lines (NCI-60) has been surface profiled using phage display selections. High throughput screenings were used to classify the cell lines according to over 25,000 tripeptide motifs. Results suggested that tumor cells can be grouped by their profiles, which lends further support to the idea that many tumor cell-surface receptors are overexpressed irrespective of tumor origin, suggesting they could be developed as broad-based tumor-targeting drugs (Kolonin et al. 2006).

2.3 Tumor Cell Specific-Targeting Peptides

Imaging agents that do not target vasculature antigens or angiogenesis markers, but tumor cell-specific antigens are also being developed. In-vivo selection schemes have been developed to isolate peptides that do not bind vasculature components, but instead extravasate the vasculature and bind tumor cells. In this way, phage peptide libraries have been selected in human PC3 prostate tumor-bearing mice, and sequences were identified that target the carcinoma, penetrate the tumor, and internalize inside the cell (Newton et al. 2006). The ability to select phage that bind specifically to a tumor in vivo has opened up new avenues for the development of cancer-targeting molecules.

Numerous recent studies with phage display technology have focused on selections performed against cultured carcinoma cell lines as well cancer-patient sera. Peptides that bind human colorectal, prostate, gastric, cervical, liver, breast, thyroid, and other carcinoma cell lines have been obtained (Aina et al. 2002; Bockmann et al. 2005; Ding et al. 2006; McGuire et al. 2006; Rasmussen et al. 2002; Robinson et al. 2005; Romanov et al. 2001) (Table 1). Screening approaches have also been developed to select endothelial cell internalizing peptides, including those that were shown to recognize vascular adhesion molecule-1 (VCAM-1) (Kelly et al. 2006b). A pool of antibodies from ovarian cancer patients were selected against a phage peptide library and revealed a consensus motif, CVPELGHEC, which enabled identification of the 90-kDa heat-shock protein (HSP90) as the native antigen mimicked by the peptide. HSP90 was found to be restricted to a subset of patients with stage IV disease and may be exploited as a new molecular target in ovarian cancer (Vidal et al. 2004).

3 Phage-display Selected Peptides as Imaging Agents

3.1 Imaging with Integrin-Targeting Peptides

There are hundreds of reports of peptides isolated from phage-display libraries that bind tumor-cell antigens or tumor-cell supporting molecules (Table 1; reviewed in Brown 2000; Landon et al. 2004b). By far the vast majority bind vascular endothelial cell components such as integrins or growth factor receptors (Arap et al. 1998, 2002b; Koivunen et al. 1999; Kolonin et al. 2001; Pasqualini and Ruoslahti 1996). A preponderance of such peptides in the literature may reflect the abundance of growth factor receptors and integrins in vivo, or the nature of the phage selection schemes employed (Arap et al. 2002b). Development of phage-selected peptide-based imaging agents has centered primarily on the $\alpha_v\beta_3$ integrin. RGD containing peptides have been most extensively employed as cancer imaging agents (Haubner and Wester 2004). Various radiolabeled linear (Sivolapenko et al. 1998), glycosylated (Haubner et al. 2001) and Cys-cyclized (Cheng et al. 2005; Janssen et al. 2002; Wang et al. 2004), RGD-containing radiolabeled peptide analogues have been examined in rodent models of human carcinoma (Chen et al. 2005b; Haubner et al. 2001; Janssen et al. 2002; Su et al. 2002). The studies showed mixed results with some radioactive peptide accumulation in tumors but high levels of renal and liver accumulation (Haubner et al. 2001; Janssen et al. 2002; Su et al. 2002). Tumor accumulation has been improved by modification of RGD sequences with polyetyhelene glycol (PEG) and use of multimeric copies of the sequence (Chen et al. 2005b). RGD peptide constructs have also been employed for the optical noninvasive imaging of tumors. Li and co-workers employed both Cy5.5 and near infrared conjugated cyclo-KRGDF peptides to image Kaposi's sarcoma and melanoma tumors expressing $\alpha_v\beta_3$ integrin in mice (Kwon et al. 2005; Wang et al. 2004). In other studies, Cy5.5 versions of monomeric, dimeric, and tetrameric

RGDyK peptides were developed to image glioblastoma xenografted mice, and results indicated that multimerization of RGD peptides resulted in moderate improvement of imaging (Cheng et al. 2005). The RGDyK peptide was labeled with a quantum dot for imaging, although significant reticuloendothelial system (RES) uptake was observed (Cai et al. 2006). Other groups have shown that not only multimerization, but spatial alignment of RGD motifs are important in $\alpha_v\beta_3$ integrin recognition (Ye et al. 2006).

3.2 Imaging with Other Types of Tumor-targeting Peptides

Few phage-selected peptides, other than RGD-based or vascular targeting peptides, have been used successfully to image tumors. In 2000, a report concluded that peptides isolated from phage display to date do not bind with high retention to tumors in vivo (Kennel et al. 2000). Since then, numerous labeling, in-vitro tumor-cell binding and biodistribution studies have been published using phage display-derived peptides. A cyclic CTTHWGFTLC peptide that targets MMP-2 and MMP-9 was radioiodinated, and biodistribution studies in Lewis lung cancer tumor-bearing mice revealed poor tumor uptake. It was speculated that poor uptake was due to low affinity of the monomeric peptide compared with the multivalent phage from which the peptide was derived (Kuhnast et al. 2004; Weber et al. 2001). Better tumor retention was observed for a radioiodinated version of peptide DUP-1 (FRPNRAQDYNTN) isolated against DU-145 human prostate cultured cell lines. The peptide exhibited 5% and 7% tumoral accumulation in DU-145 and PC-3 heterotransplanted nude mice, respectively (Zitzmann et al. 2005). A peptide selected against a neuroblastoma cell line known as p160 (VPWMEPAYQRFL), whose target antigen remains unknown, was similarly radiolabeled and shown to be taken up by neuroblastoma and breast cancer tumors to a higher extent than most organs (Askoxylakis et al. 2005, 2006). A comparison study indicated that the p160 peptide had a higher tumor-to-organ ratio than a similarly radiolabeled RGD peptide construct (Askoxylakis et al. 2005). An E-selectin binding-peptide DITWDQLWDLMK, isolated from phage display (Funovics et al. 2005; Martens et al. 1995), was conjugated to amino-CLIO (Cy5.5), a crosslinked dextran-coated iron oxide nanoparticle, and demonstrated fluorescence accumulation in Lewis lung carcinoma-xenografted mice. The peptide was used for imaging E-selectin in not only Lewis lung carcinomas but also endothelial cells and human prostate cancer specimens (Funovics et al. 2005). Our group has been able to employ ^{111}In-labeled ErbB-2 targeting KCCYSL peptide and the gal-3 targeting peptide G3-C12, for SPECT/CT imaging of human MDA-MB-435-xenografted breast tumors in mice (Kumar et al. 2007). A peptide selected from cultured human HT29 colon carcinoma cells, CPIEDRPMC, known as "RPMC" (Kelly et al. 2004; Kelly and Jones 2003), was radiolabeled with ^{111}In and showed tumor accumulation of 7% id/g versus 1% for a scrambled peptide and imaged HT29 tumors in mice. Orthotopic tumors were readily detectable by using fluorescence endoscopy with FITC-labeled RPMC peptide (Fig. 2).

White Light Fluorescence

FITC-
RPMC

FITC-
Scrambled

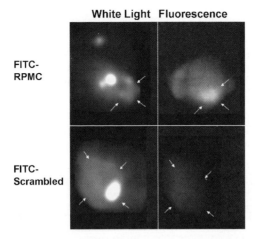

Fig. 2 Fluorescence imaging of orthotopic HT29 colon carcinomas with fluorescently labeled phage display-derived RPMC colon carcinoma targeting peptide. Fluorescence endoscopy was utilized for the detection of tumoral accumulation of FITC-labeled RPMC peptide (Kelly and Jones 2003). White light photographs of HT29 colon carcinomas were compared with fluorescent photographs to verify tumoral accumulation of the HT29 targeting peptide. Specificity of the tumor targeting peptide was confirmed by the inability of the scrambled peptide to target the orthotopic colon carcinoma. (Courtesy of K. Kelly and R. Weissleder)

4 Phage as Cancer Imaging Agents

Phage display has allowed for selection of peptides with high affinity (nanomolar) and specificity considered to be suitable for in-vivo tumor targeting and imaging. However, a comprehensive assessment of first generation or even second generation peptides obtained from phage display libraries indicates that the vast majority of peptides, while performing quite well in vitro, do not behave well in vivo (Table 1). One can argue that this discrepancy may be due to the very nature of the phage used in affinity selections. Depending on the phage and vector system utilized, typically at least five and up to thousands of copies of the peptide are displayed on the surface of each virion. Multiple display results in increased avidity of the phage for the desired target compared with the corresponding synthesized peptide (Smith 1985). Furthermore, addition of fluorophores and radiochelators to a peptide can have negative effects on the peptide's binding properties and hence imaging capabilities (Reubi 2003). Our group (Newton et al. 2006) as well as others (Hajitou et al. 2006; Souza et al. 2006) envision that peptide-displaying phage obtained from affinity selections can serve as valuable first-line agents to determine if the phage and corresponding synthesized peptides would function as efficacious tumor-targeting and imaging agents in vivo. Numerous inherent properties of fd phage support this notion. The ability to easily manipulate the phage genome as a vector allows for quick modification and introduction of a foreign sequences to be displayed on the surface of the virion, compared with the more costly and lengthy procedure of peptide synthesis. Screening of recombinant phage particles allows for more flexibility than screening of the synthesized peptides. Initial screening of phage displaying selected peptides can be accomplished biologically by tracking the phage spectrophotometrically or by monitoring infectivity of host *Escherichia coli*. More advanced screening and/or tracking of phage can be accomplished through the addition of optical or radioactive imaging tags. Phage displaying about five copies of a peptide on cpIII could be easily derivatized via modification of some of the many cpVIII protein molecules, yielding a bifunctional tumor imaging agent. Numerous labels covalently attached to the same virion would have the potential to generate signal amplification that can be exploited for in-vivo imaging. Injection of labeled phage into tumor-bearing rodents would allow for the noninvasive real-time imaging of the in-vivo biodistribution, tumor targeting propensity, and clearance rate of the labeled phage. Phage themselves are commonly found in the environment and are nonpathogenic, suggesting that phage vectors may ultimately have application to humans (Zou et al. 2004).

Initial studies with phage for in-vivo imaging centered on their obvious potential to image bacteria in mice. Biotinylated phage labelled with ^{99m}Tc successfully imaged bacterial infections in mouse models of inflammation (Edgar et al. 2006; Rusckowski et al. 2004). Kelly et al. (2006b) demonstrated that phage displaying the VHSPNKK peptide (Table 1) imaged VCAM-1-expressing endothelial cells in a murine tumor necrosis factor-α (TNFα) induced inflammatory ear model via intravital confocal microscopy (Fig. 3). In the TNFα ear model used, 24 h prior to phage injection the left ear of a mouse received a subcutaneous injection of TNFα while the right ear received no injection. VCAM-1 phage fluorescently labeled with VT680 were then injected into the mouse and imaged 6 h post injection by intravital confocal microscopy.

Phage displaying the RGD-4C peptide have been modified with gold nanoparticles and used in cultured carcinoma cell binding experiments (Souza et al. 2006). One of newest applications of phage is to integrate tumor targeting and genetic (viral) imaging in order to deliver and image specific transgenes. Pasqualini's group developed chimeric fd-tet phage (displaying RGD integrin-targeting sequences) — adeno-associated virus constructs which were evaluated for not only tumor targeting and imaging but also Herpes simplex virus thymidine kinase gene expression in mouse models of Karposi's sarcoma, and bladder and prostate carcinoma, as monitored by positron emission tomography (Hajitou et al. 2006).

We have employed our in-vivo selected prostate tumor targeting phage as optical imaging agents. The vasculature-extravasating phage were fluorescently labeled with the NIRF AF680 and allowed the successful noninvasive optical imaging of prostate tumors in immunocompromised mice (Newton et al. 2006).

While fluorescently labeled phage can be used for long-term animal imaging studies, radiolabeled phage may cause significant organ damage. Phage are very high molecular weight particles, taking ~ 48 h to clear through the RES with accumulation in the liver, spleen, and lung (Zou et al. 2004). Hence, implementation of a two-step pretargeting system could allow for the clearance of the majority of the phage before injection of an imaging label. To this end, biotinylated phage

VCAM-1 Phage   AngioSense750

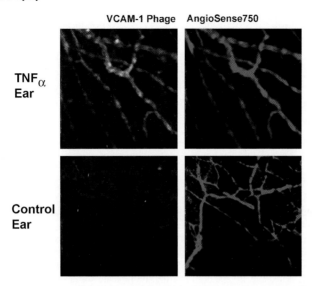

Fig. 3 Optical imaging of TNFα-induced inflammation using fluorescently labeled VCAM-1 phage. VCAM-1 expressing vascular endothelial cells were imaged using phage labeled with the fluorophore, VT680. TNF induced inflammation and VT680 labeled VCAM-1 phage vascular endothelium binding was detected with intravital confocal microscopy. AngioSense750 was used to delineate the vasculature from the surrounding tissues, and comparison of the two images was used to verify that the VCAM-1 phage were bound to the vascular endothelium. (Courtesy of K. Kelly and R. Weissleder)

Coregistered SPECT/CT   Axial SPECT/CT

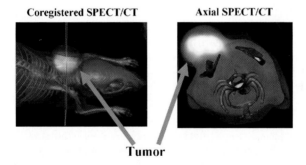

Tumor

Fig. 4 Two-step SPECT/CT imaging of B16-F1 mouse melanoma using biotinylated phage displaying an α-MSH peptide analogue in combination with an ^{111}In-DTPA-streptavidin complex. A syngeneic grafted B16-F1 melanoma tumor was imaged through the pretargeting of biotinylated MSH phage, followed by an injection of 7.40 MBq ^{111}In-DTPA-streptavidin 4 h later. The mouse was euthanized at 4 h post injection and image data was acquired using a CTI-Concorde Microsystems Micro SPECT/CT System

displaying tumor homing peptides in combination with ^{111}In-radiolabeled streptavidin have been utilized to image cancer in animals. Biotinylated phage displaying an α-MSH peptide analogue (MSH phage) were able to target the melanocortin 1 receptor (MC1R) (Martens et al. 1995) on B16-F1 mouse melanoma cells. Analysis of in-vivo distribution data demonstrated selective tumor uptake and retention within melanoma tumors in mice over a 24-h time period post injection with ^{111}In-labeled streptavidin-chelator. Specific tumor targeting was demonstrated through competition with a natural α-MSH peptide analogue. MicroSPECT/CT imaging studies clearly demonstrated the tumor targeting ability of the biotinylated MSH phage and the viability of a two-step pretargeting system incorporating biotinylated phage and radiolabeled streptavidin (Fig. 4).

References

Aina OH, Sroka TC, Chen ML, Lam KS (2002) Therapeutic cancer targeting peptides. Biopolymers 66:184–199

Arap W, Pasqualini R, Ruoslahti E (1998) Cancer treatment by targeted drug delivery to tumor vasculature in a mouse model. Science 279:377–380

Arap W, Haedicke W, Bernasconi M, Kain R, Rajotte D, Krajewski S, Ellerby HM, Bredesen DE, Pasqualini R, Ruoslahti E (2002a) Targeting the prostate for destruction through a vascular address. ProcNatl Acad Sci USA 99:1527–1531

Arap W, Kolonin M, Trepel M, Lahdenranta J, Cardo-Vila M, Giordano RJ, Mintz PJ, Ardelt PU, Yao VJ, Vidal CI, Chen L, Flamm A, Valtanen H, Weavind LM, Hicks ME, Pollock RE, Botz GH, Bucana CD, Koivunen E, Cahill D, Troncoso P, Baggerly KA, Pentz RD, Do KA, Logothetis CJ, Pasqualini R (2002b) Steps toward mapping the human vasculature by phage display. Nat Med 8:121–127

Arap MA, Lahdenranta J, Mintz PJ, Hajitou A, Sarkis AS, Arap W, Pasqualini R (2004) Cell surface expression of the stress response chaperone GRP78 enables tumor targeting by circulating ligands. Cancer Cell 6:275–284

Askoxylakis V, Zitzmann S, Mier W, Graham K, Kramer S, von Wegner F, Fink RH, Schwab M, Eisenhut M, Haberkorn U (2005) Preclinical evaluation of the breast cancer cell-binding peptide, p160. Clin Cancer Res 11:6705–6712

Askoxylakis V, Mier W, Zitzmann S, Ehemann V, Zhang J, Kramer S, Beck C, Schwab M, Eisenhut M, Haberkorn U (2006) Characterization and development of a peptide (p160) with affinity for neuroblastoma cells. J Nucl Med 47:981–988

Atwell S, Wells JA (1999) Selection for improved subtiligases by phage display. Proc Natl Acad Sci USA 96:9497–9502

Bakker WH, Krenning EP, Reubi JC, Breeman WA, Setyono-Han B, de Jong M, Kooij PP, Bruns C, van Hagen PM, Marbach P et al (1991) In vivo application of [111In-DTPA-D-Phe1]-octreotide for detection of somatostatin receptor-positive tumors in rats. Life Sci 49:1593–1601

Barbas CF 3rd, Kang AS, Lerner RA, Benkovic SJ (1991) Assembly of combinatorial antibody libraries on phage surfaces: the gene III site. Proc Natl Acad Sci USA 88:7978–7982

Behr TM, Gotthardt M, Barth A, Behe M (2001) Imaging tumors with peptide-based radioligands. Q J Nucl Med 45:189–200

Binetruy-Tournaire R, Demangel C, Malavaud B, Vassy R, Rouyre S, Kraemer M, Plouet J, Derbin C, Perret G, Mazie JC (2000) Identification of a peptide blocking vascular endothelial growth factor (VEGF)-mediated angiogenesis. EMBO J 19:1525–1533

Bockmann M, Drosten M, Putzer BM (2005) Discovery of targeting peptides for selective therapy of medullary thyroid carcinoma. J Gene Med 7:179–188

Brown KC (2000) New approaches for cell-specific targeting: identification of cell-selective peptides from combinatorial libraries. Curr Opin Chem Biol 4:16–21

Cai W, Shin DW, Chen K, Gheysens O, Cao Q, Wang SX, Gambhir SS, Chen X (2006) Peptide-labeled near-infrared quantum dots for imaging tumor vasculature in living subjects. Nano Lett 6:669–676

Chen J, Cheng Z, Hoffman TJ, Jurisson SS, Quinn TP (2000) Melanoma-targeting properties of (99m)technetium-labeled cyclic alpha-melanocyte-stimulating hormone peptide analogues. Cancer Res 60:5649–5658

Chen J, Tung CH, Allport JR, Chen S, Weissleder R, Huang PL (2005a) Near-infrared fluorescent imaging of matrix metalloproteinase activity after myocardial infarction. Circulation 111:1800–1805

Chen L, Zurita AJ, Ardelt PU, Giordano RJ, Arap W, Pasqualini R (2004) Design and validation of a bifunctional ligand display system for receptor targeting. Chem Biol 11:1081–1091

Chen X, Sievers E, Hou Y, Park R, Tohme M, Bart R, Bremner R, Bading JR, Conti PS (2005b) Integrin alpha v beta 3-targeted imaging of lung cancer. Neoplasia 7:271–9

Cheng Z, Wu Y, Xiong Z, Gambhir SS, Chen X (2005) Near-infrared fluorescent RGD peptides for optical imaging of integrin alphavbeta3 expression in living mice. Bioconjug Chem 16:1433–1441

Crameri R, Kodzius R (2001) The powerful combination of phage surface display of cDNA libraries and high throughput screening. Comb Chem High Throughput Screen 4:145–155

Ding H, Prodinger WM, Kopecek J (2006) Identification of CD21-binding peptides with phage display and investigation of binding properties of HPMA copolymer-peptide conjugates. Bioconjug Chem 17:514–523

Du B, Qian M, Zhou Z, Wang P, Wang L, Zhang X, Wu M, Zhang P, Mei B (2006) In vitro panning of a targeting peptide to hepatocarcinoma from a phage display peptide library. Biochem Biophys Res Commun 342:956–962

Edgar R, McKinstry M, Hwang J, Oppenheim AB, Fekete RA, Giulian G, Merril C, Nagashima K, Adhya S (2006) High-sensitivity bacterial detection using biotin-tagged phage and quantum-dot nanocomplexes. Proc Natl Acad Sci USA 103:4841–4845

Fan H, Duan Y, Zhou H, Li W, Li F, Guo L, Roeske RW (2002) Selection of peptide ligands binding to fibroblast growth factor receptor 1. IUBMB Life 54:67–72

Fleming TJ, Sachdeva M, Delic M, Beltzer J, Wescott CR, Devlin M, Lander RC, Nixon AE, Roschke V, Hilbert DM, Sexton DJ (2005) Discovery of high-affinity peptide binders to BLyS by phage display. J Mol Recognit 18:94–102

Fong S, Doyle MV, Goodson RJ, Drummond RJ, Stratton JR, McGuire L, Doyle LV, Chapman HA, Rosenberg S (2002) Random peptide bacteriophage display as a probe for urokinase receptor ligands. Biol Chem 383:149–158

Fukuda MN, Ohyama C, Lowitz K, Matsuo O, Pasqualini R, Ruoslahti E, Fukuda M (2000) A peptide mimic of E-selectin ligand inhibits sialyl Lewis X-dependent lung colonization of tumor cells. Cancer Res 60:450–456

Funovics M, Montet X, Reynolds F, Weissleder R, Josephson L (2005) Nanoparticles for the optical imaging of tumor E-selectin. Neoplasia 7:904–911

Giordano RJ, Cardo-Vila M, Lahdenranta J, Pasqualini R, Arap W (2001) Biopanning and rapid analysis of selective interactive ligands. Nat Med 7:1249–1253

Glinsky VV, Huflejt ME, Glinsky GV, Deutscher SL, Quinn TP (2000) Effects of Thomsen-Friedenreich antigen-specific peptide P-30 on beta-galactoside-mediated homotypic aggregation and adhesion to the endothelium of MDA-MB-435 human breast carcinoma cells. Cancer Res 60:2584–2588

Glinsky VV, Glinsky GV, Rittenhouse-Olson K, Huflejt ME, Glinskii OV, Deutscher SL, Quinn TP (2001) The role of Thomsen-Friedenreich antigen in adhesion of human breast and prostate cancer cells to the endothelium. Cancer Res 61:4851–4857

Goldenberg DM (2002) Targeted therapy of cancer with radiolabeled antibodies. J Nucl Med 43:693–713

Goldenberg MM (1999) Trastuzumab, a recombinant DNA-derived humanized monoclonal antibody, a novel agent for the treatment of metastatic breast cancer. Clin Ther 21:309–318

Goodson RJ, Doyle MV, Kaufman SE, Rosenberg S (1994) High-affinity urokinase receptor antagonists identified with bacteriophage peptide display. Proc Natl Acad Sci US A 91:7129–7133

Hajitou A, Trepel M, Lilley CE, Soghomonyan S, Alauddin MM, Marini FC, 3rd, Restel BH, Ozawa MG, Moya CA, Rangel R, Sun Y, Zaoui K, Schmidt M, von Kalle C, Weitzman MD,

Gelovani JG, Pasqualini R, Arap W (2006) A hybrid vector for ligand-directed tumor targeting and molecular imaging. Cell 125:385–398

Haubner R, Wester HJ (2004) Radiolabeled tracers for imaging of tumor angiogenesis and evaluation of anti-angiogenic therapies. Curr Pharm Des 10:1439–1455

Haubner R, Wester HJ, Burkhart F, Senekowitsch-Schmidtke R, Weber W, Goodman SL, Kessler H, Schwaiger M (2001) Glycosylated RGD-containing peptides: tracer for tumor targeting and angiogenesis imaging with improved biokinetics. J Nucl Med 42:326–336

Heppeler A, Froidevaux S, Eberle AN, Maecke HR (2000) Receptor targeting for tumor localisation and therapy with radiopeptides. Curr Med Chem 7:971–994

Hetian L, Ping A, Shumei S, Xiaoying L, Luowen H, Jian W, Lin M, Meisheng L, Junshan Y, Chengchao S (2002) A novel peptide isolated from a phage display library inhibits tumor growth and metastasis by blocking the binding of vascular endothelial growth factor to its kinase domain receptor. J Biol Chem 277:43137–43142

Houghten RA, Pinilla C, Blondelle SE, Appel JR, Dooley CT, Cuervo JH (1991) Generation and use of synthetic peptide combinatorial libraries for basic research and drug discovery. Nature 354:84–86

Houimel M, Schneider P, Terskikh A, Mach JP (2001) Selection of peptides and synthesis of pentameric peptabody molecules reacting specifically with ErbB-2 receptor. Int J Cancer 92:748–755

Janssen ML, Oyen WJ, Dijkgraaf I, Massuger LF, Frielink C, Edwards DS, Rajopadhye M, Boonstra H, Corstens FH, Boerman OC (2002) Tumor targeting with radiolabeled alpha(v)beta(3) integrin binding peptides in a nude mouse model. Cancer Res 62:6146–6151

Jaye DL, Nolte FS, Mazzucchelli L, Geigerman C, Akyildiz A, Parkos CA (2003) Use of real-time polymerase chain reaction to identify cell- and tissue-type-selective peptides by phage display. Am J Pathol 162:1419–1429

Jaye DL, Geigerman CM, Fuller RE, Akyildiz A, Parkos CA (2004) Direct fluorochrome labeling of phage display library clones for studying binding specificities: applications in flow cytometry and fluorescence microscopy. J Immunol Methods 295:119–127

Karasseva N, Glinsky VV, Chen NX, Komatireddy R, Quinn TP (2002) Identification and characterization of peptides that bind human ErbB-2 selected from a bacteriophage display library. J Protein Chem 21:287–296

Ke SH, Coombs GS, Tachias K, Corey DR, Madison EL (1997) Optimal subsite occupancy and design of a selective inhibitor of urokinase. J Biol Chem 272:20456–20462

Kelly KA, Jones DA (2003) Isolation of a colon tumor specific binding peptide using phage display selection. Neoplasia 5:437–444

Kelly K, Alencar H, Funovics M, Mahmood U, Weissleder R (2004) Detection of invasive colon cancer using a novel, targeted, library-derived fluorescent peptide. Cancer Res 64:6247–6251

Kelly KA, Clemons PA, Yu AM, Weissleder R (2006a) High-throughput identification of phage-derived imaging agents. Mol Imaging 5:24–30

Kelly KA, Nahrendorf M, Yu AM, Reynolds F, Weissleder R (2006b) In vivo phage display selection yields atherosclerotic plaque targeted peptides for imaging. Mol Imaging Biol 8:201–207

Kennel SJ, Mirzadeh S, Hurst GB, Foote LJ, Lankford TK, Glowienka KA, Chappell LL, Kelso JR, Davern SM, Safavy A, Brechbiel MW (2000) Labeling and distribution of linear peptides identified using in vivo phage display selection for tumors. Nucl Med Biol 27:815–825

Kim JW, Wang XW (2003) Gene expression profiling of preneoplastic liver disease and liver cancer: a new era for improved early detection and treatment of these deadly diseases? Carcinogenesis 24:363–369

Kim Y, Lillo AM, Steiniger SC, Liu Y, Ballatore C, Anichini A, Mortarini R, Kaufmann GF, Zhou B, Felding-Habermann B, Janda KD (2006) Targeting heat shock proteins on cancer cells: selection, characterization, and cell-penetrating properties of a peptidic GRP78 ligand. Biochemistry 45:9434–9444

Koivunen E, Arap W, Rajotte D, Lahdenranta J, Pasqualini R (1999) Identification of receptor ligands with phage display peptide libraries. J Nucl Medi 40:883–888

Kolonin M, Pasqualini R, Arap W (2001) Molecular addresses in blood vessels as targets for therapy. Curr Opin Chem Biol 5:308–313

Kolonin MG, Bover L, Sun J, Zurita AJ, Do KA, Lahdenranta J, Cardo-Vila M, Giordano RJ, Jaalouk DE, Ozawa MG, Moya CA, Souza GR, Staquicini FI, Kunyiasu A, Scudiero DA, Holbeck SL, Sausville EA, Arap W, Pasqualini R (2006) Ligand-directed surface profiling of human cancer cells with combinatorial peptide libraries. Cancer Res 66:34–40

Koolpe M, Dail M, Pasquale EB (2002) An ephrin mimetic peptide that selectively targets the EphA2 receptor. J Biol Chem 277:46974–46979

Koolpe M, Burgess R, Dail M, Pasquale EB (2005) EphB receptor-binding peptides identified by phage display enable design of an antagonist with ephrin-like affinity. J Biol Chem 280: 17301–17311

Kridel SJ, Chen E, Kotra LP, Howard EW, Mobashery S, Smith JW (2001) Substrate hydrolysis by matrix metalloproteinase-9. J Biol Chem 276:20572–20578

Kuhnast B, Bodenstein C, Haubner R, Wester HJ, Senekowitsch-Schmidtke R, Schwaiger M, Weber WA (2004) Targeting of gelatinase activity with a radiolabeled cyclic HWGF peptide. Nucl Med Biol 31:337–344

Kumada Y, Nogami M, Minami N, Maehara M, Katoh S (2005) Application of protein-coupled liposomes to effective affinity screening from phage library. J Chromatogr A 1080:22–28

Kumar S, Quinn T, Deutscher S (2007) Evaluation of an 111In-radiolabeled peptide as a targeting and imaging agent for ErbB-2 receptor expressing breast carcinomas. Clin Cancer Res 13:6070–6079

Kwon S, Ke S, Houston JP, Wang W, Wu Q, Li C, Sevick-Muraca EM (2005) Imaging dose-dependent pharmacokinetics of an RGD-fluorescent dye conjugate targeted to alpha v beta 3 receptor expressed in Kaposi's sarcoma. Mol Imaging 4:75–87

Landon LA, Harden W, Illy C, Deutscher SL (2004a) High-throughput fluorescence spectroscopic analysis of affinity of peptides displayed on bacteriophage. Anal Biochem 331:60–67

Landon LA, Zou J, Deutscher SL (2004b) Is phage display on target for developing peptide-based cancer drugs? Curr Drug Discov Technol 1:113–132

Liang S, Lin T, Ding J, Pan Y, Dang D, Guo C, Zhi M, Zhao P, Sun L, Hong L, Shi Y, Yao L, Liu J, Wu K, Fan D (2006) Screening and identification of vascular-endothelial-cell-specific binding peptide in gastric cancer. J Mol Med 84:764–773

Marik J, Lam KS (2005) Peptide and small-molecule microarrays. Methods Mol Biol 310:217–226

Martens CL, Cwirla SE, Lee RY, Whitehorn E, Chen EY, Bakker A, Martin EL, Wagstrom C, Gopalan P, Smith CW et al (1995) Peptides which bind to E-selectin and block neutrophil adhesion. J Biol Chem 270:21129–21136

Maruta F, Parker AL, Fisher KD, Hallissey MT, Ismail T, Rowlands DC, Chandler LA, Kerr DJ, Seymour LW (2002) Identification of FGF receptor-binding peptides for cancer gene therapy. Cancer Gene Therapy 9:543–552

Maruta F, Parker AL, Fisher KD, Murray PG, Kerr DJ, Seymour LW (2003) Use of a phage display library to identify oligopeptides binding to the lumenal surface of polarized endothelium by ex vivo perfusion of human umbilical veins. J Drug Target 11:53–59

McGuire MJ, Samli KN, Chang YC, Brown KC (2006) Novel ligands for cancer diagnosis: selection of peptide ligands for identification and isolation of B-cell lymphomas. Exp Hematol 34:443–452

Meredith RF, Bueschen AJ, Khazaeli MB, Plott WE, Grizzle WE, Wheeler RH, Schlom J, Russell CD, Liu T, LoBuglio AF (1994) Treatment of metastatic prostate carcinoma with radiolabeled antibody CC49. J Nucl Med 35:1017–1022

Michon IN, Penning LC, Molenaar TJ, van Berkel TJ, Biessen EA, Kuiper J (2002) The effect of TGF-beta receptor binding peptides on smooth muscle cells. Biochem Biophys Res Commun 293:1279–1286

Newton JR, Kelly KA, Mahmood U, Weissleder R, Deutscher SL (2006) In vivo selection of phage for the optical imaging PC-3 human prostate carcinoma in mice. Neoplasia 8:772–780

Nowak JE, Chatterjee M, Mohapatra S, Dryden SC, Tainsky MA (2006) Direct production and purification of T7 phage display cloned proteins selected and analyzed on microarrays. Biotechniques 40:220–227

Orlova A, Magnusson M, Eriksson TL, Nilsson M, Larsson B, Hoiden-Guthenberg I, Widstrom C, Carlsson J, Tolmachev V, Stahl S, Nilsson FY (2006) Tumor imaging using a picomolar affinity HER2 binding affibody molecule. Cancer Res 66:4339–4348

Pakkala M, Jylhasalmi A, Wu P, Leinonen J, Stenman UH, Santa H, Vepsalainen J, Perakyla M, Narvanen A (2004) Conformational and biochemical analysis of the cyclic peptides which modulate serine protease activity. J Pept Sci 10:439–447

Pan W, Arnone M, Kendall M, Grafstrom RH, Seitz SP, Wasserman ZR, Albright CF (2003) Identification of peptide substrates for human MMP-11 (stromelysin-3) using phage display. J Biol Chem 278:27820–27827

Pasqualini R, Ruoslahti E (1996) Organ targeting in vivo using phage display peptide libraries. Nature 380:364–366

Peletskaya EN, Glinsky G, Deutscher SL, Quinn TP (1996) Identification of peptide sequences that bind the Thomsen-Friedenreich cancer-associated glycoantigen from bacteriophage peptide display libraries. Mol Divers 2:13–18

Peletskaya EN, Glinsky VV, Glinsky GV, Deutscher SL, Quinn TP (1997) Characterization of peptides that bind the tumor-associated Thomsen-Friedenreich antigen selected from bacteriophage display libraries. J Mol Biol 270:374–384

Ploug M, Østergaard S, Gårdsvoll H, Kovalski K, Holst-Hansen C, Holm A, Ossowski L, Danø K (2001) Peptide-derived antagonists of the urokinase receptor. Affinity maturation by combinatorial chemistry, identification of functional epitopes, and inhibitory effect on cancer cell intravasation. Biochemistry 40:12157–12168

Popkov M, Rader C, Barbas CF, 3rd (2004) Isolation of human prostate cancer cell reactive antibodies using phage display technology. J Immunol Methods 291:137–151

Rahim A, Coutelle C, Harbottle R (2003) High-throughput pyrosequencing of a phage display library for the identification of enriched target-specific peptides. Biotechniques 35:317–320, 322, 324

Rasmussen UB, Schreiber V, Schultz H, Mischler F, Schughart K (2002) Tumor cell-targeting by phage-displayed peptides. Cancer Gene Ther 9:606–612

Reubi JC (2003) Peptide receptors as molecular targets for cancer diagnosis and therapy. Endocr Rev 24:389–427

Robinson P, Stuber D, Deryckere F, Tedbury P, Lagrange M, Orfanoudakis G (2005) Identification using phage display of peptides promoting targeting and internalization into HPV-transformed cell lines. J Mol Recognit 18:175–182

Romanov VI, Durand DB, Petrenko VA (2001) Phage display selection of peptides that affect prostate carcinoma cells attachment and invasion. Prostate 47:239–251

Rusckowski M, Gupta S, Liu G, Dou S, Hnatowich DJ (2004) Investigations of a (99m)Tc-labeled bacteriophage as a potential infection-specific imaging agent. J Nucl Med 45:1201–1208

Samoylov AM, Samoylova TI, Hartell MG, Pathirana ST, Smith BF, Vodyanoy V (2002) Recognition of cell-specific binding of phage display derived peptides using an acoustic wave sensor. Biomol Eng 18:269–272

Shukla GS, Krag DN (2005) Phage display selection for cell-specific ligands: development of a screening procedure suitable for small tumor specimens. J Drug Target 13:7–18

Sivolapenko GB, Skarlos D, Pectasides D, Stathopoulou E, Milonakis A, Sirmalis G, Stuttle A, Courtenay-Luck NS, Konstantinides K, Epenetos AA (1998) Imaging of metastatic melanoma utilising a technetium-99m labelled RGD-containing synthetic peptide. Eur J Nucl Med 25:1383–1389

Skelton NJ, Chen YM, Dubree N, Quan C, Jackson DY, Cochran A, Zobel K, Deshayes K, Baca M, Pisabarro MT, Lowman HB (2001) Structure-function analysis of a phage display-derived peptide that binds to insulin-like growth factor binding protein 1. Biochemistry 40:8487–8498

Smith GP (1985) Filamentous fusion phage: novel expression vectors that display cloned antigens on the virion surface. Science 228:1315–1317

Souza GR, Christianson DR, Staquicini FI, Ozawa MG, Snyder EY, Sidman RL, Miller JH, Arap W, Pasqualini R (2006) Networks of gold nanoparticles and bacteriophage as biological sensors and cell-targeting agents. Proc Natl Acad Sci USA 103:1215–1220

Spear MA, Breakefield XO, Beltzer J, Schuback D, Weissleder R, Pardo FS, Ladner R (2001) Isolation, characterization, and recovery of small peptide phage display epitopes selected against viable malignant glioma cells. Cancer Gene Ther 8:506–511

Stortelers C, Souriau C, van Liempt E, van de Poll ML, van Zoelen EJ (2002) Role of the N-terminus of epidermal growth factor in ErbB-2/ErbB-3 binding studied by phage display. Biochemistry 41:8732–8741

Su ZF, Liu G, Gupta S, Zhu Z, Rusckowski M, Hnatowich DJ (2002) In vitro and in vivo evaluation of a Technetium-99m-labeled cyclic RGD peptide as a specific marker of alpha(V)beta(3) integrin for tumor imaging. Bioconjugate Chem 13:561–570

Urbanelli L, Ronchini C, Fontana L, Menard S, Orlandi R, Monaci P (2001) Targeted gene transduction of mammalian cells expressing the HER2/neu receptor by filamentous phage. J Mol Biol 313:965–976

Van de Wiele C, Dumont F, Dierckx RA, Peers SH, Thornback JR, Slegers G, Thierens H (2001) Biodistribution and dosimetry of (99m)Tc-RP527, a gastrin-releasing peptide (GRP) agonist for the visualization of GRP receptor-expressing malignancies. J Nucl Med 42:1722–1727

van der Flier A, Sonnenberg A (2001) Function and interactions of integrins. Cell Tissue Res 305:285–298

Vidal CI, Mintz PJ, Lu K, Ellis LM, Manenti L, Giavazzi R, Gershenson DM, Broaddus R, Liu J, Arap W, Pasqualini R (2004) An HSP90-mimic peptide revealed by fingerprinting the pool of antibodies from ovarian cancer patients. Oncogene 23:8859–8867

Virgolini I (1997) Mack Forster Award Lecture. Receptor nuclear medicine: vasointestinal peptide and somatostatin receptor scintigraphy for diagnosis and treatment of tumour patients. Eur J Clin Invest 27:793–800

Voss SD, DeGrand AM, Romeo GR, Cantley LC, Frangioni JV (2002) An integrated vector system for cellular studies of phage display-derived peptides. Anal Biochem 308:364–372

Walter G, Konthur Z, Lehrach H (2001) High-throughput screening of surface displayed gene products. Comb Chem High Throughput Screen 4:193–205

Waltz E (2006) After criticism, more modest cancer genome project takes shape. Nat Med 12:259

Wang W, Ke S, Wu Q, Charnsangavej C, Gurfinkel M, Gelovani JG, Abbruzzese JL, Sevick-Muraca EM, Li C (2004) Near-infrared optical imaging of integrin alphavbeta3 in human tumor xenografts. Mol Imaging 3:343–351

Weber WA, Haubner R, Vabuliene E, Kuhnast B, Wester HJ, Schwaiger M (2001) Tumor angiogenesis targeting using imaging agents. Q J Nucl Med 45:179–182

Yang SQ, Craik CS (1998) Engineering bidentate macromolecular inhibitors for trypsin and urokinase-type plasminogen activator. J Mol Biol 279:1001–1011

Ye Y, Bloch S, Xu B, Achilefu S (2006) Design, synthesis, and evaluation of near infrared fluorescent multimeric RGD peptides for targeting tumors. J Med Chem 49:2268–2275

Zitzmann S, Mier W, Schad A, Kinscherf R, Askoxylakis V, Kramer S, Altmann A, Eisenhut M, Haberkorn U (2005) A new prostate carcinoma binding peptide (DUP-1) for tumor imaging and therapy. Clin Cancer Res 11:139–146

Zou J, Dickerson MT, Owen NK, Landon LA, Deutscher SL (2004) Biodistribution of filamentous phage peptide libraries in mice. Mol Biol Rep 31:121–129

Zou J, Glinsky VV, Landon LA, Matthews L, Deutscher SL (2005) Peptides specific to the galectin-3 carbohydrate recognition domain inhibit metastasis-associated cancer cell adhesion. Carcinogenesis 26:309–318

Zurita AJ, Troncoso P, Cardo-Vila M, Logothetis CJ, Pasqualini R, Arap W (2004) Combinatorial screenings in patients: the interleukin-11 receptor alpha as a candidate target in the progression of human prostate cancer. Cancer Res 64:435–439

Part V
Applications: Experimental Imaging

Molecular Imaging: Reporter Gene Imaging

Inna Serganova, Phillipp Mayer-Kukuck, Ruimin Huang,
and Ronald Blasberg(✉)

Abstract Non-invasive in-vivo molecular genetic imaging developed over the past decade and predominantly utilises radiotracer (PET, gamma camera, autoradiography), magnetic resonance and optical imaging technology. Molecular genetic imaging has its roots in both molecular biology and cell biology. The convergence of these disciplines and imaging modalities has provided the opportunity to address new research questions, including oncogenesis, tumour maintenance and progression, as well as responses to molecular-targeted therapy. Three different imaging strategies are described: (1) "bio-marker" or "surrogate" imaging; (2) "direct" imaging of specific molecules and pathway activity; (3) "indirect" reporter gene imaging. Examples of each imaging strategy are presented and discussed. Several applications of PET- and optical-based reporter imaging are demonstrated, including signal transduction pathway monitoring, oncogenesis in genetic mouse models, endogenous molecular genetic/biological processes and the response to therapy in

Ronald Blasberg
Departments of Neurology and Radiology, Memorial Sloan-Kettering Cancer Center, 1275 York Avenue, New York, NY 10021, USA
blasberg@neuro1.mskcc.org

W. Semmler and M. Schwaiger (eds.), *Molecular Imaging II.*
Handbook of Experimental Pharmacology 185/II.

167

animal models of human disease. Molecular imaging studies will compliment established ex-vivo molecular-biological assays that require tissue sampling by providing a spatial and a temporal dimension to our understanding of disease development and progression, as well as response to treatment. Although molecular imaging studies are currently being performed primarily in experimental animals, we optimistically expect they will be translated to human subjects with cancer and other diseases in the near future.

1 Introduction

Medical imaging has undergone a remarkable revolution and expansion in the past two decades, and this expansion coincides with novel molecular-based medical therapies that have emerged following the complete sequencing of the human genome. Recent progress in our understanding of the molecular genetic mechanisms in many diseases and the application of new biologically based approaches in therapy are exciting new developments. Novel "molecular therapies" have been developed that target specific oncogenic mutations in chronic myelogenous leukemia (CML) (Druker et al. 1996), gastrointestinal stromal tumours (GIST) (Tuveson et al. 2001), and lung cancer (Lynch et al. 2004). New gene-based therapies can provide control over the level, timing and duration of action of many biologically active transgene products by including specific promoter/activator regulatory elements in the genetic material that is transferred. Controlled gene delivery and gene expression systems have recently been developed for specific somatic tissues and tumours (Papadakis et al. 2004; Ray et al. 2004; Zhu et al. 2004; Sadeghi and Hitt 2005). For example, novel gene constructs that target vectors to specific tissues/organs, and for controlling gene expression using cell-specific, replication-activated and drug-controlled expression systems. In addition, small radiolabelled compounds and paramagnetic probes are being developed to image specific proteins in specific signalling cascades, and they are being applied to monitor drug response. The inclusion of non-invasive imaging of specific molecular genetic and cellular processes will accelerate our research efforts and lead to more effective therapeutic strategies (Harrington et al. 2000; Nakagawa et al. 2001).

Molecular imaging provides visualisation in space and time of normal as well as abnormal cellular processes at a molecular genetic or cellular level of function. Although the term "molecular imaging" was coined in the mid 1990s, it has its roots in molecular biology and cell biology, as well as in imaging technology and chemistry. For example, for many years researchers used reporter genes encoding enzymes, such as bacterial β-galactosidase (*lacZ* gene) (Forss-Petter et al. 1990) and chloramphenicol acetyltransferase (*CAT* gene) (Overbeek et al. 1985), to study various cellular processes. However, 'visualisation' of these enzymes required postmortem tissue sampling and processing for precise quantitative analysis. Advances in cell biology, especially the translation of these advances to clinical applications, dictate the development of novel visualisation systems that would provide accurate and sensitive measurements, as well as allow visualisation in living cells, live animals and human subjects.

Molecular imaging in living animals is the direct result of significant developments in several non-invasive, in-vivo imaging technologies: (1) magnetic resonance (MR) imaging (Ichikawa et al. 2002); (2) nuclear imaging (QAR, gamma camera and PET) (Blasberg and Gelovani 2002); (3) optical imaging of small animals (Edinger et al. 2002; Weissleder 2002; Hoffman 2005), as well as two-photon fluorescent imaging of viable cells, small organisms and embryos (Hadjantonakis et al. 2002). It should be noted that these developments occurred more or less in parallel to each other, and were largely independent of the advances that were occurring in genetics and in molecular and cell biology during the 1980s and early 1990s. However, each of these imaging technologies have had important antecedents. For example, radionuclide-based imaging is founded on the radiotracer principle, first described by George de Hevesy. In 1935, he published a letter in *Nature* on the tracer principle using ^{32}P for the study of phosphorus metabolism (Chievitz and Hevesy 1935; Myers 1979) and he was awarded the Nobel Prize in Chemistry in 1943. The tracer technique was later adapted for many applications in physiology and biochemistry, as well as in functional diagnosis and use in nuclear medicine and molecular imaging.

The convergence of the imaging and molecular/cell biology disciplines in the mid 1990s is at the heart of this success story and it is the wellspring for further advances in this new field. Although first applied to non-invasive in-vivo imaging of small animals, molecular imaging paradigms are now being translated into clinic imaging paradigms (Jacobs et al. 2001b; Penuelas et al. 2005) that will establish new standards of medical practice. The development of versatile and sensitive non-invasive assays that do *not* require tissue samples will be of considerable value for monitoring molecular-genetic and cellular processes in animal models of human disease, as well as for studies in human subjects in the future.

This new field of investigation has expanded rapidly following the establishment of "cancer imaging" as one of six "extraordinary scientific opportunities" by NCI in 1997-98. Subsequent funding initiatives have provided a major stimulus to further the development of this new discipline. Substantial resources have been made available to the research community through NCI's Small Animal Imaging Resources Program (SAIRP) and the In Vivo Cellular and Molecular Imaging Centers (ICMIC) program. Similar funding initiatives have been developed by other NIH Institutes and by the Department of Energy (DOE). In addition, a new NIH institute — the National Institute for Biomedical Imaging and Bioengineering (NIBIB) — has recently been formed to better represent the breadth of an expanding imaging community. In addition, there are two new journals devoted the field of molecular imaging — Molecular Imaging (BC Decker, Publisher; the official journal of the Society of Molecular Imaging, www.molecularimaging.org) and Molecular Imaging and Biology (Springer New York, Publisher; the official journal of the Academy of Molecular Imaging, www.ami-imaging.org), and other established imaging-related journals have added "molecular imaging" components.

2 Molecular Imaging Strategies

The most widely used molecular imaging modalities include: (1) optical (fluorescence, bioluminescence, spectroscopy, optical coherence tomography), (2) radionuclide (PET, SPECT, gamma camera, autoradiography) and (3) magnetic resonance (spectroscopy, contrast, diffusion-weighted imaging). In addition, other modalities, such as ultrasound and CT, are seeing increasing application and could be included as well. The interaction of several disciplines, including molecular cell biology and chemistry with different imaging modalities is illustrated by the Ven diagram (Fig. 1), and illustrates the theme of this presentation. Namely, a multi-modality, multi-disciplinary approach to molecular imaging provides many positive advantages. Several of the imaging modalities (fluorescence, bioluminescence, nuclear, and magnetic resonance) are illustrated in the following sections and their combined advantage are highlighted.

Before discussing specific molecular imaging issues, it would be helpful to briefly outline three currently used imaging strategies to non-invasively monitor and measure molecular events. They have been broadly defined as "biomarker", "direct" and "indirect" imaging. These strategies have been discussed previously in several recent reviews (Contag et al. 1998; Gambhir et al. 2000b; Tavitian 2000; Berger and Gambhir 2001; Ray et al. 2001; Blasberg and Gelovani 2002; Gelovani Tjuvajev and Blasberg 2003; Luker et al. 2003c; Weissleder and Ntziachristos 2003) and in other perspectives on molecular imaging (Blasberg and Gelovani 2002; Contag and Ross 2002; Gambhir 2002; Weissleder and Ntziachristos 2003; Min and Gambhir 2004; Shah et al. 2004).

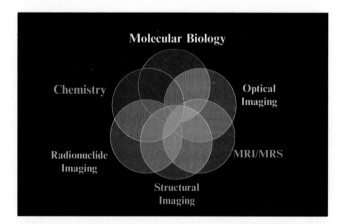

Fig. 1 Multidisciplinary approach to molecular imaging. Molecular and cell biology, along with chemistry, provide the foundation and resources for developing novel in-vivo molecular constructs and imaging paradigms. Three imaging modalities currently dominate the field, along with structural/anatomical imaging. This list will likely expand to include other modalities in the near future. The *Ven diagram* emphasizes the interaction between disciplines and different imaging modalities; it is this interaction that provides a broad new approach to the field

2.1 Biomarker Imaging

Biomarker or surrogate-marker imaging can be used to assess downstream effects of one or more endogenous molecular genetic processes. This approach is particularly attractive for potential translation into clinical studies in the short-term, because existing radiopharmaceuticals and imaging paradigms may be useful for monitoring downstream effects of changes in specific molecular genetic pathways in diseases such as cancer. For example, tumour imaging of glucose utilisation using a radiolabelled analogue of glucose (2′-fluoro-2′-deoxyglucose — [^{18}F]FDG) and positron emission tomography (PET) is based on the fact that malignant tumours frequently have high glycolytic rates (Warburg 1956). The images of increased glucose utilisation and increased glycolysis reflect increased glucose transport and hexokinase activity, as well as the pathways that regulate these processes. This imaging strategy has been recognized for nearly three decades and was initially applied to malignant brain tumours by Di Chiro et al. (1982). Only small-bore (head-only) PET tomographs were available at that time, until the introduction of commercial whole-body PET scanners in the early 1990s. Now, whole-body [^{18}F]FDG PET imaging is routinely and widely used in the clinic for tumour diagnosis and staging the extent of disease (Shreve et al. 1999), as well as for monitoring the efficacy of anti-cancer therapies (Schelling et al. 2000).

The regulation of glucose utilisation in cells is complex and reflects the sum of multiple inputs at various levels involving different signalling pathways. For example, increased glycolysis can be a response to an increase in cellular energy and substrate requirements, to an increase in cell proliferation and synthesis rates, and to the activation of specific oncogenic pathways that can occur in the presence of adequate oxygen (Warburg effect). Although glucose uptake and glycolytic enzyme activity are homeostatically regulated, glucose metabolism has also been shown to be regulated by extracellular signals mediated by cell surface receptors such as cKIT. Receptor-mediated regulation of glucose uptake is thought to involve activation of PI3 kinase, Akt, mTOR (the kinase mammalian target of rapamycin) and S6 kinase. Examples of this include the CD28 signalling pathway in T-cells and insulin receptor signalling (Frauwirth et al. 2002). A likely explanation for the dramatic effect of STI571 (Gleevec) on glucose uptake in GIST is that c-Kit receptor signalling regulates/mediates glucose uptake as well as glucose metabolism. Interestingly, in a lymphoma and a lymphocyte cell line, mTOR depletion or rapamycin treatment and glucose deprivation trigger a stress response similar to a starvation phenotype (Peng et al. 2002). In addition, various inputs that increase HIF-1α levels impact on and increase glycolysis through enhanced translation and transcription; similarly, the mutation and functional inactivation of specific proteins (e.g. VHL and p53) that results in stabilisation and reduced degradation rate of the HIF-1α protein also increase glucose transport and glycolysis.

Biomarker [^{18}F]FDG PET studies have been extensively used to assess biological effects occurring during neoplastic progression and to monitor the effects of therapy. However, biomarker imaging may be relatively "non-specific", in that it is likely to reflect effects on more than a single protein or signalling pathway. Nevertheless, it benefits from the use of radiolabelled probes that have already been developed and studied in human subjects. Thus, the translation of biomarker imaging paradigms into patients will be far easier than either the direct imaging paradigms or reporter transgene imaging paradigms outlined below. However, it remains to be shown whether there is a sufficiently high correlation between "surrogate marker" imaging and direct molecular assays that reflect the activity of a particular molecular/genetic pathway of interest.

Very few studies have attempted a rigorous correlation between biomarker imaging and transcriptional activity of a particular gene, or post-transcriptional processing of the gene product, or the activity of a specific signal transduction pathway that is targeted by a particular drug. The application of biomarker imaging for monitoring treatment response is gaining increasing attention, particularly as it relates to the development and testing of new pathway-specific drugs. One recent example of clinically useful biomarker imaging is the early (1–7 days) assessment of treatment response with [^{18}F]FDG PET imaging, as applied to gastrointestinal stromal tumours (GIST) pre- and post-imatinib mesylate (Gleevec, Glivec, STI571) treatment (Demetri et al. 2002) (Fig. 2a). This is significant because imatinib mesylate treatment specifically targets the c-Kit receptor tyrosine kinase that is mutated and constitutively over-expressed in GIST, and the metabolic response to treatment is observed within hours. [^{18}F]FDG PET imaging is also useful in monitoring patients with GIST for recurrent disease or failure of current therapy (Fig. 2b).

Several clinical cancer trials involving mTOR inhibitors have been shown sporadic anti-tumour activity, leading to uncertainty about the appropriate clinical setting for their use. Recently Thomas et al. (2006) have shown that loss of the Von Hippel-Lindau tumour suppressor gene (VHL) sensitizes kidney cancer cells to the mTOR inhibitor CCI-779, both in vitro and in mouse tumour models. Growth arrest caused by CCI-779 was shown to correlate with a block in translation of mRNA encoding the hypoxia-inducible factor (HIF-1α), and VHL-deficient tumours showed increased uptake of [^{18}F]FDG in an mTOR-dependent manner. Prior clinical PET studies in individuals with kidney cancer indicate that only a proportion ($\sim$50–70%) of these tumours accumulate FDG to high levels, consistent with the expected frequency of VHL loss (Hain and Maisey 2003). These findings provide preclinical data for prospective, [^{18}F]FDG PET biomarker-driven clinical studies of mTOR inhibitors in kidney cancer. It suggests that [^{18}F]FDG PET scans could be used as a pharmacodynamic marker of treatment potential as well as response. Whether imaging "surrogate markers" will be of value for assessing treatment directed at other molecular/genetic abnormalities in tumours (EGFR, p53, c-Met, HIF-1, etc.) remains to be demonstrated.

PET with [^{18}F]FDG is approved by the Center for Medicare and Medicaid Services in the United States for diagnosing, staging, and restaging lung cancer, colorectal cancer, lymphoma, melanoma, head and neck cancer, and esophageal cancer. Unfortunately, tumour cells are not the only cells that have high uptake of [^{18}F]FDG. Recently, Maschauer and co-workers have shown that endothelial cells within the tumours and vascular lesions exhibit high [^{18}F]FDG uptake, and that it correlates with enhanced by vascular endothelial growth factor (VEGF) expression. VEGF

a **Response: Time after Gleevec**

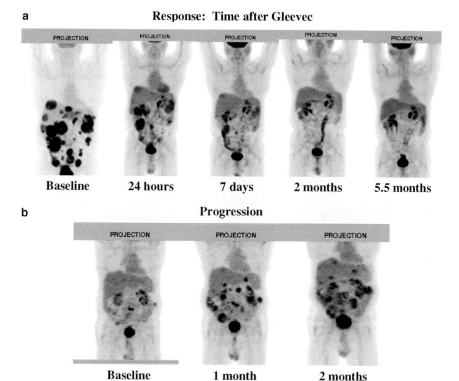

b **Progression**

Baseline   1 month   2 months

Fig. 2 [^{18}F]FDG PET imaging of GIST before and after treatment. In patients with gastrointestinal stromal tumours (GIST), tumour glucose utilisation is very high and these tumours can be readily visualised by [^{18}F]FDG PET. A striking observation in patients with GIST who are treated with STI571 (Gleevec) was the rapid and a decrease in [^{18}F]FDG uptake determined by PET scan was seen as early as 24 h after one dose of STI571, and this was sustained over many months **a**. Correspondingly, treatment failure and progression of disease can be readily monitored by [^{18}F]FDG PET **b**. The high FDG levels seen in the kidney, ureter and bladder are normal in both the pre- and post-Gleevec images. [Adapted from van den Abbeele (2001), with appreciation and permission from Dr. Annick Van den Abbeele, Dana-Farber Cancer Institute, Boston, Massachusetts]

stimulates the proliferation and migration of vascularly derived endothelial cells and it is highly expressed in a variety of tumours, including renal, breast, ovary, and colon cancer (Maschauer et al. 2004). Numerous reports have shown that lesions with a high concentration of inflammatory cells, such as neutrophils and activated macrophages, also show increased [^{18}F]FDG uptake, which can be mistaken for malignancy in patients with proven or suspected cancer (Brown et al. 1996).

[^{18}F]FDG PET has been repeatedly shown to improve staging accuracy compared with CT scanning alone, and it provides a cost-effective adjunct to the pre-operative staging of NSCLC and lung metastases (Hoekstra et al. 2003). Combined [^{18}F]FDG PET-CT imaging has been shown to be effective in demonstrating early (at 3 weeks) response (Fig. 3a) as well as failure to chemotherapy (Fig. 3b). However, in patients with adenocarcinoma and mediastinal lymph nodes of < 1 cm,

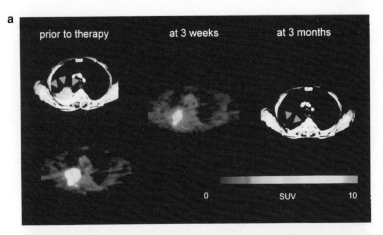

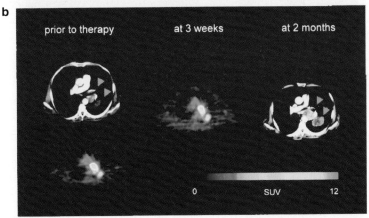

Fig. 3 [^{18}F]FDG PET imaging lung tumours before and after treatment. [^{18}F]FDG PET and CT scans of two patients with lung tumours: a responding patient **a** and a non-responding patient **b**. In the responding tumour, there is a 61% decrease in FDG uptake 3 weeks after initiation of chemotherapy. In contrast, tumour FDG uptake is essentially unchanged in the non-responding tumour. (Adapted from Weber et al. 2003)

[^{18}F]FDG PET scanning cannot yet replace mediastinoscopy (Kelly et al. 2004). This imaging modality is also having an impact on radiation therapy volume delineation in NSCLC. Radiation targeting based on fused [^{18}F]FDG PET and CT images resulted in alterations in radiation therapy planning in over 50% of patients by comparison with CT targeting (Bradley et al. 2004). [^{18}F]FDG PET is also being used to assess response to chemotherapy and may have predictive value. A reduction in metabolic activity after one cycle of chemotherapy has been shown to be correlated with final outcome of therapy (Weber et al. 2003). The use of metabolic markers to determine response may shorten the duration of phase II studies evaluating new cytotoxic drugs, and may decrease the morbidity and costs of therapy in non-responding patients.

2.2 Direct Molecular Imaging

Direct imaging strategies are usually described in terms of a specific target and a target-specific probe. This strategy has been established using nuclear, optical and MR imaging technology. The resultant image of probe localisation and concentration (signal intensity) is directly related to its interaction with the target. Imaging cell-surface-specific antigens with radiolabelled antibodies and genetically engineered antibody fragments, such as *minibodies*, are examples of direct molecular imaging that have evolved over the past 30 years. In addition, in-vivo imaging of receptor density/occupancy using small radiolabelled ligands has also been widely used, particularly in neuroscience research, over the past two decades. These examples represent some of the first molecular imaging applications used in clinical nuclear medicine research. More recent research has focused on chemistry and the synthesis of small radiolabelled or fluorescent molecules (and paramagnetic nanoparticles) that target-specific receptors (e.g. the estrogen or androgen receptors) (Dehdashti et al. 1995; Larson et al. 2004) and fluorescent probes that are activated by endogenous proteases (Jaffer et al. 2002). For example, the alpha(v)beta3 integrin is highly expressed on tumour vasculature and plays an important role in metastasis and tumour-induced angiogenesis; initial studies of targeting and imaging of the alpha(v)beta3 integrin with radiolabelled glycosylated RGD-containing peptides are very encouraging (Fig. 4) (Halbhuber and Konig 2003). Another example is direct imaging of the cell-surface-receptor tyrosine kinase HER2, which is over-expressed in many breast tumours. The level of expression of HER2 can be imaged with radiolabelled (Blend et al. 2003; Palm et al. 2003; Funovics et al. 2004) or gadolinium-chelated (Artemov et al. 2003) antibodies specific for HER2.

Other direct radiotracer imaging strategies involve the development of radiolabelled antisense and aptomer oligonucleotide probes (RASONs) that specifically hybridize to target mRNA. Some efficacy for gamma camera and PET imaging endogenous gene expression using RASONs has been reported (Dewanjee et al. 1994; Cammilleri et al. 1996; Phillips et al. 1997; Tavitian et al. 1998). Nevertheless, RASON imaging has several serious limitations, including: (1) low number of target mRNA/DNA molecules per cell; (2) limited tracer delivery (poor cell membrane, vascular and blood-brain barrier permeability); (3) poor stability; (4) slow clearance of non-bound oligonucleotides); (5) comparatively high background activity and low specificity of localisation (low target/background ratios). A further constraint limiting direct radiotracer imaging strategies is the necessity to develop a specific probe for each molecular target, and then to validate the sensitivity, specificity and safety of each probe for specific applications. This can be very time consuming and costly. For example the development, validation and regulatory approval for $[^{18}F]$FDG PET imaging of glucose utilisation in tumours has taken over 20 years.

The diagnostic potential of radiolabelled antibodies that localise specifically to tumours has been incrementally developed over three decades. Currently available antibodies (and large antibody fragments) suffer several drawbacks as radiolabelled pharmaceuticals. This is primarily related to the prolonged biological half-life of intact antibodies, leading to high background signal. A promising approach has been

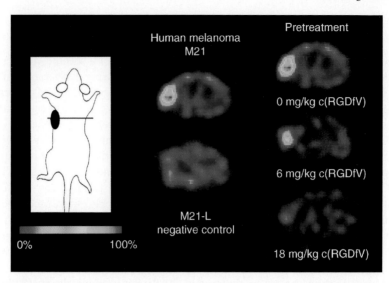

Fig. 4 Non-invasive imaging of alpha(v)beta(3) integrin expression by PET. Transaxial PET images of nude mice bearing human melanoma xenografts. Images were acquired 90 min after injection of approximately 5.5 MBq of [^{18}F]Galacto-RGD. The *top left* image shows selective accumulation of the tracer in the alpha(v)beta(3)-positve (*M21*) tumour on the left flank. No focal tracer accumulation is visible in the alpha(v)beta(3)-negative (*M21 − L*) control tumour (*bottom left image*). The three images on the *right* were obtained from serial [^{18}F]Galacto-RGD PET studies in one mouse. These images illustrate the dose-dependent blockade of tracer uptake by the alpha(v)beta(3)-selective cyclic pentapeptide cyclo (-Arg-Gly-Asp-D-Phe-Val-). (Adapted from Haubner et al. 2001)

to genetically engineer small radiolabelled antibody fragments to have high targeted localisation to a specific antigen, with low non-target binding and rapid clearance from the body. For example, a series of engineered antibody fragments was derived from the parental murine monoclonal antibody T84.66. These fragments were selected for high affinity and specificity for carcinoembryonic antigen (CEA), an antigen highly expressed in colorectal carcinoma and frequently elevated in adenocarcinomas of the lung, breast, other gastrointestinal organs, and ovary (Neumaier et al. 1990). An engineered fragment called the minibody (an scFv-C_H3 fusion protein) have been constructed, radiolabelled with ^{123}I($t_{1/2} = 13$h), and evaluated in vivo using a standard gamma camera (Wu 2004; Wu and Senter 2005). The evaluation of this minibody labelled with a positron-emitting radionuclide, copper-64 ($t_{1/2} = 6$h), was performed soon after; as expected, liver activity was elevated and this limited imaging applications to extrahepatic sites. To overcome these obstacles, later work by the same group demonstrated that radiolabelling anti-CEA minibodies and diabodies with a longer-lived positron emitter, iodine-124 ($t_{1/2} = 4$ days), resulted in excellent tumour targeting and visualisation by PET imaging at later times (1–4 days). The high target-to-background achieved in the PET images was predominantly due to low background activity following clearance of radioactivity from normal tissues (Sundaresan et al. 2003) (Fig. 5).

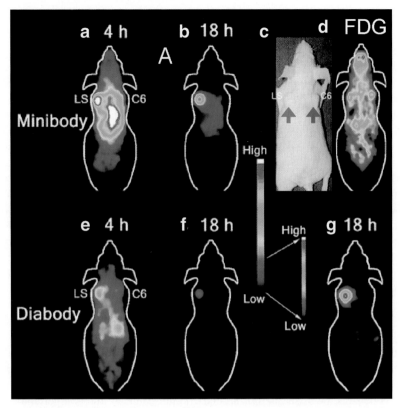

Fig. 5 Comparison of ^{124}I minibody and ^{124}I diabody by serial PET imaging. Mice bearing LS174T (LS, left shoulder) and C6 rat glioma (C6, right shoulder, negative control) xenografts were injected via tail vein with 1.9–3.1 MBq (65–85 µCi)^{124}I minibody **a, b** or diabody **e, f** and imaged at 4 and 18 h. A photograph of the mouse with *arrows* pointing to the tumours **c** and an [^{18}F]FDG microPET scan **d** show the location of the xenografts. At 18 h, background activity in the animal was minimal compared with the 4-h images, resulting in high contrast. **a, b, e** and **f** are colour-coded to the same radioactivity scale. Image **f** was rescaled in **g** to illustrate the excellent contrast achieved with the ^{124}I diabody at 18 h. (Adapted from Sundaresan et al. 2003)

Another example of this approach is the development of anti-p185^{HER2} mini-bodies. These minibodies have high specific binding to p185^{HER2}-positive cells in vitro. One variant was radioiodinated and evaluated for its blood clearance, tumour-targeting properties, and normal organ uptake of the radiolabel in nude mice bearing p185^{HER2}-positive xenografts. The anti-p185^{HER2} 10H8 minibody showed the expected blood clearance, but the tumour activity reached a maximum of only $5.6 \pm 1.7\%$ ID/g at 12 h. Tumour localisation and persistence was substantially less than that previously observed with the radioiodinated anti-CEA minibody, and illustrates the variability in the kinetics of minibody targeting and biodistribution in different tumours. These differences were thought to be partially due to some combination of internalization, metabolism and dehalogenation of the minibody fragment (Olafsen et al. 2005).

Recent developments in MR imaging have enabled direct in-vivo imaging at high resolution ($\sim 50\,\mu m$) (Johnson 1993; Jacobs 1999). This approach is largely based on labelling cells with superparamagnetic iron oxide (SPIO) particles that permit visualisation and tracking of cells using MRI based on the large suscepti- bility artefacts (T_2^*-effect) produced by iron oxide (Bulte et al. 2004). The SPIO particles range between 50 and 100 nm in diameter and two characteristics in par- ticular make superparamagnetic nanoparticle/MR imaging a technique with broad applications. First, methods have been developed for efficient SPIO cell labelling. Either nanaoparticles are being coated with a dendrimer that confers membrane permeability or a SPIO, such as Feredex, is transfected into cells by means of transfection reagents. Importantly, these passive labelling strategies are applicable to many different cell types, including resting stem cells. The utility of this ap- proach is further underscored by recent efforts at clinical development; as Arbab et al. (2004) have described, a SPIO-based labelling preparation consisting of FDA approved materials. As an alternate labelling strategy, superparamagnetic nanopar- ticles can be modified with a TAT peptide, which facilitates transport across the cell membrane (Lewin et al. 2000). Second, in most cell types there is, thus far, little ev- idence of toxicity related to labelling. Recent work, however, suggested an adverse influence of the iron oxide label specifically on chondrocyte differentiation on mes- enchymal progenitor cells, but an independent study could not confirm this finding (Kostura et al. 2004; Arbab et al. 2005). Since experimental conditions were differ- ent between those studies, no general conclusions can be derived as yet and further investigations are necessary. In addition to SPIO particles, micrometer-size particles harboring iron oxide (MPIOs) are available; they feature cell uptake through an inert divinyl benzene polymer shell of around 900-nm diameter and a larger amount of iron oxide per particle compared with SPIOs (Hinds et al. 2003).

The application of superparamagnetic nanoparticle/MR imaging is increasing and recent studies included imaging migration of locally injected iron oxide-labelled stem cells in the rat brain (Hoehn et al. 2002). Migration was also studied by Dodd et al. (2001), who imaged murine T-cells homing to the spleen. Although a clear reduction in signal intensity in the spleen was observed, the duration of the lat- ter study did not exceed a 24-h period. A similar study reported that OVA-specific T-cells labelled with iron oxide nanoparticles migrated to and accumulated in an OVA-expressing melanoma xenograft over a period of 5 days (Kircher 2003). These labelling techniques clearly improved imaging the initial phase of T-cell migration following the adoptive transfer of the labelled lymphoid cells to sites providing a supportive microenvironment. However, ex-vivo labelling of T-cells with MR con- trast is only transient and does not provide an opportunity to monitor their functional status, such as activation upon antigen recognition, cytokine secretion, proliferation and cytolytic functions. Nevertheless, MR imaging of iron oxide in general has re- cently been demonstrated to be of great clinical value (Harisinghani et al. 2003). As illustrated in Fig. 6, a clinical trial of MRI post systemic injection of lymphotropic nanocrystalline iron oxide in 33 patients affected by prostate cancer showed supe- rior detection of lymph-node metastases compared with conventional proton MRI (Harisinghani et al. 2003).

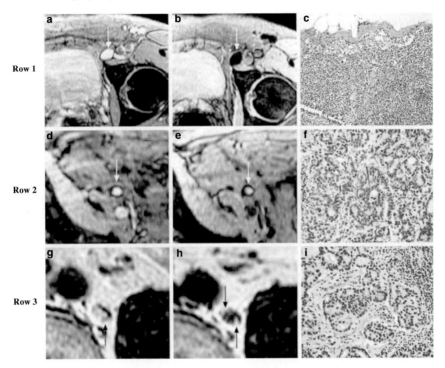

Fig. 6 a–i Non-invasive detection of clinically occult lymph-node metastases in prostate cancer by MRI using lymphotropic superparamagnetic nanoparticles. *Row 1:* Compared with conventional MRI **a**, MRI obtained 24 h after the administration of lymphotropic superparamagnetic nanoparticles **b** shows a homogeneous decrease in signal intensity due to the accumulation of lymphotropic superparamagnetic nanoparticles in a normal lymph node in the left iliac region (*arrow*). Panel **c** shows the corresponding histological findings of the normal lymph node (hematoxylin and eosin, ×125). *Row 2:* Conventional MRI shows high signal intensity in an unenlarged iliac lymph node completely replaced by tumour (*arrow* in **d**). Nodal signal intensity remains high indicated infiltration of tumour (*arrow* in **e**). Panel **f** shows the corresponding histologic findings and confirms the presence of tumour within the node (hematoxylin and eosin, ×200). *Row 3:* Conventional MRI shows high signal intensity in a retroperitoneal node with micrometastases (*arrow* in **g**). MRI with lymphotropic superparamagnetic nanoparticles demonstrates two hyperintense foci (*arrows* in **h**) within the node, corresponding to 2-mm metastases. Corresponding histological analysis confirms the presence of adenocarcinoma within the node (**i** hematoxylin and eosin, ×200). (Adapted from Harisinghani et al. 2003)

2.3 Indirect Molecular Imaging

Indirect imaging strategies are a little more complex. One example of indirect imaging that is now being widely used is reporter gene imaging. It requires "pre-targeting" (delivery) of the reporter gene to the target tissue (by transfection/transduction), and it usually includes transcriptional control components that can function as "molecular genetic sensors" that initiate reporter gene expression. This strategy has been widely applied in optical- (Contag et al. 1998; Rehemtulla et al. 2000; Hoffman 2005) and radionuclide-based imaging (Tjuvajev et al. 1995b, 1996, 1998; Gambhir et al. 1998, 1999), and to a lesser degree for MR (Weissleder et al. 1997; Louie et al. 2000) imaging. Early reporter gene imaging approaches required post-mortem tissue sampling and processing (Overbeek et al. 1985; Forss-Petter et al. 1990), but more recent studies have emphasised non-invasive imaging techniques involving live animals and human subjects (Halbhuber and Konig 2003).

A general paradigm for non-invasive reporter gene imaging using radiolabelled probes was initially described in 1995 (Tjuvajev et al. 1995b) and is shown diagrammatically in Fig. 7. A simplified cartoon of a reporter gene is shown in Fig. 7a, and a representation of different reporter genes for imaging transduced cells is shown in Fig. 7b. This paradigm requires the appropriate combination of a reporter transgene and a reporter probe. The reporter transgene can encode a receptor [e.g. hD2R (human dopamine D2 receptor; Liang et al. 2001) and hSSTR2 (human somatostatin receptors; Rogers et al. 2000)], or a transporter [e.g. hNIS (human sodium iodide symporter; Haberkorn 2001) and hNET (human norepinephrine transporter; Altmann et al. 2003)], or a fluorescent protein [e.g. eGFP (enhanced green fluorescent protein; Chishima et al. 1997)] in addition to an enzyme, such as HSV1-tk (herpes simplex virus type 1 thymidine kinase; Tjuvajev et al. 1995b) [Fig. 7a (a), (b)] or luciferase (Contag et al. 1997) [Fig. 7a (a), (c)]. The reporter transgene usually codes for an enzyme, receptor or transporter that selectively interacts with a specific

---

Fig. 7 a Structure of a reporter gene construct and the indirect reporter imaging paradigm. The basic structure of a reporter gene complex is shown, expressing either HSV1-tk or luciferase. The control and regulation of gene expression is performed through promoter and enhancer regions that are located at the 5' end ("up-stream") of the reporter gene. These promoter/enhancer elements can be "constitutive" and result in continuous gene expression ("always on"), or they can be "inducible" and sensitive to activation by endogenous transcription factors and promoters. Following the initiation of transcription and translation, the gene product — a protein — accumulates. b In this case the reporter gene product is the enzyme HSV1-tk, which phosphorylates selected thymidine analogues (e.g. FIAU or FHBG), whereas these probes are not phosphorylated by endogenous mammalian TK1. The phosphorylated probe does not cross the cell membrane readily; it is effectively "trapped" and accumulates is within transduced cells. Thus, the magnitude of probe accumulation in the cell (level of radioactivity) reflects the level of HSV1-tk enzyme activity and level of *HSV1-tk* reporter gene expression. c In this case, luciferase is the reporter gene product and expression is detected via its catalytic action resulting in production of bioluminescence. b Different reporter systems. The reporter gene complex is transfected into target cells by a vector (e.g. a virus). Inside the transfected cell, the reporter gene may or may not be integrated into the host-cell genome; transcription of the reporter gene to mRNA is initiated by "constitutive" or "inducible" promoters, and translation of the mRNA to a protein occurs on the ribosomes. The reporter gene product can be a cytoplasmic or nuclear enzyme, a transporter in the cell membrane, a receptor at the cell surface or part of cytoplasmic or nuclear complex, an artificial cell surface antigen, or a fluorescent protein. Often, a complimentary reporter probe (e.g. a radiolabelled, magnetic or bioluminescent molecule) is given and the probe concentrates (or emits light) at the site of reporter gene expression. The level of probe concentration (or intensity of light) is usually proportional to the level reporter gene product and can reflect several processes, including the level of transcription, the modulation and regulation of translation, protein-protein interactions, and post-translational regulation of protein conformation and degradation

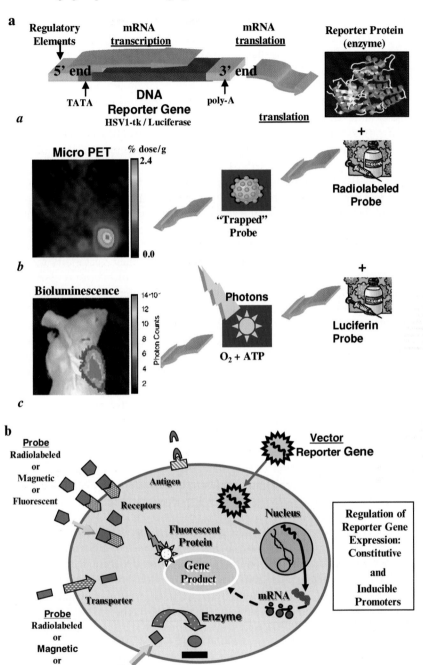

radiolabelled probe and results in its accumulation only in transduced cells. Alternatively, the enzyme (e.g. luciferase) will catalyse a reaction to yield light (photons) in the presence of substrate (e.g. luciferin, ATP and oxygen for firefly luciferase). Alternatively, the reporter gene product can be a fluorescent protein that can be imaged in vivo as well as ex vivo.

It may be helpful to consider the HSV1-tk reporter imaging paradigm as an example of an in-vivo radiotracer assay that reflects reporter gene expression [Fig. 7a (a), (b)]. Enzymatic amplification of the signal (e.g. level of radioactivity accumulation) facilitates imaging the location and magnitude of reporter gene expression. Viewed from this perspective, HSV1-tk reporter gene imaging with radiolabelled FIAU or FHBG is similar to imaging hexokinase activity with FDG. It is important to note that imaging transgene expression is largely independent of the vector used to shuttle the reporter gene into the cells of the target tissue; namely, any of several currently available vectors can be used (e.g. retrovirus, adenovirus, adeno-associated virus, lentivirus, liposomes, etc.).

A common feature of all reporter constructs (and their vectors) is the cDNA expression cassette containing the reporter transgene(s) of interest (e.g. *HSV1-tk*), which can be placed under the control of specific promoter-enhancer elements. The upstream promoter-enhancer elements can be used to regulate transcription of the reporter cDNA. The versatility of reporter constructs (and their vectors) is due in part to their modular design, since arrangements in the expression cassette can be varied to some extent. For example, reporter genes can be "always turned on" by constitutive promoters (such as *LTR, RSV, CMV, PGK, EF1*, etc.) and used to monitor cell trafficking by identifying the location, migration, targeting and proliferation of stably transduced cells. Reporter gene labelling provides the opportunity for repetitive imaging and sequential monitoring of tumour growth rate and response to treatment (Rehemtulla et al. 2000), as well as imaging metastases (Chishima et al. 1997). Alternatively, the promoter/enhancer elements can be constructed to be "inducible" and "sensitive" to activation and regulation by specific endogenous transcription factors and promoters (factors that bind to and activate specific enhancer elements in the promoter region of the reporter vector construct leading to the initiation of reporter gene transcription).

Considerable progress in reporter gene imaging has been achieved during the past 5 years. Important proof-of-principle experiments in small animals include the imaging of endogenous regulation of transcription (Doubrovin et al. 2001; Iyer et al. 2001b; Ponomarev et al. 2001), post-transcriptional modulation of translation (Mayer-Kuckuk et al. 2002), protein-protein interactions (Luker et al. 2002, 2003b; Ray et al. 2002), protein degradation and activity of the proteosomal ubiquination pathway (Luker et al. 2003a), apoptosis (Laxman et al. 2002), etc. Non-invasive imaging of viral (Gambhir et al. 1999; Tjuvajev et al. 1999), bacterial (Tjuvajev et al. 2001) and cell trafficking (Koehne et al. 2003), plus tissue-specific reporter gene imaging in prostate cancer (Zhang et al. 2002), hepatocytes (Green et al. 2002) and colorectal cancer cells have also been reported (Qiao et al. 2002).

2.3.1 Radiotracer Reporter Gene Imaging

HSV1-tk is the most widely used reporter gene for radiotracer-based molecular imaging, and has been used as a therapeutic "suicide" gene in clinical anti-cancer gene therapy trials as well as a research tool in gene targeting strategies. The HSV1-tk enzyme, like mammalian thymidine kinases, phosphorylates thymidine to thymidine-monophosphate (TdR). Unlike mammalian TK1, viral HSV1-tk can also phosphorylate modified thymidine analogues, including 2′-deoxy-2′-fluoro-5-iodo-1-[β]-D-arabinofuranosyluracil (FIAU), 2′-fluoro-5-ethyl-1-[β]-D-arabinofuranosyl-uracil (FEAU) as well as acycloguanosine analogs [e.g. acyclovir (ACV); ganciclovir (GCV); penciclovir (PCV)] that are not (or minimally) phosphorylated by eukaryotic thymidine kinases (Tjuvajev et al. 1995b). The resulting monophos-phorylated compound is subsequently diphosphorylated and triphosphorylated by cellular kinases. The triphosphorylated compound can act as an inhibitor of DNA-polymerization, resulting in chain termination during DNA replication, leading to cell death. For this reason, *HSV1-tk* has been studied extensively as a therapeutic gene and used in gene therapy clinical trials that have been performed in the United States and Europe.

Several important issues were raised during these trials, including whether the viral transduction of the target tissue has been successful; what level of transgene expression is achieved in the target tissue; and what is the optimal time for beginning ganciclovir treatment. Another important clinical issue is monitoring for potential toxicity. Imaging the distribution and expression level of the therapeutic gene in non-target normal tissues provides a level of safety in individual patients undergoing gene therapy.

In the mid 1990s, a number of potential reporter probes for imaging *HSV1-tk* gene expression were studied in our laboratory (Tjuvajev et al. 1995b, 1996, 1998). After in-vitro determinations of HSV1-tk sensitivity and selectivity for FIAU, this compound was found to have good imaging potential and can be radiolabelled with a variety of radionuclides (^{11}C, ^{124}I, ^{18}F^{131}I, ^{123}I). FIAU contains a 2′-fluoro substitu-tion in the sugar that impedes cleavage of the N-glycosidic bond by nucleoside phos-phorylases. This results in a significant prolongation of the nucleoside in plasma and an increase in delivery of non-degraded radiolabelled tracer to the target tissues. The first series of imaging experiments involving *HSV1-tk*-transduced tissue and FIAU were performed in rats bearing intracerebral (i.c.) RG2 tumours using quantitative autoradiography (QAR) techniques (Tjuvajev et al. 1995a) (Fig. 8a). This was sub-sequently followed by gamma camera, single photon emission computed tomogra-phy (SPECT) (Fig. 8b) and positron emission tomography (PET) imaging studies (Fig. 8c). Other pyrimidine nucleoside probes for imaging viral thymidine kinase acitivity have been proposed (Fig. 9a).

Investigators from UCLA have used other radiolabelled compounds for PET imaging of HSV1-tk expression with the goal of developing methods for repeti-tive imaging (every 6–8 h) of the reporter protein. Their choice of acycloguano-sine derivatives as reporter probes was based on the ability of these nucleosides to be radiolabelled with short-lived fluorine-18 $\left(t_{1/2} = 110\,\text{min}\right)$ and no affinity to

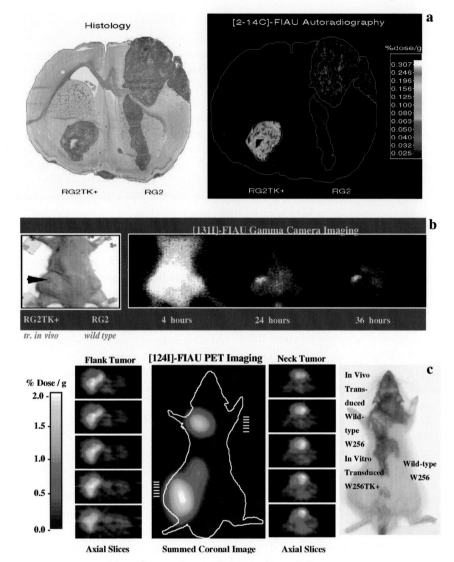

the mammalian TK-1. A list of ^{18}F-labelled acycloguanosine analogues is shown in Fig. 9b. After several years of comparative studies (Fyfe et al. 1978; Gambhir et al. 1998; Iyer et al. 2001a), a new radiolabelled acycloguanine, 9-(4-[18F]fluoro-3-hydroxymethylbutyl)guanine or [18F]FHBG (FHBG) (Alauddin and Conti 1998; Yaghoubi et al. 2001) was developed at USC. In parallel, the UCLA investigators evaluated a mutant HSV1-tk enzyme (HSV1-sr39tk) with increased acyclovir and ganciclovir suicidal efficacy. They showed higher affinity and uptake of [18F]FHBG in HSV1-sr39tk transduced cells (Gambhir et al. 2000a). The mutant, HSV1-sr39TK, enhances [18F]FHBG uptake by twofold compared with wild-type

Fig. 8 a Autoradiographic imaging HSV1-tk expression. A rat brain with a stably transduced RG2TK+ brain tumour in the left hemisphere and a wild-type (non-transduced) RG2 tumour in the right hemisphere is shown. The histology and autoradiographic images were generated from the same tissue section. Both tumours are clearly seen in the toluidine blue-stained histological section. Twenty four hours after i.v. administration of [^{14}C]FIAU, the RG2TK$^+$ tumour is clearly visualised in the autoradiographic image, whereas the RG2 tumour is barely detectable; the surrounding brain is at background levels. (Adapted from Tjuvajev et al. 1995b). **b** Gamma-camera imaging HSV1-tk expression. Gamma-camera imaging was performed at 4, 24 and 36 h after [^{131}I]FIAU injection in an animals bearing bilateral RG2 flank xenografts; all images have been normalised to a reference standard (not shown in the field of view). The site of inoculation of HSV1-*tk* retroviral vector producer cells (gp-STK-A2) into the left flank xenograft is indicated by the *arrow*. The sequential images demonstrate wash-out of radioactivity from the body, with specific retention of activity in the area of gp-STK-A2 cell inoculation and transduction of RG2 tumour cells with the HSV1-tk reporter (see the 24- and 36-h images; readjustment of the pseudocolour-intensity scale demonstrated visualisation or the gp-STK-A2 flank tumour at 4 h, although background activity was high). The non-transduced contralateral xenograft (right flank) and other tissues did not show any retention of radioactivity. This sequence of images demonstrates the advantages of a "wash-out strategy" and late imaging with [^{131}I] – or [^{124}I]-labelled FIAU. Figure adapted from Tjuvajev et al. 1996 (Tjuvajev et al. 1996). **c** PET imaging of HSV1-tk expression. Three tumours were produced in rnu rats. A W256TK$^+$ (positive control) tumour was produced from stably transduced W256TK$^+$ cells and is located in the left flank, and two wild-type W256 tumours were produced in the dorsum of the neck (test) and in the right flank (negative control). The neck tumour was inoculated with 10^6 gp-STK-A2 vector-producer cells (retroviral titre: 10^6–10^7 cfu/ml) to induce HSV1-*tk* transduction of the tumour wild-type in vivo. Fourteen days after gp-STK-A2 cell inoculation, no carrier added [^{124}I]FIAU (25 µCi) was injected i.v. and PET imaging was performed 30 h later. Localisation of radioactivity is clearly seen in left flank tumour (positive control) and in the in-vivo transduced neck tumour (test), but only low background levels of radioactivity were observed in the right flank tumour wild-type (negative control). (Adapted from Tjuvajev et al. 1998)

HSV1-tk, thus improving the imaging capabilities of the enzyme. However, differences exist between the sensitivity and specificity of [^{124}I]FIAU and [^{18}F]FHBG with respect to wild-type HSV1-tk (Tjuvajev et al. 2002) and HSV1-sr39tk (Min et al. 2003).

One example of a reporter system involving a transporter is the sodium iodide symporter (NIS). Since cloning of the *NIS* gene in 1996 (Dai et al. 1996), *NIS* was considered an attractive imaging reporter gene (Dai et al. 1996; Boland et al. 2000). There are several distinct advantages for using *NIS* as a reporter gene. First, the distribution of endogenous NIS protein is limited in the body (thyroid and stomach are major exceptions); as a result, imaging of exogenous *NIS* gene expression can be performed in a variety of tissues due to low background activity. Second, NIS mediates the uptake of simple radiopharmaceuticals; therefore, complicated syntheses and labelling of substrate molecules are not required for imaging. Third, most of the radiotracers are specific only to NIS-expressing cells; therefore, background signal is significantly reduced. Fourth, NIS-mediated radiotracer uptake in target tissue is rapid, as is the clearance of radioactivity from both target and non-target tissues; this facilitates repetitive sequential imaging. Fifth, the human and murine genes of NIS have been cloned, which provides a non-immunogenic reporter system for human as well as rodent imaging studies.

a

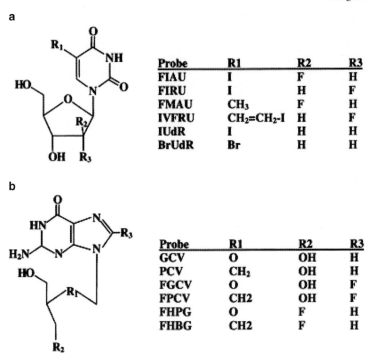

Probe	R1	R2	R3
FIAU	I	F	H
FIRU	I	H	F
FMAU	CH₃	F	H
IVFRU	CH₂=CH₂-I	H	F
IUdR	I	H	H
BrUdR	Br	H	H

b

Probe	R1	R2	R3
GCV	O	OH	H
PCV	CH₂	OH	H
FGCV	O	OH	F
FPCV	CH2	OH	F
FHPG	O	F	H
FHBG	CH2	F	H

Fig. 9 a, b Substrates for HSV1-tk phosphorylation. **a** Pyrimidine nucleosides. **b** Acycloguanosine analogues. (Adapted from Tjuvajev et al. 2002)

An application of *hNIS* as a reporter gene was demonstrated by gamma-camera imaging myocardial gene transfer in living rats using adenoviral vectors and radioiodide (Shin et al. 2004). In this study, an adenovirus that expressed both NIS protein and enhanced green fluorescent protein (EGFP) (Ad.EGFP.NIS) was injected into the myocardium of living rats. Following ^{123}I scintigraphy demonstrated clear focal myocardial uptake at the Ad.EGFP.NIS injection site. Histological analysis confirmed the co-localisation of ^{123}I radioactivity, EGFP fluorescence and NIS staining. To develop a molecular imaging method suitable for monitoring viable cancer cells, another dual-imaging reporter gene system was constructed from two individual reporter genes — sodium iodide symporter (NIS) and luciferase (Lee et al. 2005). In parallel, our group has developed a self-inactivating retroviral vector containing a dual-reporter gene cassette (*hNIS-IRES2-GFP*) with the *hNIS* and *GFP* genes, separated by an internal ribosomal entry site (IRES) element; the expression cassette was driven by a constitutive CMV promoter. A stably transduced rat glioma (RG2) cell line was generated with this construct and used for in-vitro and in-vivo imaging studies of ^{131}I-iodide and $^{99\,m}$TcO$_4$-pertechnetate accumulation, as well as GFP fluorescence. The experiments demonstrated a high correlation between the expression of hNIS and GFP. Gamma-camera imaging studies performed on RG2 *hNIS-IRES2-GFP* tumour-bearing mice revealed that the *IRES*-linked dual reporter gene is functional and stable (Che et al. 2005).

The first successful reporter gene imaging study in patients was performed in Cologne using a *HSV1-tk* liposomal vector, [^{124}I]FIAU and PET to monitor *HSV1-tk* suicide gene therapy of high-grade brain tumours (Jacobs et al. 2001b). *HSV1-tk* gene expression was visualised in only one of six patients who received an intra-tumoural injection of the vector (Fig. 10.). Later on, [^{18}F]FHBG was studied in normal human volunteers and the biodistribution, bio-safety, and dosimetry was determined; it was found to be safe and potentially useful for human applications (Yaghoubi et al. 2005). More recently, the HSV1-sr39tk/[^{18}F]FHBG PET imaging system has been used to monitor thymidine kinase gene expression after intra-tumoural injection of the first-generation recombinant adenovirus in patients with hepatocellular carcinoma (Penuelas et al. 2005). Transgene expression in the tumour was dependent on the injected dose of the adenovirus and was detectable by PET during the first hours after administration of the radiotracer in all patients, who received $\geq 10^{12}$ viral particles (Fig. 10b). Non-specific expression of the transgene was not detected in any distant organs, or in the surrounding liver tissue in any of these studied cases. These results illustrate that PET imaging may help in the design of gene-therapy strategies and in the clinical assessment of new-generation vectors. Non-invasive monitoring of the distribution of transgene expression over

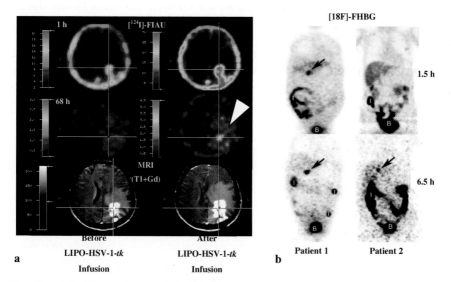

Fig. 10 a *HSV1-tk* reporter gene imaging in patients after liposome-*HSV1-tk*-complex transduction. Co-registration of [^{124}I]FIAU-PET and MRI before (*left column*) and after (*right column*) *HSV1-tk* vector application. A region of specific [^{124}I]FIAU retention (at 68 h) within the tumour is visualized (*white arrow*). This tumour region showed signs of necrosis (*cross hairs, right column*) after ganciclovir treatment. (Adapted from Jacobs et al. 2001b). **b** Adenoviral transgene (*HSV1-tksr39*) expression in patients with liver cancer. Coronal PET images 1.5 and 6.5 h after injection of [^{18}F]-FHBG (48 h after 2×10^{12} AdV-*tk*). Localisation of [^{18}F]-FHBG in the treated lesion was variable in the early images, but could be seen at 6.5 h in all patients (*arrow*). (Adapted from Penuelas et al. 2005)

time is highly desirable and will have a critical impact on the development of standardised gene therapy protocols and on efficient and safe vector applications in human beings. It is most likely that [124I]FIAU and [18F]FHBG will be the radiolabelled probes that will be introduced into the clinic for the imaging of *HSV1-tk* gene expression.

2.3.2 Optical-reporter gene imaging

Optical (bioluminescence and fluorescence) reporter systems have received increased attention recently, because of their efficiency for sequential imaging, operational simplicity, and substantial cost benefits.

Bioluminescence reporter genes

Bioluminescence reporter genes are being widely used for whole-body imaging in small animals. Luciferin and luciferase are generic terms, but not all luciferases exhibit sequence homology between the different classes. The most commonly used bioluminescence reporter systems include the firefly (FLuc) or *Renilla* (RLuc) luciferase genes (Yu et al. 2003). Useful luciferases have also been cloned from jellyfish (*Aequorea*), sea copepod (*Gaussia*; GLuc), corals (*Tenilla*), click beetle (*Pyrophorus plagiophthalamus*) and several bacterial species (*Vibrio fischeri, V. harveyi*). As with nuclear and magnetic resonance reporter systems, bioluminescence imaging depends on the delivery of a specific substrate to the reporter gene expressing cells. Further, the light emitting bioluminescence reaction catalysed by luciferases depends on the presence of oxygen (Wilson and Hastings 1998) and, for example, in the case of FLuc, additionally on the co-factor ATP. The firefly and *Renilla* luciferase reporter systems, in combination with their corresponding luminescent substrates (luciferin and coelenterazine), have several advantages for imaging small living animals. Autobioluminescence in most cases is essentially non-existent and results in very low background light emission; this contributes to the very high sensitivity and specificity of this optical imaging technique (Bhaumik and Gambhir 2002; Wu et al. 2002). Semi-quantitative accuracy and reproducibility requires that the luciferin, ATP and oxygen levels are *not* rate determining, but rather are in excess. Under these conditions, the photon emission flux (light intensity) is directly related to reporter gene expression and the level of reporter gene product; namely, luciferase. Another potential concern is the fact that the substrate for *Renilla* luciferase, coelenterazine, is a substrate for the MDR1 transporter. It has recently been shown that coelenterazine is rapidly exported from cell lines that express MDR1, and this could impact on the photon emission flux from the coelenterazine-*Renilla* luciferase reporter system in these cells (Pichler et al. 2004). In-vivo bioluminescence imaging has been successfully applied to monitor the growth of individual tumours (Fig. 11) and to assess the function of many novel reporter systems (see below). However, care must be exercised when comparing

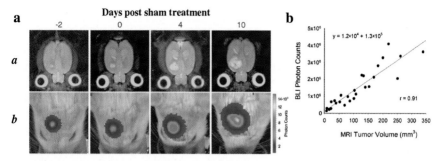

Fig. 11 a, b Kinetics of intracranial glioma growth. **a** 9L^{Luc} cells were implanted intracerebrally and tumour progression was monitored with MRI (*row a*) and BLI (*row b*). The days of post-sham treatment on which the images were obtained are indicated at the *top*. The MR images are T$_2$-weighted and are of a representative slice from the multislice dataset. **b** The *scale to the right* of the BL images describes the colour map for luminescent signal. Correlation of tumour volume with in vivo photon emission is shown where tumour volume was measured from T$_2$-weighted MR images and plotted against total measured photon counts. The relationship between the two measurements was defined by regression analysis ($r = 0.91$). (Adapted from Rehemtulla et al. 2000)

different tumours (or sites of bioluminescence) because of the significant loss of signal due to the scatter and absorption of emitted photons that can vary over several logs with distance from the surface and tissue type (e.g. lung vs liver vs bone).

Fluorescent protein-based reporter systems

Fluorescent protein-based reporter systems have also become very popular during the 1990s, especially for in-vitro and embryogenesis studies. For example, green fluorescent protein (GFP) has evolved from a little known protein to a common widely used tool in molecular biology and cell biology. It started with different spectral shifted variants of *Aequorea victoria* GFP (*GFP*), including an enhanced GFP (*eGFP*) (Levy et al. 1996; Lalwani et al. 1997; Ellenberg et al. 1999; Matz et al. 1999; Falk and Lauf 2001; Hadjantonakis and Nagy 2001; Labas et al. 2002). These GFP variants are particularly useful because of their stability and the fact that the chromophore is formed by autocatalytic cyclization. Furthermore, it appears that fusion of GFP to other proteins does not significantly alter its fluorescence properties or the intracellular location of the fusion protein (Ponomarev et al. 2003, 2004). A number of red fluorescent proteins including *Discosoma species* (*dsRed1* and *dsRed2*) (Campbell et al. 2002; Mathieu and El-Battari 2003) and *Heteractis crispa* (*HcRed*) (Gurskaya et al. 2001) have also been described. Employing DsRed as a genetically encoded fusion tag has been limited because of two critical problems: obligate tetramerization and incomplete maturation. Several attempts have been made to overcome these shortcomings, including genetic modification and creation of DsRed2 and DsRed-Express (T1) proteins. Significant progress has been achieved in resolving the problem of tetramerization by transforming DsRed

into a far-red dimer, HcRed1, which was generated on the basis of the chromopro-
tein from *Heteractis crispa* (Gurskaya et al. 2001). Roger Y. Tsien's group have
presented the step-wise evolution of DsRed to a dimer and then either to a genetic
fusion of two copies of the protein, i.e. a tandem dimer, or to a true monomer,
designated mRFP1 (monomeric red fluorescent protein) (Campbell et al. 2002). Recently, the same group has reported on the development of a novel mutant mRFP
monomeric fluorescent protein called mPlum with an emission wavelength 649 nm,
which is 37 nm longer than the peak of the original mRFP and 12 nm beyond the
previous tandem dimer t-HcRed1 (Wang et al. 2004).

Fluorescence imaging has been shown to be useful for various in-vitro applications, such as: (1) monitoring the gene expression, (2) tracking of the protein of
interest: its expression, localisation, movement, interaction and functional activity
within the cell, (3) identifying and selecting cells by FACS analysis and sorting
(e.g. expression of p53 in tissue sections at the microscopic level by in-situ fluorescence imaging (Doubrovin et al. 2001), (4) tracking the movement of labelled cells,
proteins and different organelles using photoswitchable proteins (Chudakov et al.
2004) and (5) for cost-effective in-vitro assays that can be used to validate the function and sensitivity of inducible reporter systems containing multi-modality reporter
genes (see below).

The brightness of all fluorescent proteins is determined by several variable factors, including the speed and efficiency of protein folding and maturation, the ex-
tinction coefficient, quantum yield and photostability of the protein, as well as the
optical properties of the imaging set-up and camera. Genetically modified fluorescent proteins can be optimised for mammalian cells with good expression at 37° C
(Fig. 12) (Shaner et al. 2004), whereas other proteins may fold less efficiently or
be rapidly degraded. Experiments in bacteria and mammalian cells have shown that
chaperones can have a substantial effect on the folding and maturation efficiency
of fluorescent proteins. An additional factor affecting the maturation of fluorescent proteins in living organisms is the presence or absence of molecular oxygen.
Fluorescence is usually prevented or reduced under anoxic conditions, although
fluorescence persists under hypoxia conditions (Shaner et al. 2005). Many wild-
type fluorescent proteins have tetrameric structures which can cause the protein aggregation and toxicity. More recently engineered monomers or tandem dimers of
tetrameric fluorescent proteins have been shown to be less toxic and more suitable
for mammalian cell studies. There are some genetically modified proteins that very
bright [e.g. mPlum, mCherry, and Emerald proteins (Shaner et al. 2005)]. Although
the present set of fluorescent proteins gives researchers a variety of options in their
studies, there is still room for improvement. In the future, monomeric proteins with
greater brightness and photostability will allow for more intensive imaging experiments in thick tissue and whole animals.

Limitations of fluorescence reporter imaging include the requirement for an
external source of light and the exponentially decreasing intensity of light with
increasing depth of the target. Endogenous autofluorescence of tissues frequently
results in substantial background emissions that limit the sensitivity and specificity
of fluorescence imaging techniques, and this contributes to an important advantage

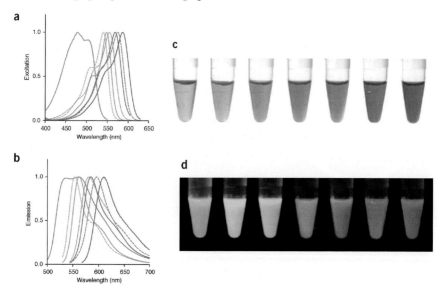

Fig. 12 a–d Excitation and emission spectra for new red fluorescent protein (RFP) variants. Spectra are normalised to the excitation and emission peak for each protein. Excitation **a** and emission **b** curves are shown as *solid or dashed lines* for monomeric variants and as a *dotted line* for dTomato and tdTomato, with colours corresponding to the colour of each variant. Purified proteins (*from left to right:* mHoneydew, mBanana, mOrange, tdTomato, mTangerine, mStrawberry, and mCherry) are shown in visible light **c** and fluorescence **d**. The fluorescence image is a composite of several images with excitation ranging from 480 to 560 nm. (Adapted from Shaner et al. 2004)

of bioluminescence over fluorescence reporters. However, the use of selective filters or the application of spectral analysis can significantly reduce the contribution of autofluorescence to the acquired images. Nevertheless, in-vivo bioluminescence reporter imaging remains more sensitive than in-vivo fluorescence reporter imaging.

Luciferase may be well suited to monitor transcription; due to its relatively fast induction (Kolb et al. 2000) and to the considerable short biological half-life of luciferin and luciferase (Thompson et al. 1991). This is an advantage compared with the longer-lived eGFP. However, short-lived (rapidly degradable) variants of eGFP have been recently developed, and eGFP can be used for higher resolution imaging in cells in vitro. Combining these reporter genes into a single gene could provide additional tools for the analysis of cancer cells in vivo and ex vivo. Such a dual-function reporter gene was created and the single encoded protein was shown to be fluorescent and bioluminescent.

Multi-modality nuclear and optical reporter imaging

The coupling of a nuclear reporter gene (e.g. *HSV1-tk*) with an optical reporter gene (e.g. *eGFP*) has been reported (Jacobs et al. 2001a). More recently, a series of HSV1-tk/eGFP mutants were developed with altered nuclear localisation

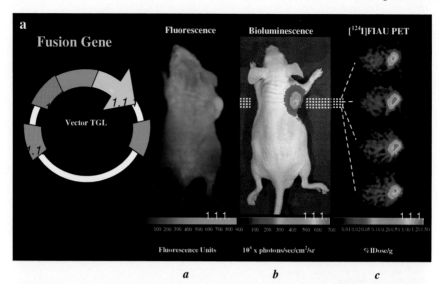

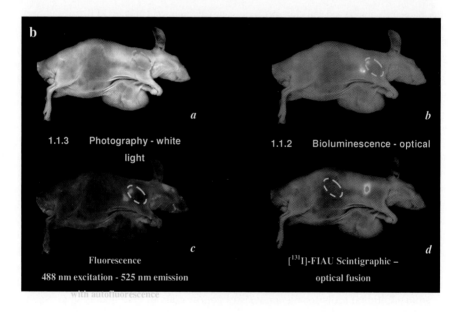

and better cellular enzymatic activity to optimise the sensitivity for imaging *HSV1-tk/eGFP* reporter gene expression (Ponomarev et al. 2003). The *HSV1-tk/eGFP* reporter gene has been introduced into several different reporter systems to assess different molecular pathways (Doubrovin et al. 2001; Ponomarev et al. 2001). Furthermore, a mutant thymidine kinase (HSV1-sr39tk)/*Renilla* luciferase (RL) fusion reporter construct $(tk_{20}rl)$ was recently developed for both nuclear and optical imaging (Ray et al. 2003). This study demonstrated the specificity and sensitivity of

Fig. 13 a, b Non-invasive multimodality imaging. **a** Non-invasive, multimodality imaging of mice bearing subcutaneous xenografts produced from nesHSV1-tk/eGFP-cmvFluc transduced U87 cells (right shoulder) and wild-type (non-transduced) U87 cells (left shoulder). Whole-body fluorescence imaging (*a*), whole-body bioluminescence imaging (*b*), and axial microPET images of [^{124}I]FIAU accumulation obtained at the levels indicated by the *dotted white lines* (*c*) are shown for the same mouse. (Adapted from Ponomarev et al. 2004). **b** Sequential images of a different mouse were obtained on a Kodak R2000MM multimodal imaging system. A white light photograph was initially obtained showing a small nesHSV1-tk/eGFP-cmvFluc transduced U87 xenograft (*dashed outline*) in the right shoulder and a large non-transduced U87MG xenograft located in the right shoulder and extending beneath the animal (*a*). This was followed by whole-body fluorescence imaging without correction for autofluorescence (*b*), whole-body bioluminescence imaging (*c*), whole-body scintigraphic imaging of [^{131}I] radioactivity, 24 h after i.v. [^{131}I]FIAU administration (*d*). All images were obtained from the same mouse at the same imaging session, and the mouse remained stationary between each imaging session. Note that (*c*) and (*d*) include optical fusion with the white-light photograph shown in (*a*)

bioluminescence imaging and showed a good correlation between the nuclear (microPET) and optical (CCD camera) read-outs of the dual reporter system.

More recently, triple-reporter constructs (e.g., HSV1-TK/eGFP/Luc or TGL), have been developed (Ray et al. 2003; Ponomarev et al. 2004). The map of the plasmid is shown in Fig. 13. A single reporter construct (vector) with a gene product(s) that can be assayed by three different imaging technologies (nuclear, fluorescence and bioluminescence) combines the benefits of each modality. Such systems facilitate the development, validation and testing of new reporter systems in small animals, as well as provide preliminary data that will facilitate the translation of such studies into humans. Using dual or triple modality reporter constructs (PET, fluorescence and bioluminescence) overcomes many of the shortcomings of each modality alone. Although optical imaging does not yet provide optimal quantitative or tomographic information, these issues are not limiting for PET-based reporter systems and PET animal studies are more easily generalised to human applications. Multi-modality reporters have been shown to facilitate the development, validation and testing of new reporter systems in small animals (Gambhir 2002; Blasberg and Tjuvajev 2003), as well as provide preliminary data that will facilitate the translation of such studies into humans.

3 Applications of Reporter Gene Imaging

Reporter gene imaging can provide non-invasive assessments of endogenous biological processes in living subjects. For example, imaging the *transcriptional regulation* of endogenous genes in living animals using non-invasive imaging techniques can provide a better understanding of normal and cancer-related biological processes. Recent papers from our group have shown that p53- and HIF-1 (hypoxia inducible factor-1)-dependent gene expression can be imaged in vivo with PET and by in-situ fluorescence (Doubrovin et al. 2001; Serganova et al. 2004). Retroviral vectors were generated by placing the *HSV1-tk/eGFP*, a dual-reporter gene, under control of a several repeats of the p53 protein (transcription factor) (Doubrovin et al. 2001), and several repeats of the hypoxia response element (HRE, a specific response element for HIF-1) (Serganova et al. 2004) (see below).

Imaging endogenous gene expression may be hampered when *weak promoters*, in their usual *cis* configuration, a re-used to activate the transcription of the reporter gene. This results in insufficient transcription of the reporter gene. To address this limitation, a "two-step transcriptional amplification" (TSTA) approach can be used to enhance transcriptional activity. TSTA was used to image activation of the androgen-responsive prostate-specific antigen promoter (PSE) with firefly luciferase and mutant herpes simplex virus type 1 thymidine kinase (HSV1-sr39tk) reporter genes in a prostate cancer cell line (LNCaP) (Zhang et al. 2002). Further improvements of the androgen-responsive TSTA system for reporter gene expression were made using a "chimeric" TSTA system that uses duplicated variants of the prostate-specific antigen (PSA) gene enhancer to express GAL4 derivatives fused to one, two, or four VP16 activation domains. A very encouraging result was the demonstration that the TSTA system was androgen concentration sensitive, suggesting a continuous rather than binary reporter response. Another study (Qiao et al. 2002) validated methods to enhance the transcriptional activity of the carcinoembryonic antigen (CEA) promoter using the TSTA principle. To increase promoter strength while maintaining tissue specificity, a recombinant adenovirus was constructed which contained a TSTA system with a tumour-specific CEA promoter driving a transcription transactivator, which then activates a minimal promoter to drive expression of the HSV1-tk suicide/reporter gene. This ADV/CEA-binary-HSV1-tk system resulted in equal or greater cell killing of transduced cells by ganciclovir in a CEA-specific manner, compared with ganciclovir killing of all cells transduced with a CEA-independent vector containing a constitutive viral promoter driving HSV1-tk expression (ADV/RSV-tk). However, as observed with the PSE-TSTA reporter system above, the in-vivo imaging comparison of the TSTA and *cis* reporter systems showed substantially less dramatic differences than that obtained by the in-vitro analyses.

Gene expression levels are also regulated by post-transcriptional modulation, including the translation of mRNA. A recent study demonstrated that imaging post-transcriptional regulation of gene expression is feasible. This was shown by exposing cells to antifolates and inducing a rapid increase in the levels of the enzyme dihydrofolate reductase (DHFR). Several studies indicated that the DHFR binds to its own mRNA in the coding region, and that inhibition of DHFR by methotrexate (MTX) releases the DHFR enzyme from its mRNA. Consequently, this release results in an increase in translation of DHFR protein. In addition to the described translational regulation of DHFR in cancer cells exposed to MTX, increased levels of DHFR also result through *DHFR* gene amplification, a common mechanism of acquired resistance to this drug. In contrast to rapid translational modulation of DHFR, gene amplification occurs in response to chronic exposure to antifolates, and elevated cellular levels of DHFR result from transcription of multiple *DHFR* gene copies. Recently, Mayer-Kuckuk et al. (2002) utilised imaging to show that the antifolate-mediated regulation of DHFR indeed occurs in vivo. For this study, a mutant DHFR was tagged with the reporter gene *HSV1-tk*; a modification that neither abolished the DHFR response to methotrexate or trimetrexate, nor compromises the activity of the robust *HSV1-tk* reporter gene. Regulation of the DHFR-HSV1-TK fusion protein could be visualised in PET imaging studies that were performed on nude rats bearing *DHFR-HSV1-tk*-transduced HCT-8 xenografts. In this model, systemic administration of antifolate results in increased accumulation of the DHFR-HSV1-TK fusion protein in tumour tissue. Positron emission tomography of this increase was achieved after injection of the HSV1-tk substrate [124I]FIAU and tracer clearance. The results of this in-vivo imaging were consistent with complementing in-vitro experiments and indicated that the increase in the fusion reporter protein DHFR-HSV1-TK was occurring at a translational level, rather than at the transcriptional level.

3.1 Tissue Hypoxia: The Biological Basis for Indirect Imaging of Hypoxia

Given the importance of hypoxia in cancer progression and therapy, there has been a long-standing interest in developing non-invasive imaging methodologies to detect and assess tumour hypoxia. However, tumour hypoxia is a spatially and temporally heterogeneous phenomenon, resulting from the combined effect of many factors, including tumour type and volume, disease site (specific organ or tissue), regional microvessel density, blood flow, oxygen diffusion and consumption rates, etc. The most important regulatory factor of the hypoxia signalling pathway in cells is hypoxia-inducible transcription factor-1 (HIF-1). HIF-1 mediates adaptive responses to reduced O_2 availability. HIF-1 is a heterodimeric protein consisting of an oxygen-regulated α-subunit and a stable β-subunit (Wang and Semenza 1995). HIF-1α undergoes rapid turnover (half-life is less than 5 min) in the presence of oxygen, being degraded by the ubiquitin-proteasome pathway through the interaction with the VHL (von Hippel-Lindau) protein (Ivan et al. 2001). VHL recognition of the HIF-1α subunit is dependent on the hydroxylation of conserved proline residues within HIF-1α, that occurs only when oxygen is available (Salceda and Caro 1997; Kaelin 2005).

We developed an inducible reporter system that was sensitive to hypoxia and could be monitored by non-invasive imaging (Serganova et al. 2004). Up-regulation of the HIF-1 transcriptional factor was demonstrated and correlated with the expression of dependent downstream genes (e.g. *VEGF*) (Fig. 14). PET imaging of HIF-1 transcriptional activity in tumours using this reporter system was developed and validated (Serganova et al. 2004), and this reporter system could be used to assess the effects of radiation, new drugs or other novel therapeutic paradigms that impact on the HIF-1 signalling pathways.

In the absence of an imaging technique to directly determine the partial oxygen pressure (pO_2) in tissue, current non-invasive methodologies must be corroborated.

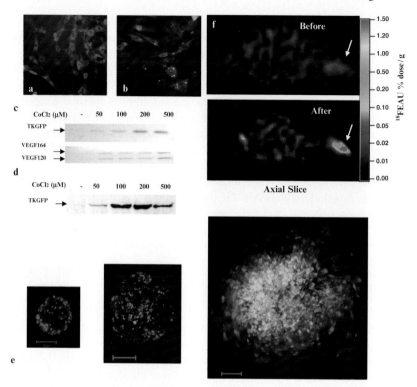

Fig. 14 a–f Characterisation of a hypoxia-sensitive specific reporter system. Fluorescence microscopy of #4C6 reporter cells (cells were transduced with a double reporter vector bearing a constitutively expressed reporter fusion *dsRed2/XPRT* and a hypoxia regulated *HSV1-tk/GFP* fusion gene) under base-line conditions **a** and following exposure to 200 μM CoCl₂ for 24 h **b**. VEGF and HSV1-tk/GFP expression in response to hypoxic conditions. **c** Agarose-gel electrophoresis of the RT-PCR products was performed to validate a hypoxia dependent reporter system (HSV1-tk/GFP). **d** Western blotting of the expression level of HSV1-tk/GFP confirms the integrity of the reporter system. Assays were performed 24 h after exposure to different concentrations of CoCl₂. **e** Sequential confocal microscopic images of the multi-cellular spheroid from reporter #4C6 cells during different phases of growth (*bar* 200 μm). Normoxic cells (small spheroid and periphery of larger spheroids) show only red-fluorescing cells and demonstrate no HIF1 transcriptional activity. Hypoxic TKGFP-fluorescing cells are clearly detectable within the central region when the spheroid grows to 350–400 μm in diameter. At a significantly larger size, this central region becomes necrotic as evidenced by the absence of cell fluorescence. In-vivo microPET imaging of ischemia-reperfusion injury-induced HIF-1 transcriptional activity. **f** Axial PET images of HIF-1-mediated HSV1-TK/GFP expression in s.c. #4C6 xenografts growing in both anterior limbs of the same mouse before and after tourniquet application to the left anterior limb proximal to tumour. The s.c. #4C6 tumour xenograft growing in the right limb was not affected and served as a control. (Adapted from Serganova et al. 2004)

Validation experiments are frequently performed by comparisons with direct pO₂ probe measurement (considered the "gold standard") or by immunohistochemical techniques, which provide detailed microdistribution data of relative (not absolute) pO₂ level. Physical measurement of pO₂ levels using polarographic oxygen electrodes (Brizel et al. 1996; Hockel et al. 1996; Nordsmark et al. 1996) have been shown to be of prognostic value. These devices provide a direct measure of pO_2 at a specific, but this method is invasive and provides selected pO_2 data along a series of individual sampling tracks with an inherent limitation of tumour sampling. Immunohistochemical (IHC) methods are based on antibody detection of exogenous hypoxia markers, such as pimonidazole (Nordsmark et al. 2003) or EF5 (Koch and Evans 2003; Evans et al. 2004), that are injected into the patient prior to surgical resection of tissue (tumour). IHC methods yield microscopic information on hypoxia in relation to tumour histology. However, such data requires the acquisition of tissue specimens by invasive time-consuming IHC techniques and provides only relative pO_2 information. In addition, only a small number of sections can be realistically processed per patient; thus, immunohistochemical methods are inherently limited and subject to sampling errors. These limitations have spurred enthusiasm for the development of non-invasive imaging methods that provide tomographic visualisation of tissue hypoxia in tumours and can be repeated. Endogenous molecular markers of tumour oxygenation have been suggested and studied. In patients with cervical cancer patients HIF-1 might represent a reliable intrinsic marker for tumour hypoxia and prognosis (Bachtiary et al. 2003). GLUT-1 has also been shown to be an endogenous marker of hypoxia for oral squamous cell carcinoma and rectal carcinoma (Cooper et al. 2003; Oliver et al. 2004). Another a much cited endogenous marker of tumour oxygenation is carbonic anhydrase 9 (CA9) (Giatromanolaki et al. 2001). It was shown, that it can be a prognostic indicator in cervical cancer (Loncaster et al. 2001), and in invasive breast cancer studies (Colpaert et al. 2003). However, none of these markers can be universally used across many tumour types, because they are likely cell-type specific and are not reliable for the reasons discussed above.

The principal non-invasive approaches to imaging tumour hypoxia include magnetic resonance and radionuclide (PET and SPECT) imaging, but other techniques such as optical imaging or electron spin resonance are under investigation. For example, near-infrared (NIR) imaging detects tissue hypoxia as a decrease in the local blood pool oxyhemoglobin-deoxyhemoglobin ratio but with poor spatial resolution (Brun et al. 1997). Electron paramagnetic resonance imaging (EPRI) is a newly emerging MR imaging technology which can produce images of oxygen levels in normal and tumour tissues (Elas et al. 2003) and may soon develop into a more widely used method in studies of hypoxia. More conventional MR techniques include blood-oxygen-level-dependent (BOLD) imaging, which detects a change in tissue perfusion by the amount of oxygenated blood (Krishna et al. 2001), and has become widely used in fMRI applications (Hennig et al. 2003). However, BOLD cannot be used to determine the level of oxygen in tissues or characterise the molecular-genetic changes in tumour cells. NMR spectroscopy can detect increased lactate (a product of anaerobic glycolysis) and decreased ATP levels in ^{1}H and ^{31}P spectra, respectively, as well as tissue pH, but has poor sensitivity (in mmol range) and poor spatial resolution ($\sim 1\,cm^3$) (Gillies et al. 2002).

Radionuclide-based imaging approaches, using a direct imaging strategy, claim a detection sensitivity which is several orders of magnitude higher than MR-based techniques. However, the resolution of modern whole-body PET and SPECT systems ranges from 4 to 10 mm. PET can provide quantitative images of a variety of processes that are related to hypoxia (Lewis and Welch 2001). Using $^{15}O_2$ inhalation (Iida et al. 1996), parametric PET images of tissue oxygenation levels, regional oxygen extraction fraction and metabolic rate can be generated with much higher accuracy than with invasive measurements of oxygen tension in tissues (Gupta et al. 2002). PET imaging with $^{15}O_2$ is currently the "gold standard" for non-invasive imaging of tissue oxygen levels. However, it is not widely used for experimental or clinical imaging, due to the very short half-life of $^{15}O_2(t_{1/2} \approx 2 \min)$, which renders such studies (both animal and clinical) logistically and technically complex as well as expensive.

The more widely used clinical studies to image hypoxia using PET are based on 2-nitroimidazole halogenated tracers, such as ^{18}F-labeled misonidazole ([^{18}F]-FMISO) (Rasey et al. 1996). The nitroimidazoles become reduced in a hypoxic environment and then covalently bind to intra- and extracellular molecules, and the magnitude of their accumulation has been shown to be proportional to the level of hypoxia (Chapman et al. 1983). Several nitroimidozole compounds have been radiolabelled and studied as potential hypoxia imaging agents. Lehtio et al. (2004) evaluated the use of ^{18}F-fluoro-erythronitroimidazole (FETNIM) and tested it as a predictor of radiotherapy outcome. They reported that the data of [^{18}F]-FETNIM was suggestive but inconclusive. Another 2-nitroimidazole, 2-(2-nitro-1H-imidazol-1-yl)-N-(2,2,3,3,3-pentafluoropropyl) acetamide (EF5), has been successfully used as an immunohistochemical marker of hypoxia in surgical trials. PET images have been obtained with EF5 (Evans et al. 2000).

3.2 Imaging Adoptive Therapies

A non-invasive method for repetitive evaluation of adoptively administered cells benefits the assessment of current adoptive therapies in clinical use (e.g. bone marrow transplantation, immune cell and blood-derived progenitor cell-based therapies) as well as future adoptive therapies using stem cells. Individual patient monitoring would contribute to patient management by visualising the trafficking, homing-targeting and persistence of adoptively administered cells, as well as assess their functional activation, proliferation and cytokine expression. Such studies would significantly aid in the clinical implementation and management of new therapeutic approaches based on the adoptive transfer of immune cells, progenitor cells and stem cells.

In this section we will focus on adoptive T-cell monitoring, although the methods for non-invasive monitoring can be readily transferred other systems (e.g. bone marrow stromal cells or endothelial precursor cell). Non-invasive imaging of lymphocyte trafficking dates back to the early 1970s, when the first experiments were performed with extracorporeal labelling of lymphocytes using various metallic radioisotopes and chelation attachments to the cell surface (e.g. ^{111}In, ^{67}Co, ^{64}Cu, ^{51}Cr, $^{99\,m}$Tc) (Papierniak 1976; Gobuty 1977; Rannie 1977; Korf 1998; Adonai

2002). A major limitation of ex-vivo labelling of lymphocytes with radionuclides is the relatively low level of radioactivity per cell that can be attained by labelling cells. The exposure of cells to higher doses of radioactivity during labelling is also limited by radiotoxicity. Another shortcoming of ex-vivo radiolabelling is the short period for cell monitoring, which is limited by radioactivity decay and biological clearance.

The genetic labelling of cells for adoptive therapy monitoring provides substantial advantages for long-term monitoring and for assessing the functional status of the adoptively transferred cells. Retroviral-mediated transduction has proven to be one of the most effective means to deliver transgenes into T-cells and results in high levels of sustained transgene expression (Gallardo et al. 1997; Hagani 1999). Genetic labelling of lymphocytes with the luciferase (*FLuc*) reporter gene and non-invasive bioluminescence imaging (BLI) of mice has been reported (Hardy 2001; Zhang 2001). Costa et al. (2001) showed the migration of myelin basic protein specific, Luc-transduced CD4$^+$ T-cells in the central nervous system. The distribution of cytotoxic T-lymphocytes (CTL) can also be followed throughout the organism and monitored over time using BLI of Luc-expressing CTLs. The variable optical characteristics of tissue at different depths from the surface on the emitted photons must be recognised in any BLI assessment of cell trafficking. Nevertheless, BLI based on Luc expression has great potential in preclinical mouse-model studies, where high sensitivity, low cost, and technical simplicity are important for rapid screening.

The long-term trafficking and localisation of T-lymphocytes is an important component of the immune response, and in the elimination of abnormal cells and infectious agents from the body. Passive (ex vivo) labelling of T-cells with radioisotopes or magnetic labels can be unstable, is limited in long-term assessments and does not account for proliferation of activated T-cells in the body. Our group demonstrated the feasibility of long-term in-vivo monitoring of adoptively transferred antigen-specific T cells that were transduced to express a radiotracer-based reporter gene for non-invasive in-vivo PET imaging (Koehne 2003). EBV-specific T cells (CTLs) were obtained and stably transduced with a constitutively expressed dual reporter gene (*HSV1-tk/GFP* fusion gene). SCID mice bearing four tumours [(1) autologous HLA-A0201$^+$ EBV-transformed B cells (EBV BLCL); (2) allogeneic EBV BLCL expressing HLA-A0201 allele; (3) allogeneic HLA mismatched EBV BLCL; (4) EBV-negative HLA-A0201$^+$ B-cell acute lymphoblastic leukemia (B-ALL)] were treated with *HSV1-tk/GFP*-transduced EBV-specific CTLs. Specific accumulation and localisation of radioactivity was observed only in the autologous and allogeneic HLA-A0201$^+$ EBV-BLCL; no T-cell infiltration was seen in the allogeneic HLA-A0201-matched, EBV-negative B-ALL or HLA-mismatched EBV BLCL xenografts (Fig. 15). Sequential imaging over 15 days after T-cell injection permitted long-term monitoring of the *HSV1-tk/GFP*-transduced cells and demonstrated tumour-specific migration and targeting of the CTLs. Infusion of EBV-specific cytotoxic T-cells (CTLs) led to the elimination of subcutaneous autologous EBV-BLCL tumour and HLA-A0201$^+$ allogenic EBV-BLCL xenografts. This tumour rejection was abolished by administration of ganciclovir, which eliminated

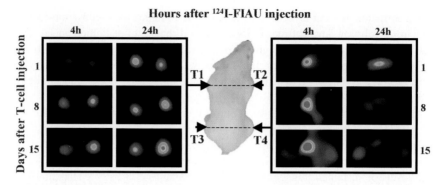

Fig. 15 MicroPET imaging of T-cell migration and targeting. Sequential axial images through the shoulders (*left panel*) and thighs (*right panel*) of mice bearing autologous BLCL (*T*1), HLA-A0201 matched BLCL (*T*2), HLA-mismatched BLCL (*T*3), and HLA-A0201 ALL (*T*4) tumours in the left and right shoulders and the left and right thighs, respectively after i.v injection of [^{124}I]FIAU 1, 8 and 15 days post T-cell infusion. All images are from a single representative animal. (Adapted from Koehne et al. 2003)

the *HSV1-tk*-transduced T-cells (our unpublished data). These studies demonstrate the feasibility of long-term in-vivo monitoring of targeting and migration of antigen-specific CTLs that are transduced to constitutively express a radionuclide-based reporter gene. This paradigm provides the opportunity for repeated visualisation of transferred T-cells within the same animal over time using non-invasive reporter gene PET imaging and it is potentially transferable to clinical studies in patients with EBV+ cancer.

The potential of PET imaging for quantifying cell signals in regions of anatomic interest exists. However, little is known about the constraints and parameters for using PET signal detection to establish cell numbers in different regions of interest. Su et al. (2004) determined the correlation of PET signal to cell number, and characterised the cellular limit of detection for PET imaging. These studies using human T-cells transduced with the *HSV1-tk* reporter gene revealed a cell number-dependent signal, with a limit of detection calculated as 10^6 cells in a region of interest of 0.1 ml volume. Quantitatively similar parameters were observed with stably transduced N2a glioma cells and primary T-lymphocytes.

An essential component of the immune response in many normal and disease states is T-cell activation. Our group has monitored and assessed T-cell receptor (TCR) -dependent activation in vivo using non-invasive PET imaging (Ponomarev et al. 2001). TCR interactions with MHC-peptide complexes expressed on antigen-presenting cells initiate T-cell activation, resulting in transcription that is mediated by several factors. Several of these factors, including IL-2 and other cytokines, contribute to the regulation of a number of target genes through several activating pathways and involve several transcription factors such as nuclear factor of activated T-cells (NFAT) (Li W 1996). Furthermore, this activation can be arrested clinically by the use calcineurin inhibitors such as cyclosporin A and FK506 (Kiani A 2000).

When combined with imaging of NFAT-mediated activation of T-cells, non-invasive PET imaging should allow for monitoring the trafficking, proliferation and antigen-specific activation of T-cells in anti-tumour vaccination trials.

3.3 Imaging the Trafficking of Bone Marrow-derived Cells

Imaging the trafficking of bone marrow-derived cells has also been performed using optical-, MR- and PET-based imaging studies. The use of PET for monitoring bone marrow and progenitor (stem) cell transplantation has lagged behind optical and MR techniques (Kiani et al. 2000; Wang et al. 2003). In most cases, PET imaging has been applied to monitoring bone marrow transplantation (BMT), to assess for residual disease (Hill et al. 2003), or BMT conditioning regimen related toxicities (Vose et al. 1996). Monitoring the fate of bone marrow stem cells with PET following direct labelling with [^{18}F]fluorobenzoate and transplantation was first reported by Olasz et al. (Olasz et al. 2002). Direct labelling of bone marrow-derived cells is limited by the half-life and quantity of isotope used in the labelling. Reporter gene technology precludes this limitation, and allows for extended monitoring of stem cell engraftment (Mayer-Kuckuk et al. 2004). Recently, Cao et al. (2004) reported luciferase bioluminescence imaging of hematopoietic stem cells following transplantation into irradiated recipient mice. Donor stem cells were derived either from a luciferase or luciferase/GFP transgenic mouse and purified through cell sorting. After systemic administration, repeated optical imaging was used to detect the sites and kinetics of hematopoietic stem cell engraftment. The data suggest that the stem cells initially home to the bone marrow or spleen, while little specificity for a particular bone marrow compartment exists. Interestingly, different subsets of progenitor cells, such as short- or long-term repopulating cells, showed comparable homing profiles but differences in their proliferative potential. The potential of bioluminescence imaging to monitor engraftment of hematopoietic progenitor cells was previously shown in a mouse model of xenotransplantation of human hematopoietic stem cell populations (Wang et al. 2003). We have applied reporter gene technology to image the trafficking and distribution of bone marrow cells using a multiple-modality reporter gene approach (Mayer-Kuckuk et al. 2006). Co-registration of microPET and microCT images facilitated interpretation of the PET signal and allowed localisation of radioactive foci to specific anatomical structures (Fig. 16). Others have studied effects of the bone marrow transplanted cells on the reconstruction of the ischemic myocardium (Tomita et al. 2002; Stamm et al. 2003).

3.4 Imaging Oncogenesis and Signalling Pathways in Genetic Modified Mouse Models

Genetic modified mouse models take advantage of the fact that cancer results from mutations in proto-oncogenes and tumour suppressor genes. They allow examination

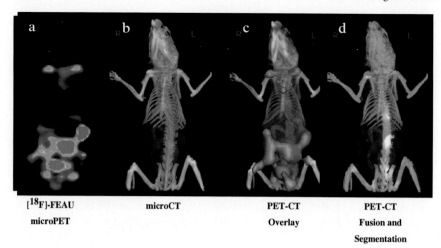

[^{18}F]-FEAU   microCT   PET-CT   PET-CT

microPET   Overlay   Fusion and

                                                                     Segmentation

Fig. 16 a–d Multi-modality imaging of autologous bone marrow-derived cells targeting bone. Multi-modality imaging: microPET **a**; microCT **b**; microPET-CT overlay **c**; microPET-CT registration, segmentation and fusion **d**. Bone marrow-derived cells were transduced with a constitutively expressing triple-modality reporter (Ponomarev et al. 2004). The images show targeting of bone and 6 days after i.v. administration. Note that the tomographic display **d** confirms the targeting of transduced cells to bone; a future objective is to perform microPET-MR acquisitions and a similar tomographic microPET-MR registration and fusion to identify soft tissue structures that are targeted or are involved in trafficking of transduced reporter cells. It is also expected that some time in the near future that tomographic bioluminescence and fluorescence images can be obtained, and that these images will be registered with currently available CT, MR and PET tomographic images. [These images were obtained by Philipp Mayer-Kukuck and Debabrata Banerjee, in collaboration with others; the image fusion and segmentation was performed by Dr. Luc Bidault, MSKCC (Mayer-Kuckuk et al. 2006)]

of the consequence of a specific gene alteration on the formation of tumours in their physiological environment. Important for the interpretation of data obtained from mouse models is the ability to accurately detect the consequences that arise from the generated genetic alteration. In most circumstances, onset and temporal dynamics of tumour growth will be a critical assessment. Mouse modelling of cancer (Holland 2004b) and the genetic alterations in mouse models of gliomagenesis have recently been reviewed (Holland 2004a). Since these mouse models require gene manipulation, it is useful to use reporter genes for the non-invasive detection and assessment of tumour growth.

A proof-of-principle study that utilises bioluminescence imaging to detect and measure K-Ras-dependent lung tumour genesis has been reported by Lyons et al. (2003). Mice engineered to induce lung tumours following Cre recombinase-mediated activation of K-Ras over-expression were crossed with animals which provide Cre controlled luciferase expression. Following adenoviral delivery of Cre to the lungs, the formation of multiple lung tumours was observed. Optical bioluminescence imaging using the luciferase reporter gene was capable of monitoring the temporal dynamics of tumour development and progression in the lung of an individual animal (Fig. 17).

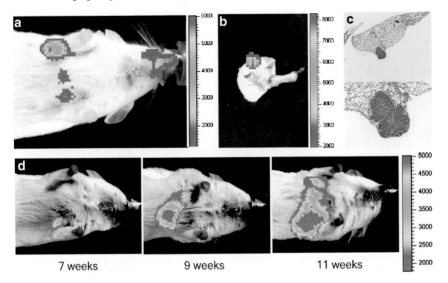

Fig. 17 a–d Bioluminescence imaging of spontaneous lung tumorigenesis and tumour progression. Tumours arising from LucRep/conditional $Kras2^{v12}$ mice were visualised non-invasively. **a** IVIS bioluminescence image of a compound LucRep/conditional $Kras2^{v12}$ mouse 13 weeks after AdCre intubation shows a bright focal region of luminescence originating from the thorax. **b** IVIS image of the lungs dissected from the mouse depicted in **a** also shows a single origin of light. **c** The same lungs after H&E processing (at $\times 2.5$ and $\times 10$ magnification) showing that the light detected in **a** and **b** originated from a single lesion measuring between 1 and 2 mm in diameter. **d** Longitudinal measurement of $Kras2^{v12}$-induced lung tumour growth in an individual mouse imaged sequentially at 2-week intervals. (Adapted from Lyons et al. 2003)

An important aspect of the report by Lyons et al. (2003) is their methodological approach. Imaging oncogenesis was accomplished by combining a conditional transgenic mouse model of tumour genesis with a conditional transgenic reporter gene mouse. This approach is highly versatile and easily translatable to other mouse models of cancer. However, reporter gene imaging was restricted to monitor tumour development and, therefore, activation of the reporter was only indirectly related to the activation of oncogenic pathways. Furthermore, all non-invasive in-vivo imaging systems have defined limits with respect to image resolution and sensitivity. Hence, it can be anticipated that only established tumours of a minimum size and with an established blood supply can be efficiently monitored by our molecular imaging techniques (e.g. microPET, bioluminescence, fluorescence). It is, therefore, unlikely that the very early events which lead to the formation of cancer can be imaged using some of our currently available molecular imaging techniques, and that further developments in imaging technology will be required to image very small populations of cells. Nevertheless, as described in the next section, reporter gene imaging has a great potential to directly assess the molecular changes that occur during oncogenesis.

The signalling pathways mediated by receptor tyrosine kinase (RTK), including PDGF, EGF and HER2 receptor, are important for oncogenesis and tumour development. These receptors have been shown to be are frequently mutated, amplified or over-expressed in tumours (Lazar-Molnar et al. 2000; Dai et al. 2001; Holland 2004b; Lyons et al. 2006). RTKs signal through several effector arms, including Ras/MAPK (MAP kinase), PI3K (phosphoinositide 3-kinase), PLC-g (phospholipase C), and JAK-STAT (signal transducers and activators of transcription), which regulate cellular proliferation, migration and invasion, and cytokine stimulation. Furthermore, the PI3K-PKB/Akt signalling pathway plays a critical role in mediating survival signals in a wide range of cell types. The binding of growth factors to specific receptor tyrosine kinases activates the phosphoinositide 3-kinase (PI3K) and the serine-threonine kinase Akt (also called protein kinase B or PKB). Akt has been shown to be activated in many tumours and up-regulation of Akt activity is consistently observed in PTEN-mutant gliomas. Activated forms of Akt substitute for IL-2 signals that phosphorylate Rb and activate E2F during G1 progression (Brennan et al. 1997). Because E2F can up-regulate the expression of c-myc (Moberg et al. 1992; Oswald et al. 1994; Wong et al. 1995), c-myc induction by Akt may be mediated, at least in part, via E2F. In addition, recent experiments suggest that Akt may also use metabolic pathways to regulate cell survival. Given the scope of biological effects from RTK stimulation, it is reasonable to investigate how the dysregulation of these pathways drives malignant transformation, progression and maintenance of these tumours.

Holland et al used the RCAS/TVA system to induce PDGF-driven gliomas in a transgenic mouse model (Dai et al. 2001; Holland 2004b). This system is comprised of two components: (1) an avian retroviral vector referred to as RCAS, (2) an avian tv-a receptor for the RCAS vector (Dai et al. 2001; Sherr and McCormick 2002). They developed an N-tv-a transgenic mouse line, expressing tv-a from the nestin promoter. Infection of RCAS-PDGFB to neural progenitors in N-tv-a mice induced the formation of gliomas in about 60% of mice (Dai et al. 2001) (Fig. 18a).

To monitor the proliferative activity of PDGF-induced gliomas by bioluminescence imaging, they also generated a transgenic reporter mouse using the human E2F1 promoter, which is strictly regulated by RB in cell-cycle progression (Dai et al. 2001; Sherr and McCormick 2002), to drive expression of the firefly luciferase gene (E2F-luc) (Dai et al. 2001; Uhrbom et al. 2004). The E2F-luc transgenic mouse line was then crossbred with the N-tv-a mouse strain. The luciferase activity of PDGF-induced gliomas could be detected in the double transgenic 4 weeks after RCAS-PDGF injection. The time-dependent increase in light production represents the sum of the tumour cells' capacity to proliferate and the overall size of the tumour (Fig. 18a).

3.5 Imaging Drug Treatment in Mouse Tumour Models

A currently applied variant of reporter imaging, particularly in the pharmaceutical industry, is to monitor tumour or xenograft growth using bioluminescence imaging. In this system, the desired cell lines are stably transduced with a luciferase reporter gene that is constitutively expressed. The transduced cells are selected and used to

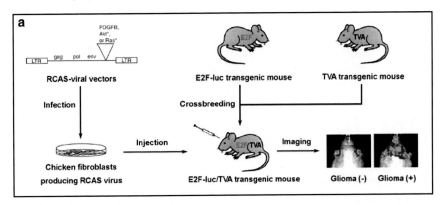

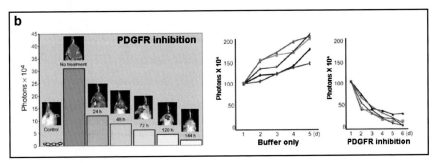

Fig. 18 a, b Bioluminescence imaging of PDGFB-induced glioma in E2F-luc/TVA transgenic mouse model. **a** Generation of PDGFB-induced glioma model in E2F-luc/TVA transgenic mice. PDGFB is inserted into the viral genome, and the modified RCAS virus is propagated in avian cells in vitro. Then the virus-producing cells are injected into the brain of the E2F-luc/TVA double transgenic mice expressing both tv-a (the RCAS receptor) under the nestin promoter and the firefly luciferase under the E2F1 promoter. After 4 weeks of injection, proliferative activity of the induced glioma has been increased and light production has been elevated. **b** Preclinical trials of PDGFB-induced gliomas-bearing E2F-luc/TVA transgenic mouse model. *Left panel:* longitudinal imaging of one tumour-bearing mouse treated with PDGFR inhibitor daily, PTK787/ZK222584, for 6 days. *Middle and right panels:* longitudinal study with five E2F-luc/TVA transgenic mice in each cohort: buffer treated (*middle panel*) or treated daily with PTK787/ZK222584 (*right panel*). (Adapted from Uhrbom et al. 2004)

produce s.c. or orthotopic xenografts. The growth and response to treatment can be monitored effectively in mice by sequential bioluminescence imaging, over time (Rehemtulla et al. 2000) (Fig. 19). The intensity of bioluminescence at a particular site in the animal is directly related to size (number of transduced cells expressing luciferase) of the tumour (Figs. 11, 17,19). The popularity and wide use of bioluminescence reporter imaging is due to its relative simplicity, low cost, high sensitivity and high throughput.

There is a strong rational to assess the effects of drugs that target PDGF/EGFR/ HER2 signalling or Ras/Raf/MEK/Erk- and PKB/Akt/mTOR-mediated pathways by non-invasive imaging. The application of biomarker or surrogate imaging using

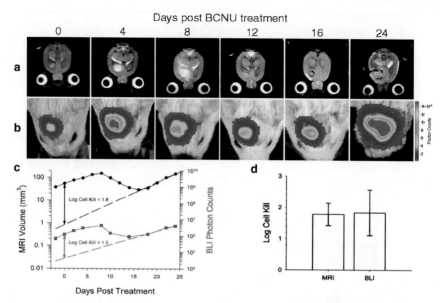

Fig. 19 a–d Temporal analysis of the response of 9LLuc tumour to BCNU chemotherapy. Tumour cells were implanted 16 days before treatment. Tumour volume was monitored with T2-weighted MRI **a** and intra-tumoural luciferase activity was monitored with BLI **b**. The days post-BCNU therapy on which the images were obtained are indicated *at the top*. The *scale to the right* of the BL images describes the colour map for the photo count. **c** Quantitative analysis of tumour progression and response to BCNU treatment. Tumour volumes and total tumour photon emission obtained by T2-weighted MRI and BLI, respectively, are plotted versus days post-BCNU treatment. The *dashed lines* are the regression fits of exponential tumour repopulation following therapy. The *solid vertical lines* denote the apparent tumour-volume and photon-production losses elicited by BCNU on the day of treatment from which log cell-kill values were calculated as previously described (Nakagawa et al. 2001). **d** Comparison of log cell-kill values determined from MRI and BLI measurements. Log cell-kill elicited by BCNU chemotherapy was calculated using MRI (1.78 + 0.36) and BLI (1.84 + 0.73). Data are represented as mean + SEM for each animal ($n = 5$). There was no statistically significant difference between the log kills calculated using the MRI abd BLI data ($P = 0.951$). (Adapted from Rehemtulla et al. 2000)

FDG and PET has been discussed above. The development and use of reporter- and direct-imaging paradigms to evaluate the efficacy of molecular-targeted therapies is now being pursued by many groups. Specific drugs that are known (or thought) to target specific signalling pathways and down-stream effectors can be assessed in the reporter-xenografts or transgenic/oncogenic reporter-animals. Namely, the effects of treatment targeted to a particular signalling pathway can be assessed by non-invasive imaging.

For example, the E2F-reporter mouse model, that monitors the proliferative activity, was used by the Holland laboratory in longitudinal preclinical studies to study the effects of treatment with a drug, PTK787/ZK222584, that inhibits the PDGF receptor. Compared with the buffer-treated control group animals, mice treated with PTK787/ZK222584 showed a clear reduction in light emission from the brain area

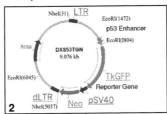

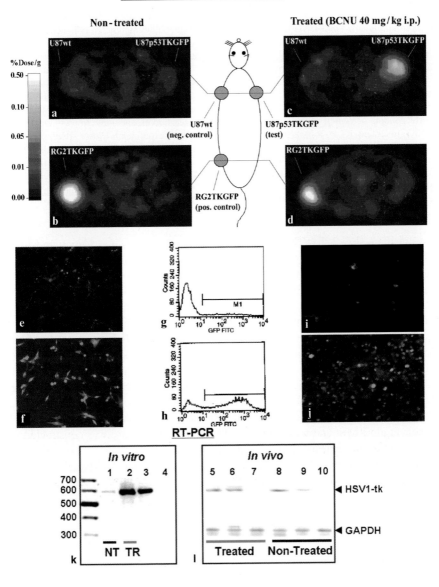

Fig. 20 a–l Imaging BCNU activation of p53. The p53-sensitive, dual-modality reporter vector (*top panel*) contains an artificial p53 specific enhancer element that activates expression of the *HSV1-TK/eGFP* reporter gene. A constitutively expressed neomycin selection gene is also included in the retroviral vector construct. Transaxial PET images (GE Advance tomograph) through the shoulder **a, c** and pelvis **b, d** of two rats are shown (*second panel*); the images are colour-coded to the same radioactivity scale (*% dose/g*). An untreated animal is shown on the *left* **a, b**, and a BCNU-treated animal, which is known to activate the p53 pathway, is shown on the *right* **c, d**. Both animals have three s.c. xenografts: a U87p53TKGFP (*test*) in the right shoulder, a U87 wild-type (*negative control*) in the left shoulder, and a RG2TKGFP (*positive control*) in the left thigh. The non-treated animal on the left shows localisation of radioactivity only in the positive control tumour (*RG2TKGFP*); the test (*U87p53TKGFP*) and negative control (*U87wt*) xenografts are at background levels. The BCNU-treated animal on the right shows significant radioactivity localisation in the test tumour (right shoulder) and in the positive control (left thigh), but no radioactivity above background in the negative control (left shoulder). Fluorescence microscopy and FACS analysis (*third panel*) of a transduced U87p53/TKGFP cell population in the non-induced (control) state **e, g**, and 24 h after a 2-h treatment with BCNU 40 mg/ml **f, h** are shown. Fluorescence microscopic images of post-motem U87p53/TKGFP s.c. tumour samples obtained from non-treated rats **i** and rats treated with 40 mg/kg BCNU i.p. **j** are also shown. These results **f–j** demonstrate a corresponding activation of the reporter system (increased fluorescence) due to p53 induction by BCNU treatment. RT-PCR blots from in-vitro **k** and in-vivo **l** experiments (*lower panel*) show very low HSV1-tk expression in non-treated U87p53TKGFP transduced cells and xenografts-bearing animals, respectively, and no HSV1-tk expression in wild-type U87 cells and tumour tissue, respectively. When U87p53TKGFP transduced cells and xenografts-bearing animals are treated with BCNU, there is a marked increase in HSV1-tk expression, comparable to that in constitutively HSV1-tk-expressing RG2TK$^+$ cells and xenografts. (Adapted from Doubrovin et al. 2001)

over 5 days (Fig. 18b). The reduction in light production was also found to be proportional to the cell proliferation index. The E2F-reporter mouse model makes it possible to investigate the importance of PDGF-related signalling pathways in glioma maintenance. The non-invasive imaging allows for dynamic in-vivo monitoring of a specific signal transduction pathway activity and precludes the animal euthanasia that is usually required to obtain tissue samples for molecular assays. It is also a valuable tool to obtain the more accurate and detailed measurement of biological processes during tumour treatment by the pathway specific/targeting drugs. Based on the strategy of construction of reporter-bearing mouse model, the activation of a specific oncogene during tumorigenesis has also been monitored through an oncogene promoter that controls the expression of a reporter gene. For example, the PSA-luc reporter mouse was used in prostate cancer model (Dai et al. 2001; Lyons et al. 2006), and the pVEGF-TSTA-luc reporter mouse was constructed for mammary tumorigenesis model (Wang et al. 2006).

As discussed above, and this has been developed and validated for several transcriptional-sensitive reporter systems (Doubrovin et al. 2001; Serganova et al. 2004). Up-regulation of these transcription factors was demonstrated and correlated with the expression of downstream-dependent genes [e.g. p21, vascular endothelial growth factor (VEGF), respectively]. Imaging BCNU activation of p53 is shown in Fig. 20. Such assays can be applied to tumours or xenografts that have been transduced with the appropriate reporter construct, or in appropriate transgenic reporter-animal models of cancer.

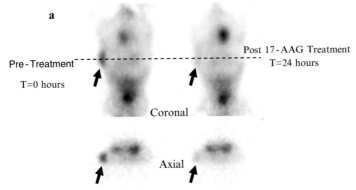

Images obtained 4 hours after ^{68}Ga - F(ab)$_2$ - Herceptin injection

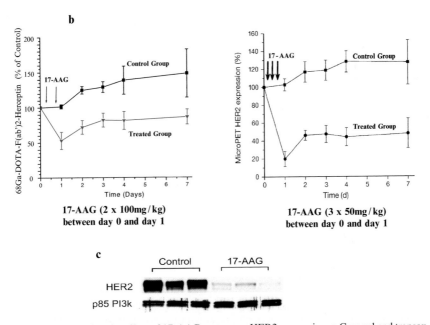

Fig. 21 a–c Monitoring the effect of 17-AAG on tumour HER2 expression. **a** Coronal and transaxial MicroPET images of [^{68}Ga]-F(ab)$_2$-Herceptin in a single nude mouse bearing a single BT 474 xenograft (*arrow*). Both image sets were acquired 3 h after i.v. injection of approximately 5 MBq of [^{68}Ga]-F(ab)$_2$-herceptin. The pre-treatment images are shown on the *left*; the post-treatment images are shown on the *right*. Treatment involved 17-AAG administered 3×50 mg/kg over 24 h, followed by imaging 24 h later. **b** The pharmacodynamics and pharmacokinetcs of HER2 expression levels following two different 17-AAG treatment schedules. MicroPET determinations of average HER2 expression in two groups of mice ($n = 5$) over a 1-week period. One treatment group (a) of mice received 2×100 mg/kg 17-AAG over 24 h, and the other treatment group (b) received 3×50 mg/kg 17-AAG over 24 h after the initial microPET scan; the control animals in each group received vehicle only. The data are normalised to the initial pretreatment uptake value. A significant difference in treatment effect on HER2 expression levels is seen between the two schedules of 17-AAG administration. **c** Western blot analysis of HER2 and the 85-kDa regulatory subunit of P13 kinase expression in BT-474 tumours from control mice and from mice 24 H treatment with 17-AAG. (Adapted from Smith-Jones et al. 2004)

In a recent study, imaging was used to sequentially monitor the pharmacodynamics of HER2 degradation in response to treatment with a HER2-chaperone protein (HSP90) inhibitor (17-AAG) (Smith-Jones et al. 2004). This study demonstrates that a highly specific, small $F(ab')_2$ antibody fragment can be diolabeled with a short-lived nuclide and used for repetitive non-invasive imaging of HER2 degradation and recovery (Fig. 21). What was novel in this study was the ability to image the target of therapy, HER2, through the effects of a drug on the HER2 chaperone protein (HSP90) rather than through an inhibition of HER2 function. The ansamycin class of antibiotics, including geldanamycin and its derivative 17-AAG, bind to the ATP-binding pocket of HSP90 and inhibit its chaperone function. The HSP90 chaperone is required for conformational maturation and stability of a number of key signalling molecules, including HER2, AKT, RAF, cdk4 serine kinases, and results in their proteosomal degradation (Neckers 2002). Since HER2 is dependent on HSP90 and is particularly sensitive to 17-AAG treatment, Smith-Jones et al. (2004) exploited this mechanism of action to image the pharmacodynamic effects of 17-AAG on HER2 (through the drug's effect on the chaperone protein) (Fig. 21). This approach could be extended to other targets of drug therapy, such as MET, IGF-1 and other RTKs that are HSP90 chaperone-dependent and could easily be adapted to human studies to provide the opportunity to non-invasively image the pharmacodynamics of drug action by repetitive imaging over time using short-lived radionuclides. The ability to image drug pharmacodynamic effects addresses a major impediment to the development of rational therapeutic strategies; namely, the determination of whether the drug treatment protocol (dose and schedule) is actually inhibiting the target and whether the level of inhibition is sufficient. Furthermore, it is not inconceivable that non-invasive imaging of drug pharmacodynamic effects could be applied to individual patients, in order to optimise dose and administration schedule.

4 Conclusions

Molecular genetic studies of disease and our understanding of the multiple and converging pathways that are involved in disease development (e.g. oncogenesis and tumour progression) have expanded rapidly over the past decade. The era of molecular medicine has begun and the benefits to individual patients are widely expected to be realised in the near future. For example, the formerly unresponsive and rapidly fatal gastrointestinal stromal tumours (GIST) and chronic myelogenous leukemia (CML) have shown remarkable responses to imatinib mesylate (Gleevac) treatment, a drug that targets several receptor tyrosine kinases (cKit and Bcr-Abl, respectively) that are mutated or constitutively over-expressed.

Biomarker or surrogate imaging that reflects endogenous molecular/genetic processes is particularly attractive for expansion and translation into clinical studies in the short-term. This is because existing radiopharmaceuticals and imaging paradigms may be useful for monitoring down-stream changes of specific molecular/genetic pathways in diseases such as cancer (e.g. FDG PET). Biomarker imaging is very likely to be less specific and more limited with respect to the number of molecular genetic processes that can be imaged. Nevertheless, it benefits from the use of radiopharmaceuticals that have already been developed and are currently being used in human subjects. Thus, the translation and application of biomarker imaging paradigms into patient studies will be far easier than either the direct imaging or reporter transgene imaging paradigms.

The "direct" molecular imaging motif builds on established chemistry and radiochemistry relationships. Bioconjugate chemistry linking specific binding motifs and bioactive molecules to paramagnetic particles for MR imaging or to radionuclides for PET and gamma camera imaging is rapidly expanding. This has occurred largely through the development of new relationships and focused interactions between molecular/cellular biologists, chemists, radiochemists, imagers and clinicians. The next generation of direct molecular imaging probes will come from better interactions between pharmaceutical companies, academia and hospitals. Such interactions are now being pursued with the objective to develop and evaluate new compounds for imaging; compounds that target specific molecules (e.g. DNA, mRNA, proteins) or activated enzyme systems in specific signal transduction pathways. However, a constraint limiting direct imaging strategies is the necessity to develop a specific probe for each molecular target, and then to validate the sensitivity, specificity and safety of each probe for specific applications prior to their introduction into the clinic.

Reporter gene imaging studies will be more limited in patients compared with that in animals, due to the necessity of transducing the target tissue or cells with specific reporter constructs, or the production of transgenic animals bearing the reporter constructs. Ideal vectors for targeting specific organs or tissue (tumours) do not exist at this time, although this is a very active area of human gene therapy research. Each new vector requires extensive and time-consuming safety testing prior to regulatory approval for human administration. Nevertheless, the reporter gene imaging, particularly the genetic labelling of cells with reporter constructs, has several advantages. For example, it is possible to develop and validate "indirect" imaging strategies more rapidly and at considerably lower cost than "direct" imaging strategies. This is because only a small number of well characterised and validated reporter gene-reporter probe pairs need to be established. For example, there are now four well-defined human genes (*hNIS, hNET, hD2R* and *hSSTR2*) with complimentary, clinically approved, radiopharmaceuticals for PET or gamma-camera imaging in patients. These four complimentary pairs (gene + probe) are excellent candidates for future reporter gene imaging in patients. Importantly, these human genes are less likely to be immunogenic compared with the reporter genes currently used in animals (e.g. viral thymidine kinases, luciferases, fluorescent proteins). It should also be noted that a single reporter gene-reporter probe pair can be used in different reporter constructs to image many different biological and molecular genetic processes. Once a complimentary reporter-pair (gene + probe) has been approved for human studies, the major regulatory focus will shift to the particular backbone and regulatory sequence of the reporter construct and to the vector used to target reporter transduction to specific cells or tissue, both ex vivo and in vivo.

The major factor limiting translation of reporter gene imaging studies to patients is the "transduction requirement"; target tissue or adoptively administered cells must be transduced (usually with viral vectors to achieve high transduction efficiency) with reporter constructs for reporter gene imaging studies. At least *two* different reporter constructs will be required in most future applications of reporter gene imaging. One will be a "constitutive" reporter that will be used to identify the site, extent and duration of vector delivery and tissue transduction or for identifying the distribution/trafficking, homing/targeting and persistence of adoptively administered cells (the "normalising" or denominator term). The second one will be an "inducible" reporter that is sensitive to endogenous transcription factors, signalling pathways or protein-protein interactions that monitor the biological activity and function of the transduced cells (the "sensor" or numerator term). The initial application of such double-reporter systems in patients will most likely be performed as part of a gene therapy protocol or an adoptive therapy protocol where the patients own cells are harvested (e.g. lymphocytes, T-cells or blood-derived progenitor cells), transduced with the reporter systems and expanded ex vivo, and then adoptively re-administered to the patient. For example, adoptive T-cell therapy could provide a venue for imaging T-cell trafficking, targeting, activation, proliferation and persistence. These issues could be addressed in a quantitative manner by repetitive PET imaging of the double-reporter system described above in the same subject over time.

We remain optimistic; the tools and resources largely exist and we should be able to perform limited gene imaging studies in patients in the near future. The advantages and benefits of non-invasive imaging to monitor transgene expression in gene therapy protocols are obvious. The ability to visualise transcriptional and post-transcriptional regulation of endogenous target gene expression, as well as specific intracellular protein-protein interactions in patients will provide the opportunity for new experimental venues in patients. They include the potential to image the malignant phenotype of an individual patient's tumour at a molecular level and to monitor changes in the phenotype over time. The potential to image a drug's effect on a specific signal transduction pathway in an individual patient's tumour provides the opportunity for monitoring treatment response at the molecular level. At the moment this requires the use of "diagnostic" reporter gene transduction vectors that target specific organs or tissue (tumours), and this will initially limit the translation and application of reporter gene technology to patients. However, direct and surrogate molecular imaging may begin to fill this gap over the next decade.

References

Adonai N NK, Walsh J, Iyer M, Toyokuni T, Phelps ME, McCarthy T, McCarthy DW, Gambhir SS (2002) Ex vivo cell labeling with 64Cu-pyruvaldehyde-bis(N4-methylthiosemicarbazone) for imaging cell trafficking in mice with positron-emission tomography. Proc Natl Acad Sci USA 99:3030–3035

Alauddin MM, Conti PS (1998) Synthesis and preliminary evaluation of 9-(4-[18F]-fluoro-3-hydroxymethylbutyl)guanine ([18F]FHBG): a new potential imaging agent for viral infection and gene therapy using PET. Nucl Med Biol 25:175–180

Altmann A, Kissel M, Zitzmann S, Kubler W, Mahmut M, Peschke P, Haberkorn U (2003) Increased MIBG uptake after transfer of the human norepinephrine transporter gene in rat hepatoma. J Nucl Med 44:973–980

Arbab AS, Yocum GT, Rad AM, Khakoo AY, Fellowes V, Read EJ, Frank JA (2005) Labeling of cells with ferumoxides-protamine sulfate complexes does not inhibit function or differentiation capacity of hematopoietic or mesenchymal stem cells. NMR Biomed 18:553–559

Arbab AS, Yocum GT, Kalish H, Jordan EK, Anderson SA, Khakoo AY, Read EJ, Frank JA (2004) Efficient magnetic cell labeling with protamine sulfate complexed to ferumoxides for cellular MRI. Blood 104:1217–1223

Artemov D, Mori N, Ravi R, Bhujwalla ZM (2003) Magnetic resonance molecular imaging of the HER-2/neu receptor. Cancer Res 63:2723–2727

Bachtiary B, Schindl M, Potter R, Dreier B, Knocke TH, Hainfellner JA, Horvat R, Birner P (2003) Overexpression of hypoxia-inducible factor 1alpha indicates diminished response to radiotherapy and unfavorable prognosis in patients receiving radical radiotherapy for cervical cancer. Clin Cancer Res 9:2234–2240

Berger F, Gambhir SS (2001) Recent advances in imaging endogenous or transferred gene expression utilizing radionuclide technologies in living subjects: applications to breast cancer. Breast Cancer Res 3:28–35

Bhaumik S, Gambhir SS (2002) Optical imaging of Renilla luciferase reporter gene expression in living mice. Proc Natl Acad Sci USA 99:377–382

Blasberg RG, Gelovani J (2002) Molecular-genetic imaging: a nuclear medicine-based perspective. Mol Imaging 1:280–300

Blasberg RG, Tjuvajev JG (2003) Molecular-genetic imaging: current and future perspectives. J Clin Invest 111:1620–1629

Blend MJ, Stastny JJ, Swanson SM, Brechbiel MW (2003) Labeling anti-HER2/neu monoclonal antibodies with 111In and 90Y using a bifunctional DTPA chelating agent. Cancer Biother Radiopharm 18:355–363

Boland A, Ricard M, Opolon P, Bidart JM, Yeh P, Filetti S, Schlumberger M, Perricaudet M (2000) Adenovirus-mediated transfer of the thyroid sodium/iodide symporter gene into tumors for a targeted radiotherapy. Cancer Res 60:3484–3492

Bradley J, Thorstad WL, Mutic S, Miller TR, Dehdashti F, Siegel BA, Bosch W, Bertrand RJ (2004) Impact of FDG-PET on radiation therapy volume delineation in non-small-cell lung cancer. Int J Radiat Oncol Biol Phys 59:78–86

Brennan P, Babbage JW, Burgering BM, Groner B, Reif K, Cantrell DA (1997) Phosphatidylinositol 3-kinase couples the interleukin-2 receptor to the cell cycle regulator E2F. Immunity 7:679–689

Brizel DM, Scully SP, Harrelson JM, Layfield LJ, Bean JM, Prosnitz LR, Dewhirst MW (1996) Tumor oxygenation predicts for the likelihood of distant metastases in human soft tissue sarcoma. Cancer Res 56:941–943

Brown RS, Leung JY, Fisher SJ, Frey KA, Ethier SP, Wahl RL (1996) Intratumoral distribution of tritiated-FDG in breast carcinoma: correlation between Glut-1 expression and FDG uptake. J Nucl Med 37:1042–1047

Brun NC, Moen A, Borch K, Saugstad OD, Greisen G (1997) Near-infrared monitoring of cerebral tissue oxygen saturation and blood volume in newborn piglets. Am J Physiol 273:H682–H686

Bulte JW, Arbab AS, Douglas T, Frank JA (2004) Preparation of magnetically labeled cells for cell tracking by magnetic resonance imaging. Methods Enzymol 386:275–299

Cammilleri S, Sangrajrang S, Perdereau B, Brixy F, Calvo F, Bazin H, Magdelenat H (1996) Biodistribution of iodine-125 tyramine transforming growth factor alpha antisense oligonucleotide in athymic mice with a human mammary tumour xenograft following intratumoral injection. Eur J Nucl Med 23:448–452

Campbell RE, Tour O, Palmer AE, Steinbach PA, Baird GS, Zacharias DA, Tsien RY (2002) A monomeric red fluorescent protein. Proc Natl Acad Sci USA 99:7877–7882

Cao YA, Wagers AJ, Beilhack A, Dusich J, Bachmann MH, Negrin RS, Weissman IL, Contag CH (2004) Shifting foci of hematopoiesis during reconstitution from single stem cells. Proc Natl Acad Sci USA 101:221–226

Chapman JD, Baer K, Lee J (1983) Characteristics of the metabolism-induced binding of misonidazole to hypoxic mammalian cells. Cancer Res 43:1523–1528

Che J, Doubrovin M, Serganova I, Ageyeva L, Zanzonico P, Blasberg R (2005) hNIS-IRES-eGFP dual reporter gene imaging. Mol Imaging 4:128–136

Chievitz O and Hevesy G (1935) Radioactive indicators in the study of phosphorous metabolism in rats. Nature 136:754–755

Chishima T, Miyagi Y, Wang X, Yamaoka H, Shimada H, Moossa AR, Hoffman RM (1997) Cancer invasion and micrometastasis visualized in live tissue by green fluorescent protein expression. Cancer Res 57:2042–2047

Chudakov DM, Verkhusha VV, Staroverov DB, Souslova EA, Lukyanov S, Lukyanov KA (2004) Photoswitchable cyan fluorescent protein for protein tracking. Nat Biotechnol 22:1435–1439

Colpaert CG, Vermeulen PB, Fox SB, Harris AL, Dirix LY, Van Marck EA (2003) The presence of a fibrotic focus in invasive breast carcinoma correlates with the expression of carbonic anhydrase IX and is a marker of hypoxia and poor prognosis. Breast Cancer Res Treat 81:137–147

Contag CH, Spilman SD, Contag PR, Oshiro M, Eames B, Dennery P, Stevenson DK, Benaron DA (1997) Visualizing gene expression in living mammals using a bioluminescent reporter. Photochem Photobiol 66:523–531

Contag PR, Olomu IN, Stevenson DK, Contag CH (1998) Bioluminescent indicators in living mammals. Nat Med 4:245–247

Contag CH, Ross BD (2002) It's not just about anatomy: in vivo bioluminescence imaging as an eyepiece into biology. J Magn Reson Imaging 16:378–387

Cooper R, Sarioglu S, Sokmen S, Fuzun M, Kupelioglu A, Valentine H, Gorken IB, Airley R, West C (2003) Glucose transporter-1 (GLUT-1): a potential marker of prognosis in rectal carcinoma? Br J Cancer 89:870–876

Costa GL SM, Nakajima A, Nguyen EV, Taylor-Edwards C, Slavin AJ, Contag CH, Fathman CG, Benson JM (2001) Adoptive immunotherapy of experimental autoimmune encephalomyelitis via T cell delivery of the IL-12 p40 subunit. J Immunol 167:2379–2387

Dai C, Celestino JC, Okada Y, Louis DN, Fuller GN, Holland EC (2001) PDGF autocrine stimulation dedifferentiates cultured astrocytes and induces oligodendrogliomas and oligoastrocytomas from neural progenitors and astrocytes in vivo. Genes Dev 15:1913–1925

Dai G, Levy O, Carrasco N (1996) Cloning and characterization of the thyroid iodide transporter. Nature 379:458–460

Dehdashti F, Mortimer JE, Siegel BA, Griffeth LK, Bonasera TJ, Fusselman MJ, Detert DD, Cutler PD, Katzenellenbogen JA, Welch MJ (1995) Positron tomographic assessment of estrogen receptors in breast cancer: comparison with FDG-PET and in vitro receptor assays. J Nucl Med 36:1766–1774

Demetri GD, von Mehren M, Blanke CD, Van den Abbeele AD, Eisenberg B, Roberts PJ, Heinrich MC, Tuveson DA, Singer S, Janicek M, Fletcher JA, Silverman SG, Silberman SL, Capdeville R, Kiese B, Peng B, Dimitrijevic S, Druker BJ, Corless C, Fletcher CD, Joensuu H (2002) Efficacy and safety of imatinib mesylate in advanced gastrointestinal stromal tumors. N Engl J Med 347:472–480

Dewanjee MK, Ghafouripour AK, Kapadvanjwala M, Dewanjee S, Serafini AN, Lopez DM, Sfakianakis GN (1994) Noninvasive imaging of c-myc oncogene messenger RNA with indium-111-antisense probes in a mammary tumor-bearing mouse model. J Nucl Med 35:1054–1063

Di Chiro G, DeLaPaz RL, Brooks RA, Sokoloff L, Kornblith PL, Smith BH, Patronas NJ, Kufta CV, Kessler RM, Johnston GS, Manning RG, Wolf AP (1982) Glucose utilization of cerebral gliomas measured by [18F] fluorodeoxyglucose and positron emission tomography. Neurology 32:1323–1329

Dodd CH, Hsu HC, Chu WJ, Yang P, Zhang HG, Mountz JD Jr, Zinn K, Forder J, Josephson L, Weissleder R, Mountz JM, Mountz JD (2001) Normal T-cell response and in vivo magnetic resonance imaging of T cells loaded with HIV transactivator-peptide-derived superparamagnetic nanoparticles. J Immunol Methods 256:89–105

Doubrovin M, Ponomarev V, Beresten T, Balatoni J, Bornmann W, Finn R, Humm J, Larson S, Sadelain M, Blasberg R, Gelovani Tjuvajev J (2001) Imaging transcriptional regulation of p53-dependent genes with positron emission tomography in vivo. Proc Natl Acad Sci USA 98:9300–9305

Druker BJ, Tamura S, Buchdunger E, Ohno S, Segal GM, Fanning S, Zimmermann J, Lydon NB (1996) Effects of a selective inhibitor of the Abl tyrosine kinase on the growth of Bcr-Abl positive cells. Nat Med 2:561–566

Edinger M, Cao YA, Hornig YS, Jenkins DE, Verneris MR, Bachmann MH, Negrin RS, Contag CH (2002) Advancing animal models of neoplasia through in vivo bioluminescence imaging. Eur J Cancer 38:2128–2136

Elas M, Williams BB, Parasca A, Mailer C, Pelizzari CA, Lewis MA, River JN, Karczmar GS, Barth ED, Halpern HJ (2003) Quantitative tumor oxymetric images from 4D electron paramagnetic resonance imaging (EPRI): methodology and comparison with blood oxygen level-dependent (BOLD) MRI. Magn Reson Med 49:682–691

Ellenberg J, Lippincott-Schwartz J, Presley JF (1999) Dual-colour imaging with GFP variants. Trends Cell Biol 9:52–56

Evans SM, Kachur AV, Shiue CY, Hustinx R, Jenkins WT, Shive GG, Karp JS, Alavi A, Lord EM, Dolbier WR, Jr., Koch CJ (2000) Noninvasive detection of tumor hypoxia using the 2-nitroimidazole [18F]EF1. J Nucl Med 41:327–336

Evans SM, Judy KD, Dunphy I, Jenkins WT, Nelson PT, Collins R, Wileyto EP, Jenkins K, Hahn SM, Stevens CW, Judkins AR, Phillips P, Geoerger B, Koch CJ (2004) Comparative measurements of hypoxia in human brain tumors using needle electrodes and EF5 binding. Cancer Res 64:1886–1892

Falk MM, Lauf U (2001) High resolution, fluorescence deconvolution microscopy and tagging with the autofluorescent tracers CFP, GFP, and YFP to study the structural composition of gap junctions in living cells. Microsc Res Tech 52:251–262

Forss-Petter S, Danielson PE, Catsicas S, Battenberg E, Price J, Nerenberg M, Sutcliffe JG (1990) Transgenic mice expressing beta-galactosidase in mature neurons under neuron-specific enolase promoter control. Neuron 5:187–197

Frauwirth KA, Riley JL, Harris MH, Parry RV, Rathmell JC, Plas DR, Elstrom RL, June CH, Thompson CB (2002) The CD28 signaling pathway regulates glucose metabolism. Immunity 16:769–777

Funovics MA, Kapeller B, Hoeller C, Su HS, Kunstfeld R, Puig S, Macfelda K (2004) MR imaging of the her2/neu and 9.2.27 tumor antigens using immunospecific contrast agents. Magn Reson Imaging 22:843–850

Fyfe JA, Keller PM, Furman PA, Miller RL, Elion GB (1978) Thymidine kinase from herpes simplex virus phosphorylates the new antiviral compound, 9-(2-hydroxyethoxymethyl)guanine. J Biol Chem 253:8721–8727

Gallardo HF, Tan C, Ory D, Sadelain M (1997) Recombinant retroviruses pseudotyped with the vesicular stomatitis virus G glycoprotein mediate both stable gene transfer and pseudotransduction in human peripheral blood lymphocytes. Blood 90:952–957

Gambhir SS (2002) Molecular imaging of cancer with positron emission tomography. Nat Rev Cancer 2:683–693

Gambhir SS, Barrio JR, Wu L, Iyer M, Namavari M, Satyamurthy N, Bauer E, Parrish C, MacLaren DC, Borghei AR, Green LA, Sharfstein S, Berk AJ, Cherry SR, Phelps ME, Herschman HR (1998) Imaging of adenoviral-directed herpes simplex virus type 1 thymidine kinase reporter gene expression in mice with radiolabeled ganciclovir. J Nucl Med 39:2003–2011

Gambhir SS, Barrio JR, Phelps ME, Iyer M, Namavari M, Satyamurthy N, Wu L, Green LA, Bauer E, MacLaren DC, Nguyen K, Berk AJ, Cherry SR, Herschman HR (1999) Imaging adenoviral-directed reporter gene expression in living animals with positron emission tomography. Proc Natl Acad Sci USA 96:2333–2338

Gambhir SS, Bauer E, Black ME, Liang Q, Kokoris MS, Barrio JR, Iyer M, Namavari M, Phelps ME, Herschman HR (2000a) A mutant herpes simplex virus type 1 thymidine kinase reporter gene shows improved sensitivity for imaging reporter gene expression with positron emission tomography. Proc Natl Acad Sci USA 97:2785–2790

Gambhir SS, Herschman HR, Cherry SR, Barrio JR, Satyamurthy N, Toyokuni T, Phelps ME, Larson SM, Balatoni J, Finn R, Sadelain M, Tjuvajev J, Blasberg R (2000b) Imaging transgene expression with radionuclide imaging technologies. Neoplasia 2:118–138

Gelovani Tjuvajev J, Blasberg RG (2003) In vivo imaging of molecular-genetic targets for cancer therapy. Cancer Cell 3:327–332

Giatromanolaki A, Koukourakis MI, Sivridis E, Pastorek J, Wykoff CC, Gatter KC, Harris AL (2001) Expression of hypoxia-inducible carbonic anhydrase-9 relates to angiogenic pathways and independently to poor outcome in non-small cell lung cancer. Cancer Res 61:7992–7998

Gillies RJ, Raghunand N, Karczmar GS, Bhujwalla ZM (2002) MRI of the tumor microenvironment. J Magn Reson Imaging 16:430–450

Gobuty AH RR, Barth RF (1977) Organ distribution of 99mTc- and 51Cr-labeled autologous peripheral blood lymphocytes in rabbits. J Nucl Med 18: 141–146

Green LA, Yap CS, Nguyen K, Barrio JR, Namavari M, Satyamurthy N, Phelps ME, Sandgren EP, Herschman HR, Gambhir SS (2002) Indirect monitoring of endogenous gene expression by positron emission tomography (PET) imaging of reporter gene expression in transgenic mice. Mol Imaging Biol 4:71–81

Gupta AK, Hutchinson PJ, Fryer T, Al-Rawi PG, Parry DA, Minhas PS, Kett-White R, Kirkpatrick PJ, Mathews JC, Downey S, Aigbirhio F, Clark J, Pickard JD, Menon DK (2002) Measurement of brain tissue oxygenation performed using positron emission tomography scanning to validate a novel monitoring method. J Neurosurg 96:263–268

Gurskaya NG, Fradkov AF, Terskikh A, Matz MV, Labas YA, Martynov VI, Yanushevich YG, Lukyanov KA, Lukyanov SA (2001) GFP-like chromoproteins as a source of far-red fluorescent proteins. FEBS Lett 507:16–20

Haberkorn U (2001) Gene therapy with sodium/iodide symporter in hepatocarcinoma. Exp Clin Endocrinol Diabetes 109:60–62

Hadjantonakis AK, Nagy A (2001) The color of mice: in the light of GFP-variant reporters. Histochem Cell Biol 115:49–58

Hadjantonakis AK, Macmaster S, Nagy A (2002) Embryonic stem cells and mice expressing different GFP variants for multiple non-invasive reporter usage within a single animal. BMC Biotechnol 2:11

Hagani AB RI, Tan C, Krause A, Sadelain M (1999) Activation conditions determine susceptibility of murine primary T-lymphocytes to retroviral infection. J Gene Med 1:341–351

Hain SF, Maisey MN (2003) Positron emission tomography for urological tumours. BJU Int 92:159–164

Halbhuber KJ, Konig K (2003) Modern laser scanning microscopy in biology, biotechnology and medicine. Ann Anat 185:1–20

Hardy J EM, Bachmann MH, Negrin RS, Fathman CG, Contag CH (2001) Bioluminescence imaging of lymphocyte trafficking in vivo. Exp Hematol 29:1353–1360

Harisinghani MG, Barentsz J, Hahn PF, Deserno WM, Tabatabaei S, van de Kaa CH, de la Rosette J, Weissleder R (2003) Noninvasive detection of clinically occult lymph-node metastases in prostate cancer. N Engl J Med 348:2491–2499

Harrington KJ, Linardakis E, Vile RG (2000) Transcriptional control: an essential component of cancer gene therapy strategies? Adv Drug Deliv Rev 44:167–184

Haubner R, Wester HJ, Weber WA, Mang C, Ziegler SI, Goodman SL, Senekowitsch-Schmidtke R, Kessler H, Schwaiger M (2001) Noninvasive imaging of alpha(v)beta3 integrin expression using 18F-labeled RGD-containing glycopeptide and positron emission tomography. Cancer Res 61:1781–1785

Hennig J, Speck O, Koch MA, Weiller C (2003) Functional magnetic resonance imaging: a review of methodological aspects and clinical applications. J Magn Reson Imaging 18:1–15

Hill JM, Dick AJ, Raman VK, Thompson RB, Yu ZX, Hinds KA, Pessanha BS, Guttman MA, Varney TR, Martin BJ, Dunbar CE, McVeigh ER, Lederman RJ (2003) Serial cardiac magnetic resonance imaging of injected mesenchymal stem cells. Circulation 108:1009–1014

Hinds KA, Hill JM, Shapiro EM, Laukkanen MO, Silva AC, Combs CA, Varney TR, Balaban RS, Koretsky AP, Dunbar CE (2003) Highly efficient endosomal labeling of progenitor and stem cells with large magnetic particles allows magnetic resonance imaging of single cells. Blood 102:867–872

Hockel M, Schlenger K, Aral B, Mitze M, Schaffer U, Vaupel P (1996) Association between tumor hypoxia and malignant progression in advanced cancer of the uterine cervix. Cancer Res 56:4509–4515

Hoehn M, Kustermann E, Blunk J, Wiedermann D, Trapp T, Wecker S, Focking M, Arnold H, Hescheler J, Fleischmann BK, Schwindt W, Buhrle C (2002) Monitoring of implanted stem cell migration in vivo: a highly resolved in vivo magnetic resonance imaging investigation of experimental stroke in rat. Proc Natl Acad Sci U S A 99:16267–16272

Hoekstra CJ, Stroobants SG, Hoekstra OS, Vansteenkiste J, Biesma B, Schramel FJ, van Zandwijk N, van Tinteren H, Smit EF (2003) The value of [18F]fluoro-2-deoxy-D-glucose positron emission tomography in the selection of patients with stage IIIA-N2 non-small cell lung cancer for combined modality treatment. Lung Cancer 39:151–157

Hoffman RM (2005) The multiple uses of fluorescent proteins to visualize cancer in vivo. Nat Rev Cancer 5: 796–806

Holland E (2004a) Mouse models of human cancer. Wiley-Liss, New York

Holland EC (2004b) Mouse models of human cancer as tools in drug development. Cancer Cell 6:197–198

Ichikawa T, Hogemann D, Saeki Y, Tyminski E, Terada K, Weissleder R, Chiocca EA, Basilion JP (2002) MRI of transgene expression: correlation to therapeutic gene expression. Neoplasia 4:523–530

Iida H, Rhodes CG, Araujo LI, Yamamoto Y, de Silva R, Maseri A, Jones T (1996) Noninvasive quantification of regional myocardial metabolic rate for oxygen by use of 15O2 inhalation and positron emission tomography. Theory, error analysis, and application in humans. Circulation 94:792–807

Ivan M, Kondo K, Yang H, Kim W, Valiando J, Ohh M, Salic A, Asara JM, Lane WS, Kaelin WG, Jr. (2001) HIFalpha targeted for VHL-mediated destruction by proline hydroxylation: implications for O2 sensing. Science 292:464–468

Iyer M, Barrio JR, Namavari M, Bauer E, Satyamurthy N, Nguyen K, Toyokuni T, Phelps ME, Herschman HR, Gambhir SS (2001a) 8-[18F]Fluoropenciclovir: an improved reporter probe for imaging HSV1-tk reporter gene expression in vivo using PET. J Nucl Med 42:96–105

Iyer M, Wu L, Carey M, Wang Y, Smallwood A, Gambhir SS (2001b) Two-step transcriptional amplification as a method for imaging reporter gene expression using weak promoters. Proc Natl Acad Sci USA 98:14595–14600

Jacobs A, Tjuvajev JG, Dubrovin M, Akhurst T, Balatoni J, Beattie B, Joshi R, Finn R, Larson SM, Herrlinger U, Pechan PA, Chiocca EA, Breakefield XO, Blasberg RG (2001a) Positron emission tomography-based imaging of transgene expression mediated by replication-conditional, oncolytic herpes simplex virus type 1 mutant vectors in vivo. Cancer Res 61:2983–2995

Jacobs A, Voges J, Reszka R, Lercher M, Gossmann A, Kracht L, Kaestle C, Wagner R, Wienhard K, Heiss WD (2001b) Positron-emission tomography of vector-mediated gene expression in gene therapy for gliomas. Lancet 358:727–729

Jacobs RE AE, Meade TJ, Fraser SE (1999) Looking deeper into vertebrate development. Trends Cell Biol 9:73–76

Jaffer FA, Tung CH, Gerszten RE, Weissleder R (2002) In vivo imaging of thrombin activity in experimental thrombi with thrombin-sensitive near-infrared molecular probe. Arterioscler Thromb Vasc Biol 22:1929–1935

Johnson GA BH, Black RD, Hedlund LW, Maronpot RR, Smith BR (1993) Histology by magnetic resonance microscopy. Magn Reson Q 9:1–30

Kaelin WG Jr (2005) The von Hippel-Lindau protein, HIF hydroxylation, and oxygen sensing. Biochem Biophys Res Commun 338:627–638

Kelly RF, Tran T, Holmstrom A, Murar J, Segurola RJ, Jr. (2004) Accuracy and cost-effectiveness of [18F]-2-fluoro-deoxy-D-glucose-positron emission tomography scan in potentially resectable non-small cell lung cancer. Chest 125:1413–1423

Kiani A RA, Aramburu J (2000) Manipulating immune responses with immunosuppressive agents that target NFAT. Immunity 12:359–372

Kircher MF AJ, Graves EE, Love V, Josephson L, Lichtman AH, Weissleder R (2003) In vivo high resolution three-dimensional imaging of antigen-specific cytotoxic T-lymphocyte trafficking to tumors. Cancer Res 63:6838–6846

Koch CJ, Evans SM (2003) Non-invasive PET and SPECT imaging of tissue hypoxia using isotopically labeled 2-nitroimidazoles. Adv Exp Med Biol 510:285–292

Koehne G, Doubrovin, M, Doubrovina, E, Zanzonico, P, Gallardo, HF, Ivanova, A, Balatoni, J, Teruya-Feldstein, J, Heller, G, May, C, Ponomarev, V, Ruan, S, Finn, R, Blasberg, RG, Bornmann, W, Riviere, I, Sadelain, M, O'Reilly, RJ, Larson, SM, Gelovani Tjuvajev, JG. (2003) Serial in vivo imaging of the targeted migration of human HSV-TK-transduced antigen-specific lymphocytes. Nat Biotechnol 21:405–413

Kolb VA, Makeyev EV, Spirin AS (2000) Co-translational folding of an eukaryotic multidomain protein in a prokaryotic translation system. J Biol Chem 275:16597–16601

Korf J V-vdDL, Brinkman-Medema R, Niemarkt A, de Leij LF (1998) Divalent cobalt as a label to study lymphocyte distribution using PET and SPECT. J Nucl Med 39:836–841

Kostura L, Kraitchman DL, Mackay AM, Pittenger MF, Bulte JW (2004) Feridex labeling of mesenchymal stem cells inhibits chondrogenesis but not adipogenesis or osteogenesis. NMR Biomed 17:513–517

Krishna MC, Subramanian S, Kuppusamy P, Mitchell JB (2001) Magnetic resonance imaging for in vivo assessment of tissue oxygen concentration. Semin Radiat Oncol 11:58–69

Labas YA, Gurskaya NG, Yanushevich YG, Fradkov AF, Lukyanov KA, Lukyanov SA, Matz MV (2002) Diversity and evolution of the green fluorescent protein family. Proc Natl Acad Sci USA 99:4256–4261

Lalwani AK, Han JJ, Walsh BJ, Zolotukhin S, Muzyczka N, Mhatre AN (1997) Green fluorescent protein as a reporter for gene transfer studies in the cochlea. Hear Res 114:139–147

Larson SM, Morris M, Gunther I, Beattie B, Humm JL, Akhurst TA, Finn RD, Erdi Y, Pentlow K, Dyke J, Squire O, Bornmann W, McCarthy T, Welch M, Scher H (2004) Tumor localization of 16beta-18F-fluoro-5alpha-dihydrotestosterone versus 18F-FDG in patients with progressive, metastatic prostate cancer. J Nucl Med 45:366–373

Laxman B, Hall DE, Bhojani MS, Hamstra DA, Chenevert TL, Ross BD, Rehemtulla A (2002) Noninvasive real-time imaging of apoptosis. Proc Natl Acad Sci USA 99:16551–16555

Lazar-Molnar E, Hegyesi H, Toth S, Falus A (2000) Autocrine and paracrine regulation by cytokines and growth factors in melanoma. Cytokine 12:547–554

Lee KH, Kim HK, Paik JY, Matsui T, Choe YS, Choi Y, Kim BT (2005) Accuracy of myocardial sodium/iodide symporter gene expression imaging with radioiodide: evaluation with a dual-gene adenovirus vector. J Nucl Med 46:652–657

Lehtio K, Eskola O, Viljanen T, Oikonen V, Gronroos T, Sillanmaki L, Grenman R, Minn H (2004) Imaging perfusion and hypoxia with PET to predict radiotherapy response in head-and-neck cancer. Int J Radiat Oncol Biol Phys 59:971–982

Levy JP, Muldoon RR, Zolotukhin S, Link CJ, Jr. (1996) Retroviral transfer and expression of a humanized, red-shifted green fluorescent protein gene into human tumor cells. Nat Biotechnol 14:610–614

Lewin M, Carlesso N, Tung CH, Tang XW, Cory D, Scadden DT, Weissleder R (2000) Tat peptide-derivatized magnetic nanoparticles allow in vivo tracking and recovery of progenitor cells. Nat Biotechnol 18 410–414

Lewis JS, Welch MJ (2001) PET imaging of hypoxia. Q J Nucl Med 45:183–188

Li W HR (1996) Regulation of the nuclear factor of activated T cells in stably transfected Jurkat cell clones. Biochem Biophys Res Commun 219:96–99

Liang Q, Satyamurthy N, Barrio JR, Toyokuni T, Phelps MP, Gambhir SS, Herschman HR (2001) Noninvasive, quantitative imaging in living animals of a mutant dopamine D2 receptor reporter gene in which ligand binding is uncoupled from signal transduction. Gene Ther 8:1490–1498

Loncaster JA, Harris AL, Davidson SE, Logue JP, Hunter RD, Wycoff CC, Pastorek J, Ratcliffe PJ, Stratford IJ, West CM (2001) Carbonic anhydrase (CA IX) expression, a potential new intrinsic marker of hypoxia: correlations with tumor oxygen measurements and prognosis in locally advanced carcinoma of the cervix. Cancer Res 61:6394–6399

Louie AY, Huber MM, Ahrens ET, Rothbacher U, Moats R, Jacobs RE, Fraser SE, Meade TJ (2000) In vivo visualization of gene expression using magnetic resonance imaging. Nat Biotechnol 18:321–325

Luker GD, Sharma V, Pica CM, Dahlheimer JL, Li W, Ochesky J, Ryan CE, Piwnica-Worms H, Piwnica-Worms D (2002) Noninvasive imaging of protein-protein interactions in living animals. Proc Natl Acad Sci USA 99:6961–6966

Luker GD, Pica CM, Song J, Luker KE, Piwnica-Worms D (2003a) Imaging 26S proteasome activity and inhibition in living mice. Nat Med 9:969–973

Luker GD, Sharma V, Pica CM, Prior JL, Li W, Piwnica-Worms D (2003b) Molecular imaging of protein-protein interactions: controlled expression of p53 and large T-antigen fusion proteins in vivo. Cancer Res 63:1780–1788

Luker GD, Sharma V, Piwnica-Worms D (2003c) Visualizing protein-protein interactions in living animals. Methods 29:110–122

Lynch TJ, Bell DW, Sordella R, Gurubhagavatula S, Okimoto RA, Brannigan BW, Harris PL, Haserlat SM, Supko JG, Haluska FG, Louis DN, Christiani DC, Settleman J, Haber DA (2004) Activating mutations in the epidermal growth factor receptor underlying responsiveness of non-small-cell lung cancer to gefitinib. N Engl J Med 350:2129–2139

Lyons SK, Meuwissen R, Krimpenfort P, Berns A (2003) The generation of a conditional reporter that enables bioluminescence imaging of Cre/loxP-dependent tumorigenesis in mice. Cancer Res 63:7042–7046

Lyons SK, Lim E, Clermont AO, Dusich J, Zhu L, Campbell KD, Coffee RJ, Grass DS, Hunter J, Purchio T, Jenkins D (2006) Noninvasive bioluminescence imaging of normal and spontaneously transformed prostate tissue in mice. Cancer Res 66:4701–4707

Maschauer S, Prante O, Hoffmann M, Deichen JT, Kuwert T (2004) Characterization of 18F-FDG uptake in human endothelial cells in vitro. J Nucl Med 45:455–460

Mathieu S, El-Battari A (2003) Monitoring E-selectin-mediated adhesion using green and red fluorescent proteins. J Immunol Methods 272:81–92

Matz MV, Fradkov AF, Labas YA, Savitsky AP, Zaraisky AG, Markelov ML, Lukyanov SA (1999) Fluorescent proteins from nonbioluminescent Anthozoa species. Nat Biotechnol 17:969–973

Mayer-Kuckuk P, Banerjee D, Malhotra S, Doubrovin M, Iwamoto M, Akhurst T, Balatoni J, Bornmann W, Finn R, Larson S, Fong Y, Gelovani Tjuvajev J, Blasberg R, Bertino JR (2002) Cells exposed to antifolates show increased cellular levels of proteins fused to dihydrofolate reductase: a method to modulate gene expression. Proc Natl Acad Sci USA 99:3400–3405

Mayer-Kuckuk P, Menon LG, Blasberg RG, Bertino JR, Banerjee D (2004) Role of reporter gene imaging in molecular and cellular biology. Biol Chem 385:353–361

Mayer-Kuckuk P, Doubrovin M, Bidaut L, Budak-Alpdogan T, Cai S, Hubbard V, Alpdogan O, van den Brink M, Bertino JR, Blasberg RG, Banerjee D, Gelovani J (2006) Molecular imaging reveals skeletal engraftment sites of transplanted bone marrow cells. Cell Transplant 15:75–82

Min JJ, Gambhir SS (2004) Gene therapy progress and prospects: noninvasive imaging of gene therapy in living subjects. Gene Ther 11:115–125

Min JJ, Iyer M, Gambhir SS (2003) Comparison of [18F]FHBG and [14C]FIAU for imaging of HSV1-tk reporter gene expression: adenoviral infection vs stable transfection. Eur J Nucl Med Mol Imaging 30:1547–1560

Moberg KH, Logan TJ, Tyndall WA, Hall DJ (1992) Three distinct elements within the murine c-myc promoter are required for transcription. Oncogene 7:411–421

Myers WG (1979) Georg Charles de Hevesy: the father of nuclear medicine. J Nucl Med 20:590–594

Nakagawa S, Massie B, Hawley RG (2001) Tetracycline-regulatable adenovirus vectors: pharmacologic properties and clinical potential. Eur J Pharm Sci 13:53–60

Neckers L (2002) Hsp90 inhibitors as novel cancer chemotherapeutic agents. Trends Mol Med 8:S55–S61

Neumaier M, Shively L, Chen FS, Gaida FJ, Ilgen C, Paxton RJ, Shively JE, Riggs AD (1990) Cloning of the genes for T84.66, an antibody that has a high specificity and affinity for carcinoembryonic antigen, and expression of chimeric human/mouse T84.66 genes in myeloma and Chinese hamster ovary cells. Cancer Res 50:2128–2134

Nordsmark M, Overgaard M, Overgaard J (1996) Pretreatment oxygenation predicts radiation response in advanced squamous cell carcinoma of the head and neck. Radiother Oncol 41:31–39

Nordsmark M, Loncaster J, Aquino-Parsons C, Chou SC, Ladekarl M, Havsteen H, Lindegaard JC, Davidson SE, Varia M, West C, Hunter R, Overgaard J, Raleigh JA (2003) Measurements of hypoxia using pimonidazole and polarographic oxygen-sensitive electrodes in human cervix carcinomas. Radiother Oncol 67:35–44

Olafsen T, Kenanova VE, Sundaresan G, Anderson AL, Crow D, Yazaki PJ, Li L, Press MF, Gambhir SS, Williams LE, Wong JY, Raubitschek AA, Shively JE, Wu AM (2005) Optimizing radiolabeled engineered anti-p185HER2 antibody fragments for in vivo imaging. Cancer Res 65:5907–5916

Olasz EB, Lang L, Seidel J, Green MV, Eckelman WC, Katz SI (2002) Fluorine-18 labeled mouse bone marrow-derived dendritic cells can be detected in vivo by high resolution projection imaging. J Immunol Methods 260:137–148

Oliver RJ, Woodwards RT, Sloan P, Thakker NS, Stratford IJ, Airley RE (2004) Prognostic value of facilitative glucose transporter Glut-1 in oral squamous cell carcinomas treated by surgical resection; results of EORTC Translational Research Fund studies. Eur J Cancer 40:503–507

Oswald F, Lovec H, Moroy T, Lipp M (1994) E2F-dependent regulation of human MYC: transactivation by cyclins D1 and A overrides tumour suppressor protein functions. Oncogene 9:2029–2036

Overbeek PA, Chepelinsky AB, Khillan JS, Piatigorsky J, Westphal H (1985) Lens-specific expression and developmental regulation of the bacterial chloramphenicol acetyltransferase gene driven by the murine alpha A-crystallin promoter in transgenic mice. Proc Natl Acad Sci USA 82:7815–7819

Palm S, Enmon RM, Jr., Matei C, Kolbert KS, Xu S, Zanzonico PB, Finn RL, Koutcher JA, Larson SM, Sgouros G (2003) Pharmacokinetics and Biodistribution of (86)Y-Trastuzumab for (90)Y dosimetry in an ovarian carcinoma model: correlative MicroPET and MRI. J Nucl Med 44:1148–1155

Papadakis ED, Nicklin SA, Baker AH, White SJ (2004) Promoters and control elements: designing expression cassettes for gene therapy. Curr Gene Ther 4:89–113

Papierniak CK BR, Kretschmer RR, Gotoff SP, Colombetti LG (1976) Technetium-99m labeling of human monocytes for chemotactic studies. J Nucl Med 17:988–992

Peng T, Golub TR, Sabatini DM (2002) The immunosuppressant rapamycin mimics a starvationlike signal distinct from amino acid and glucose deprivation. Mol Cell Biol 22:5575–5584

Penuelas I, Mazzolini G, Boan JF, Sangro B, Marti-Climent J, Ruiz M, Ruiz J, Satyamurthy N, Qian C, Barrio JR, Phelps ME, Richter JA, Gambhir SS, Prieto J (2005) Positron emission tomography imaging of adenoviral-mediated transgene expression in liver cancer patients. Gastroenterology 128:1787–1795

Phillips JA, Craig SJ, Bayley D, Christian RA, Geary R, Nicklin PL (1997) Pharmacokinetics, metabolism, and elimination of a 20-mer phosphorothioate oligodeoxynucleotide (CGP 69846A) after intravenous and subcutaneous administration. Biochem Pharmacol 54:657–668

Pichler A, Prior JL, Piwnica-Worms D (2004) Imaging reversal of multidrug resistance in living mice with bioluminescence: MDR1 P-glycoprotein transports coelenterazine. Proc Natl Acad Sci USA 101:1702–1707

Ponomarev V, Doubrovin M, Lyddane C, Beresten T, Balatoni J, Bornman W, Finn R, Akhurst T, Larson S, Blasberg R, Sadelain M, Tjuvajev JG (2001) Imaging TCR-dependent NFAT-mediated T-cell activation with positron emission tomography in vivo. Neoplasia 3:480–488

Ponomarev V, Doubrovin M, Serganova I, Beresten T, Vider J, Shavrin A, Ageyeva L, Balatoni J, Blasberg R, Tjuvajev JG (2003) Cytoplasmically retargeted HSV1-tk/GFP reporter gene mutants for optimization of noninvasive molecular-genetic imaging. Neoplasia 5:245–254

Ponomarev V, Doubrovin M, Serganova I, Vider J, Shavrin A, Beresten T, Ivanova A, Ageyeva L, Tourkova V, Balatoni J, Bornmann W, Blasberg R, Gelovani Tjuvajev J (2004) A novel triple-modality reporter gene for whole-body fluorescent, bioluminescent, and nuclear noninvasive imaging. Eur J Nucl Med Mol Imaging 31:740–751

Qiao J, Doubrovin M, Sauter BV, Huang Y, Guo ZS, Balatoni J, Akhurst T, Blasberg RG, Tjuvajev JG, Chen SH, Woo SL (2002) Tumor-specific transcriptional targeting of suicide gene therapy. Gene Ther 9: 168–175

Rannie GH TM, Ford WL (1977) An experimental comparison of radioactive labels with potential application to lymphocyte migration studies in patients. Clin Exp Immunol 29: 509–514

Rasey JS, Koh WJ, Evans ML, Peterson LM, Lewellen TK, Graham MM, Krohn KA (1996) Quantifying regional hypoxia in human tumors with positron emission tomography of [18F]fluoromisonidazole: a pretherapy study of 37 patients. Int J Radiat Oncol Biol Phys 36:417–428

Ray P, Bauer E, Iyer M, Barrio JR, Satyamurthy N, Phelps ME, Herschman HR, Gambhir SS (2001) Monitoring gene therapy with reporter gene imaging. Semin Nucl Med 31:312–320

Ray P, Pimenta H, Paulmurugan R, Berger F, Phelps ME, Iyer M, Gambhir SS (2002) Noninvasive quantitative imaging of protein-protein interactions in living subjects. Proc Natl Acad Sci USA 99:3105–3110

Ray P, Wu AM, Gambhir SS (2003) Optical bioluminescence and positron emission tomography imaging of a novel fusion reporter gene in tumor xenografts of living mice. Cancer Res 63:1160–1165

Ray S, Paulmurugan R, Hildebrandt I, Iyer M, Wu L, Carey M, Gambhir SS (2004) Novel bidirectional vector strategy for amplification of therapeutic and reporter gene expression. Hum Gene Ther 15:681–690

Rehemtulla A, Stegman LD, Cardozo SJ, Gupta S, Hall DE, Contag CH, Ross BD (2000) Rapid and quantitative assessment of cancer treatment response using in vivo bioluminescence imaging. Neoplasia 2:491–495

Rogers BE, Zinn KR, Buchsbaum DJ (2000) Gene transfer strategies for improving radiolabeled peptide imaging and therapy. Q J Nucl Med 44:208–223

Sadeghi H, Hitt MM (2005) Transcriptionally targeted adenovirus vectors. Curr Gene Ther 5: 411–427

Salceda S, Caro J (1997) Hypoxia-inducible factor 1alpha (HIF-1alpha) protein is rapidly degraded by the ubiquitin-proteasome system under normoxic conditions. Its stabilization by hypoxia depends on redox-induced changes. J Biol Chem 272:22642–22647

Schelling M, Avril N, Nahrig J, Kuhn W, Romer W, Sattler D, Werner M, Dose J, Janicke F, Graeff H, Schwaiger M (2000) Positron emission tomography using [(18)F]Fluorodeoxy-glucose for monitoring primary chemotherapy in breast cancer. J Clin Oncol 18:1689–1695

Serganova I, Doubrovin M, Vider J, Ponomarev V, Soghomonyan S, Beresten T, Ageyeva L, Serganov A, Cai S, Balatoni J, Blasberg R, Gelovani J (2004) Molecular imaging of temporal dynamics and spatial heterogeneity of hypoxia-inducible factor-1 signal transduction activity in tumors in living mice. Cancer Res 64:6101–6108

Shah K, Jacobs A, Breakefield XO, Weissleder R (2004) Molecular imaging of gene therapy for cancer. Gene Ther 11:1175–1187

Shaner NC, Steinbach PA, Tsien RY (2005) A guide to choosing fluorescent proteins. Nat Methods 2:905–909

Shaner NC, Campbell RE, Steinbach PA, Giepmans BN, Palmer AE, Tsien RY (2004) Improved monomeric red, orange and yellow fluorescent proteins derived from Discosoma sp. red fluorescent protein. Nat Biotechnol 22:1567–1572

Sherr CJ, McCormick F (2002) The RB and p53 pathways in cancer. Cancer Cell 2:103–112

Shin JH, Chung JK, Kang JH, Lee YJ, Kim KI, So Y, Jeong JM, Lee DS, Lee MC (2004) Noninvasive imaging for monitoring of viable cancer cells using a dual-imaging reporter gene. J Nucl Med 45:2109–2115

Shreve PD, Anzai Y, Wahl RL (1999) Pitfalls in oncologic diagnosis with FDG PET imaging: physiologic and benign variants. Radiographics 19:61–77; quiz 150–151

Smith-Jones PM, Solit DB, Akhurst T, Afroze F, Rosen N, Larson SM (2004) Imaging the pharma-codynamics of HER2 degradation in response to Hsp90 inhibitors. Nat Biotechnol 22:701–706

Stamm C, Westphal B, Kleine HD, Petzsch M, Kittner C, Klinge H, Schumichen C, Nienaber CA, Freund M, Steinhoff G (2003) Autologous bone-marrow stem-cell transplantation for myocardial regeneration. Lancet 361:45–46

Su H FA, Gambhir SS, Braun J (2004) Quantitation of cell number by a positron emission tomography reporter gene strategy. Mol Imaging Biol 6:139–148

Sundaresan G, Yazaki PJ, Shively JE, Finn RD, Larson SM, Raubitschek AA, Williams LE, Chatziioannou AF, Gambhir SS, Wu AM (2003) 124I-labeled engineered anti-CEA minibodies and diabodies allow high-contrast, antigen-specific small-animal PET imaging of xenografts in athymic mice. J Nucl Med 44:1962–1969

Tavitian B (2000) In vivo antisense imaging. Q J Nucl Med 44:236–255

Tavitian B, Terrazzino S, Kuhnast B, Marzabal S, Stettler O, Dolle F, Deverre JR, Jobert A, Hinnen F, Bendriem B, Crouzel C, Di Giamberardino L (1998) In vivo imaging of oligonu-cleotides with positron emission tomography. Nat Med 4:467–471

Thomas GV, Tran C, Mellinghoff IK, Welsbie DS, Chan E, Fueger B, Czernin J, Sawyers CL (2006) Hypoxia-inducible factor determines sensitivity to inhibitors of mTOR in kidney cancer. Nat Med 12:122–127

Thompson JF, Hayes LS, Lloyd DB (1991) Modulation of firefly luciferase stability and impact on studies of gene regulation. Gene 103:171–177

Tjuvajev J, Gansbacher B, Desai R, Beattie B, Kaplitt M, Matei C, Koutcher J, Gilboa E, Blasberg R (1995a) RG-2 glioma growth attenuation and severe brain edema caused by local production of interleukin-2 and interferon-gamma. Cancer Res 55:1902–1910

Tjuvajev JG, Stockhammer G, Desai R, Uehara H, Watanabe K, Gansbacher B, Blasberg RG (1995b) Imaging the expression of transfected genes in vivo. Cancer Res 55:6126–6132

Tjuvajev JG, Finn R, Watanabe K, Joshi R, Oku T, Kennedy J, Beattie B, Koutcher J, Larson S, Blasberg RG (1996) Noninvasive imaging of herpes virus thymidine kinase gene transfer and expression: a potential method for monitoring clinical gene therapy. Cancer Res 56:4087–4095

Tjuvajev JG, Avril N, Oku T, Sasajima T, Miyagawa T, Joshi R, Safer M, Beattie B, DiResta G, Daghighian F, Augensen F, Koutcher J, Zweit J, Humm J, Larson SM, Finn R, Blasberg R (1998) Imaging herpes virus thymidine kinase gene transfer and expression by positron emission tomography. Cancer Res 58:4333–4341

Tjuvajev JG, Chen SH, Joshi A, Joshi R, Guo ZS, Balatoni J, Ballon D, Koutcher J, Finn R, Woo SL, Blasberg RG (1999) Imaging adenoviral-mediated herpes virus thymidine kinase gene transfer and expression in vivo. Cancer Res 59:5186–5193

Tjuvajev J, Blasberg R, Luo X, Zheng LM, King I, Bermudes D (2001) Salmonella-based tumor-targeted cancer therapy: tumor amplified protein expression therapy (TAPET) for diagnostic imaging. J Control Release 74:313–315

Tjuvajev JG, Doubrovin M, Akhurst T, Cai S, Balatoni J, Alauddin MM, Finn R, Bornmann W, Thaler H, Conti PS, Blasberg RG (2002) Comparison of radiolabeled nucleoside probes (FIAU, FHBG, and FHPG) for PET imaging of HSV1-tk gene expression. J Nucl Med 43:1072–1083

Tomita S, Mickle DA, Weisel RD, Jia ZQ, Tumiati LC, Allidina Y, Liu P, Li RK (2002) Improved heart function with myogenesis and angiogenesis after autologous porcine bone marrow stromal cell transplantation. J Thorac Cardiovasc Surg 123:1132–1140

Tuveson DA, Willis NA, Jacks T, Griffin JD, Singer S, Fletcher CD, Fletcher JA, Demetri GD (2001) STI571 inactivation of the gastrointestinal stromal tumor c-KIT oncoprotein: biological and clinical implications. Oncogene 20:5054–5058

Uhrbom L, Nerio E, Holland EC (2004) Dissecting tumor maintenance requirements using biolu-minescence imaging of cell proliferation in a mouse glioma model. Nat Med 10:1257–1260

van den Abbeele A (2001) F18-FDG-PET provides early evidence of biological response to ST1571 pateins with malignant gastointestinal stromal tumors (GIST). Proc Am Soc Clin Oncol 20:362a

Vose JM, Bierman PJ, Anderson JR, Harrison KA, Dalrymple GV, Byar K, Kessinger A, Armitage JO (1996) Single-photon emission computed tomography gallium imaging versus computed tomography: predictive value in patients undergoing high-dose chemotherapy and autologous stem-cell transplantation for non-Hodgkin's lymphoma. J Clin Oncol 14:2473–2479

Wang GL, Semenza GL (1995) Purification and characterization of hypoxia-inducible factor 1. J Biol Chem 270:1230–1237

Wang L, Jackson WC, Steinbach PA, Tsien RY (2004) Evolution of new nonantibody proteins via iterative somatic hypermutation. Proc Natl Acad Sci USA 101:16745–16749

Wang X, Rosol M, Ge S, Peterson D, McNamara G, Pollack H, Kohn DB, Nelson MD, Crooks GM (2003) Dynamic tracking of human hematopoietic stem cell engraftment using in vivo bioluminescence imaging. Blood 102:3478–3482

Wang Y, Iyer M, Annala A, Wu L, Carey M, Gambhir SS (2006) Noninvasive indirect imaging of vascular endothelial growth factor gene expression using bioluminescence imaging in living transgenic mice. Physiol Genomics 24:173–180

Warburg O (1956) On the origin of cancer cells. Science 123:309–314

Weber WA, Petersen V, Schmidt B, Tyndale-Hines L, Link T, Peschel C, Schwaiger M (2003) Positron emission tomography in non-small-cell lung cancer: prediction of response to chemotherapy by quantitative assessment of glucose use. J Clin Oncol 21:2651–2657

Weissleder R (2002) Scaling down imaging: molecular mapping of cancer in mice. Nat Rev Cancer 2:11–18

Weissleder R, Ntziachristos V (2003) Shedding light onto live molecular targets. Nat Med 9: 123–128

Weissleder R, Simonova M, Bogdanova A, Bredow S, Enochs WS, Bogdanov A Jr (1997) MR imaging and scintigraphy of gene expression through melanin induction. Radiology 204: 425–429

Wilson T, Hastings JW (1998) Bioluminescence. Annu Rev Cell Dev Biol 14:197–230

Wong KK, Zou X, Merrell KT, Patel AJ, Marcu KB, Chellappan S, Calame K (1995) v-Abl activates c-myc transcription through the E2F site. Mol Cell Biol 15:6535–6544

Wu AM (2004) Engineering multivalent antibody fragments for in vivo targeting. Methods Mol Biol 248:209–225

Wu AM, Senter PD (2005) Arming antibodies: prospects and challenges for immunoconjugates. Nat Biotechnol 23:1137–1146

Wu JC, Inubushi M, Sundaresan G, Schelbert HR, Gambhir SS (2002) Optical imaging of cardiac reporter gene expression in living rats. Circulation 105:1631–1634

Yaghoubi S, Barrio JR, Dahlbom M, Iyer M, Namavari M, Satyamurthy N, Goldman R, Herschman HR, Phelps ME, Gambhir SS (2001) Human pharmacokinetic and dosimetry studies of [(18)F]FHBG: a reporter probe for imaging herpes simplex virus type-1 thymidine kinase reporter gene expression. J Nucl Med 42:1225–1234

Yaghoubi SS, Barrio JR, Namavari M, Satyamurthy N, Phelps ME, Herschman HR, Gambhir SS (2005) Imaging progress of herpes simplex virus type 1 thymidine kinase suicide gene therapy in living subjects with positron emission tomography. Cancer Gene Ther 12:329–339

Yu YA, Timiryasova T, Zhang Q, Beltz R, Szalay AA (2003) Optical imaging: bacteria, viruses, and mammalian cells encoding light-emitting proteins reveal the locations of primary tumors and metastases in animals. Anal Bioanal Chem 377:964–972

Zhang L, Adams JY, Billick E, Ilagan R, Iyer M, Le K, Smallwood A, Gambhir SS, Carey M, Wu L (2002) Molecular engineering of a two-step transcription amplification (TSTA) system for transgene delivery in prostate cancer. Mol Ther 5:223–232

Zhang W FJ, Harris SE, Contag PR, Stevenson DK, Contag CH (2001) Rapid in vivo functional analysis of transgenes in mice using whole body imaging of luciferase expression. Transgenic Res 10:423-434

Zhu ZB, Makhija SK, Lu B, Wang M, Kaliberova L, Liu B, Rivera AA, Nettelbeck DM, Mahasreshti PJ, Leath CA, 3rd, Yamamoto M, Alvarez RD, Curiel DT (2004) Transcriptional targeting of adenoviral vector through the CXCR4 tumor-specific promoter. Gene Ther 11: 645–648

The Use of Ultrasound in Transfection and Transgene Expression

Claire Rome, Roel Deckers, and Chrit T.W. Moonen(✉)

Abstract The interaction of ultrasound with tissue leads to radiation pressure, heat generation, and cavitation. These phenomena have been utilised for local gene delivery, transfection and control of expression. Specially designed nanocarriers or adapted ultrasound contrast agents can further enhance local delivery by: (1) increased permeability of cell membranes; (2) local release of genes. Biological carriers may also be used for local gene delivery. Stem cells and immune cells appear especially promising because of their homing capabilities to lesion sites. Imaging methods can be employed for pharmacodistribution and pharmacokinetics. MRI contrast agents can serve as non-invasive reporters on gene distribution

Chrit T.W. Moonen

Laboratory for Molecular and Functional Imaging: From Physiology to Therapy, UMR5231 CNRS, Université Victor Segalen Bordeaux 2, Bordeaux, France
chrit.moonen@imf.u-bordeaux2.fr

W. Semmler and M. Schwaiger (eds.), *Molecular Imaging II.*
Handbook of Experimental Pharmacology 185/II.
© Springer-Verlag Berlin Heidelberg 2008

when co-delivered with the gene. They can be used to label nanocarriers and cellular transport systems in gene therapy strategies such as those based on stem cells. Finally, ultrasound heating together with the use of a temperature sensitive promoter allows a local, physical, spatio-temporal control of transgene expression, in particular when combined with MRI temperature mapping for monitoring and even controlling ultrasound heating.

1 Introduction

Ultrasound is a form of mechanical energy that is propagated as a vibrational wave of particles within the medium at a frequency between about 20 kHz and 200 MHz. The oscillatory displacement of particles is associated with a pressure wave. The behaviour of ultrasound waves in medium may be described in a similar way to that in optics. At tissue interfaces reflection of the wave occurs according to Snell's law, depending on the wave velocity and the incident angle. The speed of ultrasound is about $1,550 \, \mathrm{ms}^{-1}$ for soft tissue, independent of the ultrasound frequency. In fatty tissue the average speed is only slightly lower $(1,480 \, \mathrm{ms}^{-1})$, whereas in air spaces a value of $600 \, \mathrm{ms}^{-1}$ is found. In bone, the speed is much higher (between $1,800$ and $3,700 \, \mathrm{ms}^{-1}$). Ultrasound beams are usually generated electrically using piezoceramic plates outside the body and propagate inwards either longitudinally or transversely (called shear waves).

Ultrasound waves can be concentrated in a focal point of dimensions of the ultrasound wavelength (of the order of 1 mm for a frequency 1.5 MHz). Ultrasound has long been considered as a way to alter tissue permeability, to increase DNA uptake, and affect gene expression (Fechheimer et al. 1987). The concept of sonoporation has been introduced in which the presence of ultrasound contrast agent and ultrasound tissue exposure is combined to create small holes in the cell membrane allowing extravasation of drugs and/or DNA fragments into the cell depending on several parameters: frequency and intensity of ultrasound, characteristics of ultrasound contrast agents and their influence on cavitation.

This review will first give an overview of the interaction of ultrasound with tissue. Then, gene microcarriers are described. MR contrast agents can be used during gene delivery to report on pharmacokinetics and pharmacodistribution. Finally, transgene delivery and transgene expression control with (focused) ultrasound is described. How MRI can be used to monitor ultrasound heating of tissue and even control the heating by feedback coupling with US is also considered.

2 Interaction of Ultrasound with Tissue

It is well known that the interaction of ultrasound with tissue can produce a wide variety of biological effects. The mechanisms underlying the many biological effects of ultrasound include acoustic heat generation, radiation pressure and, with respect to local gene delivery perhaps most importantly, cavitation. Below, the physical principles that are associated with these three mechanisms and their bioeffects are discussed in more detail.

2.1 Heat Generation

The intensity of an ultrasonic wave travelling through a medium may be attenuated. Part of this attenuation is due to absorption. During absorption, the mechanical energy of the acoustic wave (micrometre displacements with a frequency in the MHz range) is converted into heat (atomic vibrations with sub-nanometre displacements with frequencies well above 1 GHz). There are several mechanisms by which absorption can occur. For example, the viscosity of the medium tends to oppose the vibrational motion of the particles of the wave and some of this energy is converted into heat (Hueter and Bolt 1955). Ultrasound absorption in tissue is much more efficient than in free liquids or in blood. The exact mechanisms by which ultrasound is absorbed by biological materials are rather complicated. It has been observed that within the frequency range used for medical ultrasonic imaging most tissues have an attenuation coefficient that is linearly proportional to the frequency (Dunn and O'Brien 1976). Overall, the attenuation of a plane wave may be described by an exponentially decaying function. The intensity I_x at depth x with respect to that at the original position (I_0) is given by

$$I_x = I_0 e^{-2\alpha x} \tag{1}$$

where α represents the attenuation coefficient of the wave amplitude per unit path length. For 1.5-MHz ultrasound waves, the intensity in soft tissues will drop to about 50% at 50-mm penetration.

2.2 Cavitation

Acoustic cavitation is defined as the formation and/or activity of gas-filled bubbles in a medium exposed to ultrasound. The sustained growth of cavitation bubbles and their oscillations over several acoustic cycles is known as stable or non-inertial cavitation (Leighton 1994). In contrast, when a cavitation bubble grows violently and collapses in less than a cycle this is called transient or inertial cavitation (Leighton 1994). Figure 1 gives an example of a microbubble oscillating over several cycles and then collapsing in smaller fragments. In general, the likelihood and intensity of transient cavitation increases at higher pressures (p) and lower frequencies (f) (Brennen 1995). These two exposure parameters have been combined in a single mechanical index (MI) defined as:

$$MI = \frac{p}{\sqrt{f}} \tag{2}$$

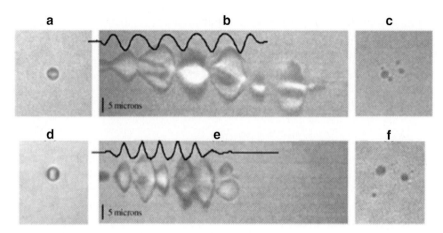

Fig. 1 a–f Optical images of triacetin-shelled AALs with an initial radius near or below the resonance size, insonified at 1.5 MHz and 2.5 MHz. Resonance radius for 1.5 MHz is approximately 2.2 μm, resonance radius for 2.5 MHz is approximately 1.6 μm. **a** A two-dimensional image of a 1.7-μm radius AAL before insonation; **b** a streak image of the same AAL under insonation at 1.6 MPa and 1.5 MHz, with overlay of hydrophone recording of transmitted pulse; **c** image of fragments after insonation. **d** A two-dimensional image of a 1.7-μm radius AAL before insonation; **e** a streak image of same AAL under insonation at 1.6 MPa and 2.5 MHz, with overlay of hydrophone recording of transmitted pulse; **f** image of fragments remaining after insonation. (Figure taken from May et al. 2002)

The cavitation process will also be affected by the number and size of the cavitation bubbles and its physical properties (Leighton 1994). In some in-vitro situations cavitation can occur at modest intensity, because of the presence of suitably sized bubbles. In contrast, cavitation nuclei are typically minimised for in-vivo conditions in mammals owing to active filtering and sterilization by physiological processes, with the exception of lungs and intestine. Besides these parameters there are other parameters that influence the effects of cavitation, like exposure time, pulse repetition frequency and duty cycle.

Both stable and transient cavitation may induce membrane permeabilization, as is demonstrated in Fig. 2. Several investigators (Everbach et al. 1997; Miller et al. 1996) argue that transient cavitation is the cause of cell damage, at least in vitro. On the other hand, other investigators advocate the idea that disruption of cell membranes is caused by stable cavitation (Liu et al. 1998). Since cavitation leads to the generation of harmonics of the basic ultrasound frequency, and ultrasound absorption is more efficient at higher frequencies, it is clear that cavitation also leads to more efficient ultrasound absorption and heating.

2.2.1 Transient Cavitation

Several physical phenomena are associated with transient cavitation. During the rapid collapse of the gas bubble, the inward moving wall of fluid has sufficient

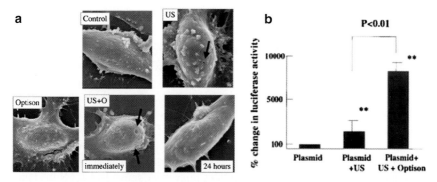

Fig. 2 a Electron microscopic views of endothelial cells transfected with naked plasmid DNA by means of ultrasound with Optison. *Control* indicates untransfected cells; *US* ultrasound alone; *Optison* Optison alone; *US+O immediately* immediately after transfection by means of ultrasound with Optison; *24 hours* 24 h after transfection by means of ultrasound with Optison. *Arrows* point out holes. **b** Comparison of luciferase activity after transfection by means of naked plasmid DNA alone, naked plasmid DNA with ultrasound, and naked plasmid DNA with ultrasound and Optison in human cultured endothelial cells 1 day after transfection. *Plasmid* indicates plasmid DNA alone; *plasmid+US* ultrasound alone; *plasmid+US+Optison* ultrasound and Optison. Values are expressed as percent increase in luciferase activity compared with plasmid; $n = 8$ for each group calculated from eight independent experiments. $^{**}P = 0.01$ vs plasmid. (Figure adapted from Taniyama et al. 2002)

inertia to not reverse direction when the acoustic pressure reverses direction, but continues to compress the gas in the bubble to a very small volume. During this process the pressure and temperature can reach thousands of bars and degrees Kelvin (Suslick 1989). This can lead to emission of light (sonoluminescence) and production of free radicals (sonochemistry). The collapse of the bubble also generates shock waves that spherically diverge in the surrounding environment of the bubble. When collapsing bubbles are in the vicinity of solid boundaries (e.g. cell membranes), the collapse will be asymmetrical and can result in the formation of high speed, fluid microjets (Blake and Gibson 1987). Lokhandwalla and Sturtevant describe how shock waves, bubble wall motion (i.e. bubble expansion and collapse) and microjets may affect membrane permeability. They show that these mechanisms can cause the membrane to deform beyond the threshold strain for rupture (Lokhandwalla et al. 2001). The critical values of area strain and critical tension for membrane disruption have been reported to be, respectively, 2–3% and $10\,\mathrm{mN\ m^{-1}}$ (Evans et al. 1976). Lokhandwalla calculated an inertial force due to shock waves of $64\,\mathrm{mN\ m^{-1}}$, for a duration of 3 ns, which is sufficient to induce pores in the membrane. For the inertial force induced by bubble wall motion a magnitude of $100\,\mathrm{mN\ m^{-1}}$ that lasted for a duration of $1\,\mu s$ was calculated, which is sufficient to cause membrane rupture.

2.2.2 Stable Cavitation

Rectified diffusion, heat production and microstreaming are physical phenomena that can be associated with stable cavitation. Rectified diffusion describes the slow growth of an oscillating bubble related to a net inflow of gas into the bubble over successive cycles, until it reaches a resonant size. At resonant size the bubble will show stable, low amplitude oscillations. These oscillations induce inhomogeneous cyclic field around the bubbles, which cause small flows in the bubble-surrounding fluid, a process known as microstreaming (Nyborg 1996). Marmottant and Hilgenfeldt (2003) showed that linear oscillations (i.e. stable cavitation) can be sufficient to rupture single cells. The microstreaming creates high shear stresses $(10^{-2}\,\mathrm{N\,m^{-1}})$ near the bubble surface that cause the strain in the membrane of cells in the neighborhood to exceed the critical strain for membrane rupture. Transient cavitation effects have to be used with caution in vivo. Vessel walls may break up leading to haemorrhage (Dalecki et al. 1997a). It has been shown that red blood cells may collapse (Miller et al. 1996; Dalecki et al. 1997b; Rooney 1970).

2.3 Radiation Force

Although the use of ultrasound in combination with ultrasound contrast agents to deliver gene by the physical process known as cavitation is well established, researchers have investigated other means of using ultrasound in drug delivery, e.g. radiation force in absence of cavitation nuclei. The radiation force is a result of the transfer of momentum when an ultrasonic wave is absorbed by a particle. The magnitude of the radiation force depends on the tissue absorption, speed of sound and the intensity of the acoustic beam. It has also been shown that it is possible to use radiation force to direct delivery vehicles near the blood vessel wall, which will increase the probability of targeted adhesion by up to 30-fold (Lum et al. 2006; Shortencarier et al. 2004). Recently, Frenkel and Li (2006) showed how non-uniform displacements caused by radiation force can induce shear forces in tissues and, as a consequence, enhance the cell permeability (*see*, for example, Fig. 3).

3 Nanoparticles for Ultrasound-mediated Gene Delivery

Research in the field of nanoparticles for local gene delivery is very active. The principles are similar for drug and gene delivery. Upon collapse of the nanoparticle, subsequent local release of the gene or drug leads to high local drug/gene concentrations while limiting toxicity effects due to high systemic concentrations for conventional ways of administering drugs/genes. Local release of genes/drugs may be triggered by natural processes, such as membrane fusion, phagocytosis and pinocytosis, but may also be triggered by external physical means. With respect to the use of ultrasound, nanoparticles may be designed specifically to enhance ultrasound-induced bio-effects.

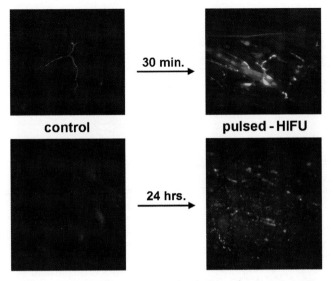

Fig. 3 Pulsed-HIFU exposures, followed by systemic administration, have been shown to improve the uptake of fluorescent nanoparticles. The enhanced delivery is the result of increased extravasation from the vasculature and improved diffusion in the interstitium. (Figure taken from Frenkel et al. 2005)

3.1 Microbubbles

As was described above, microbubbles can drastically enhance ultrasound bio-effects, notably cavitation. Microbubbles, either non-specific or targeted, may also be used as gene carriers and the increased ultrasound bio-effects can lead to enhanced transfection efficiency. Most microbubbles consist of air- or perfluorocarbon-filled microspheres stabilized by an albumin or lipid shell, with a size in the range of 1–10 µm (Grayburn 2002). There are several different approaches to how microbubbles can transport genes and drugs. An outline of common carriers for gene/drug delivery is given in Fig. 4. They can be attached to the membrane surrounding the microbubble (Frenkel et al. 2002), a drug can be imbedded within the membrane itself, genes can be bound non-covalently to the surface of the microbubble (Shohet et al. 2000) and the drug can be loaded to the interior of the microbubble, either in an oil or aqueous phase (Lum et al. 2006; Shohet et al. 2000). These microbubbles loaded with drugs/genes can be targeted to specific (pathologic) sites using different targeting ligands incorporated into bioconjugates (Unger et al. 2002). Bekeredjian et al. (2005) gave a broad overview of in-vitro and in-vivo studies of microbubbles for delivery of substances. Because of their size, microbubbles are mainly applicable for targeting intravascular targets. For extravascular targeting nanobubbles and perfluorocarbon emulsions are needed with much smaller diameters.

Thus, the use of microbubbles as gene carriers has two components. First, the transported substances may be released from the microbubbles by destruction in

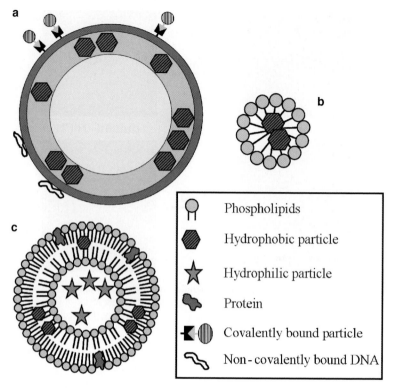

Fig. 4 a–c Overview of different nanoparticles used for gene and drug delivery. **a** Particles can be bound covalently and non-covalently to the membrane of the microbubble or the particle can be loaded to the interior of the microbubble. **b** Hydrophobic particles can be loaded inside the hydrophobic centre of micelles. **c** Liposomes can be loaded with both hydrophobic and hydrophilic particles because of their bilayer membrane

a temporally and spatially controlled manner, increasing the local concentration. Second, the destruction of microbubbles by ultrasound may cause cavitation effects in the surrounding tissue, which increases extravasation of the released substances.

3.2 Micelles

Micelles are often used as carrier of drugs (Gao et al. 2005). Micelles are built of amphiphilic molecules, molecules that contain both a hydrophobic and hydrophilic part. Because of this dual character and the energetically unfavourable contact between water and the hydrophobic part, amphiphiles self-assemble into aggregates with the hydrophilic parts facing the water and the hydrophobic parts clustering together. The hydrophobic centre of the micelles can be loaded with hydrophobic drugs. The diameters of micelles range between 5 and 30 nm, large enough to escape renal excretion and small enough to extravasate at the tumour site. Furthermore, micelles are not recognised by cells of the reticulo endothelial system. According to Husseini et al. (2000) transient cavitation plays an important role in triggering drug release from micelles. However, micelles lack a gas-filled nucleus and cannot take advantages of cavitation effects for increased delivery of the substances to surrounding tissue; therefore, the co-administration of cavitation ultrasound contrast agents may be necessary.

3.3 Liposomes

The concept of using thermosensitive liposomes in combination with local hyperthermia for drug delivery was proposed more than 25 years ago by Weinstein et al. (1979). Liposomes remain relatively stable in the circulation at temperatures well below the phase transition temperature (T_c) of the liposome membrane. At T_c distinctive structural changes occur in the lipid bilayer, resulting in increased membrane permeability and the accompanying release of the liposomes' content (Bos et al. 2005; Fossheim et al. 2000; Frenkel et al. 2006). Liposomes exhibit the possibility of carrying both hydrophilic and hydrophobic drugs in their aqueous interior and lipid bilayer membrane, respectively. In contrast to micelles, liposomes are recognised and cleared by the cells of the reticulo endothelial system due to their larger size (150–200 nm), but it is possible to increase the circulation half-lives by incorporating polyethylene glycol (PEG)-lipids into the bilayer. The PEG-lipids increase the "stealth" properties of the liposomes. The recent developments of measuring and controlling temperature with MRI (*see* 5.2.1) should lead to improved control of locally release drugs with temperature-sensitive nanocarriers.

3.4 Biological Carriers: Viruses, Stem Cells and Immune Cells

Viral-mediated gene transfer is efficient but safety aspects have limited therapeutic applications (Newman et al. 1995). Stem cells and immune cells have a particular advantage as gene delivery systems since they have been shown to home to lesions by the action of chemokines. Stem cells and progenitor cells constitute nature's repair shop and have shown great therapeutic potential in animal models following transplantation. Injection of stem cells has already been applied in clinical research in order to assess its potential following cardiac ischemia (Schachinger et al. 2004; Strauer et al. 2002). In the scope of this review, the use of stem cells is evaluated for the development of improved gene therapy strategies. Techniques have been developed to isolate stem cells, grow them in cell culture, label them with iron particles, and re-inject them into the tissue or into the bloodstream to permit tracking with MRI (Bulte et al. 2004; Hoehn et al. 2002). It has been shown in animal models that stem cells can home to the lesion site (Hoehn et al. 2002; Hauger et al. 2006). Stem cells can also be labelled with the marker gene coding for luciferase and tracked using bioluminescence imaging (Cao et al. 2004). Immune cells such as genetically modified lymphocytes have been used in advanced cancer therapies (de Vries et al. 2005).

4 Image-based Analysis of Pharmacodistribution and Pharmacokinetics

A thorough analysis of pharmacodistribution and pharmacokinetics is a mandatory aspect of pharmacology. Similarly, the field of local gene delivery requires such an evaluation. Using most of the methods described above, genes are delivered within the vascular system, and its local distribution and temporal evolution are a function of the local perfusion, uptake by surrounding cells, metabolism, and release. Therefore, it may be argued that such local gene delivery must be accompanied by evaluation of pharmacodistribution and pharmacokinetics, in order to predict outcome. Imaging may provide a non-invasive assessment of such parameters. Two methods are described below using MRI contrast agents. In addition, imaging biomarkers may provide physiological read-outs for indirect evaluation.

4.1 Pharmacokinetics with MR Contrast Agents

Similar to the encapsulation of drugs in nanocarriers, contrast agents can be included that report on the local release of drugs and subsequent tissue distribution. In this regard, MR contrast agents affecting T1 and T2 relaxation parameters are particularly useful, since they are not visualised directly in MR but their effect on the MR signal depends on the interaction with tissue water. Thus, such MR contrast agents have a negligible role when encapsulated (preventing interaction with tissue water) and lead to MR signal change related to their local concentration upon release. If the distribution of contrast agent is identical to that of the drug, MRI can be used for pharmacodistribution and pharmacokinetics. Ideally, such contrast agents would be directly linked with the drugs. However, in many cases such co-released MR contrast agents may provide useful data related to pharmacodistribution even when they are not linked.

4.2 Labelling with MR Contrast Agents to Allow Tracking

As previously discussed, T1 and T2 MRI contrast agents can be used to report on pharmacodistribution when they are co-released with the drug/gene. In addition, contrast agents may be used that allow tracking of the drug/gene carriers. In order to allow their use as T1 and T2 relaxation agents, they should be at the outside of the carriers. If their action is via increased local magnetic field inhomogeneity (and visualised through the $T2^*$ mechanism), they may be concentrated in the particle interior.

5 Gene Therapy: Ultrasound-guided Gene Delivery and Gene Expression

The prospect of safe and efficient gene therapy for diseases that are difficult to treat with conventional therapies, including genetic disorders and cancer, is clearly an attractive one. The goal of gene therapy is to treat disease by introducing a recombinant gene into somatic cells. Several strategies have been developed to transfect target cells. Viral-mediated gene transfer is efficient but safety aspects have limited therapeutic applications (Newman et al. 1995). Non-viral methods (electroporation, liposomes-mediated transfection) are safer but lead to poor transfection rates (Baek and March 1998). Novel approaches to improve the safety and efficiency of non-viral DNA delivery and subsequent transgene expression are clearly required. As discussed above, ultrasound exposure combines many favourable characteristics for gene therapy, including minimal invasiveness, spatial specificity, low toxicity, no immunogenicity, repeatable applicability, and low costs. The use of ultrasound in gene transfection in vivo and in vitro has been reported by many investigators. Below, a brief overview is given of the major findings. In addition, a novel approach is described for ultrasound-induced control of transgene expression.

5.1 Ultrasound Exposure and Transfection

Ultrasound exposure leads to permeabilisation of plasma membranes, also known as sonoporation, and should increase DNA uptake by the cells. According to most researchers, the physical source of sonoporation is attributed to cavitation. Because cavitation activity is highly localised, the combination of ultrasound and microbubble contrast agents provides a means for non-invasive, site-specific therapies. Many efforts to develop more efficient non-viral techniques for gene delivery have been reported where ultrasound exposure has been shown to enhance transgene expression (Unger et al. 1997; Lawrie et al. 1999; Schratzberger et al. 2002; Lee et al. 2005; Lee and Peng 2005; Hou et al. 2005). Examples can be found in many research areas. Since microbubble cavitation effects primarily originate in the vasculature, vascular therapy is an important field of applications. In primary porcine vascular smooth muscle cells following naked DNA transfection by up to 300-fold (Lawrie et al. 1999, 2000). Similar effects have also been reported by other groups, using a variety of immortalized cell lines and primary cultures of non-vascular cells: an effect of ultrasound exposure, and transfection rates of up to 15% using naked DNA and two- to 1,000-fold enhancements in reporter gene expression after lipofection have been reported (Kim et al. 1996; Bao et al. 1997; Tata et al. 1997; Unger et al. 1997; Greenleaf et al. 1998; Huber and Pfisterer 2000; Mukherjee et al. 2000; Newman et al. 2001; Porter and Xie 2001; Pislaru et al. 2003). Furthermore, there are reports of successful ultrasound-enhanced marker and/or therapeutic gene delivery in intact blood vessels ex vivo (Teupe et al. 2002) and normal skeletal and cardiac muscle, animal models of vascular disease and cancer and, most recently, in tissues in vivo like skeletal muscle (*see*, for example, Figs. 2 and 5) (Schratzberger et al. 2002; Taniyama et al. 2002; Lu et al. 2003), pancreatic islets (Chen et al. 2006), diverse tumour cells (Bao et al. 1998; Huber and Pfisterer 2000; Manome et al. 2000; Miller et al. 2002), arterial wall (Amabile et al. 2001) or dental pulp stem cells (Nakashima et al. 2003). Ultrasound transfection with microbubbles significantly enhanced transfection efficiency of plasmid DNA for intervertebral disc cells in vivo. Furthermore, the sustained transgene expression in vivo was possible for up

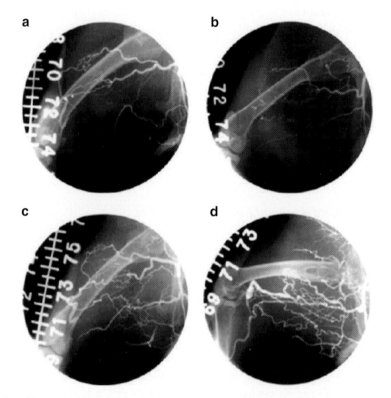

Fig. 5 a–d Representative images of selective internal iliac angiography at day 30 after treatment. **a** Control rabbit, saline injection, no ultrasound. **b** Saline-injected rabbit with ultrasound exposure shows no obvious increase in collateral development, as compared with **a. c** This hind limb was transfected with 500 g i.m. of *phVEGF165* and shows extensive collateral artery formation. **d** When VEGF transfection was followed by ultrasound exposure, collateral formation was most abundant. (Figure taken from Schratzberger et al. 2002)

to 24 weeks. The long-term gene expression mediated by this simple and safe procedure may have important clinical applications (Nishida et al. 2006). Ultrasound-microbubble-mediated gene therapy was used to inhibit renal inflammation by transfection of *smad7* gene in vivo (Ng et al. 2005).

Gene therapy with ultrasound may be an important tool in future medicine because of the demonstrated efficacy in a large variety of organs/diseases where this non-invasive gene transfer method is applicable. As discussed in the preceding text, an important role for acoustic cavitation has been established. However, these studies did not elucidate the relative roles of other mechanical effects (microjets, microstreaming and radiation pressure) and even the possible sonochemical effects (free radical production) of microbubble oscillation and collapse. These questions are important because knowledge of the key attributes of the incident ultrasound beam could facilitate optimisation of ultrasound exposure conditions to maximise gene delivery and minimise associated toxic effects (Lawrie et al. 2003).

5.2 Gene Expression Control with MR-guided Focused Ultrasound and Temperature-sensitive Promoters

Among the key challenges in gene therapy are the method of gene delivery and the spatial and temporal control of therapeutic (trans)gene expression in the targeted tissue. The ability of high-intensity focused ultrasound (HIFU) to heat tissue deep inside the body can be used to control transgene expression when the gene is placed under control of a heat-sensitive promoter. Such promoters exist widely in nature. For example, all mammals use such promoters when they have a fever in order to produce protecting proteins, the so-called heat-shock proteins. The use of such promoters for the control of expression of therapeutic genes requires tight temperature control in the region of interest. The heat-shock promoters, and especially the *hsp70* promoters, have been used quite often in gene therapy strategies because they are both heat inducible and efficient. The promoter for one of the inducible heat-shock protein systems, HSP70, can activate gene expression several-thousand-fold in response to hyperthermia (Dreano et al. 1986). The natural role of the HSP70 protein is to protect the tissue from stress from hyperthermia, pH and other stress factors. The minimal *hsp70* promoter is almost exclusively sensitive to temperature (for a review *see* Rome et al. 2005). It has been suggested to use the *hsp70* promoter and local hyperthermia to control transgene expression (Madio et al. 1998). The feasibility of the approach has been demonstrated both in vitro (Blackburn et al. 1998; Arai et al. 1999; Huang et al. 2000) and in vivo (Smith et al. 2002) for the expression of suicide genes in an implanted mammary cancer cell line (Braiden et al. 2000) and the expression of a reporter gene in transected muscle (Xu et al. 2004) or in implanted C6 cells (Guilhon et al. 2003a, b). MRI can be used for rapid temperature mapping and has, therefore, been utilised for feedback control of the heating procedure (see below). It has been demonstrated that local over-expression of a marker gene in a modified glioma cell line is feasible using this technology. Local control of the transgenic expression has recently been combined with modified stem cells. Mesenchymal stem cells from the bone marrow of rats were transfected with *hsp-luc* expressing the *luciferase* gene under control of an *hsp70* promoter. Transformed mesenchymal stem cells were injected in the left renal artery and transgenic expression was induced by MRI-controlled HIFU hyperthermia (Letavernier et al. 2008).

The use of MR imaging for monitoring ultrasound to induce gene expression has been demonstrated in other organs. The feasibility of using ultrasonic heating to control transgene expression spatially using a minimally invasive approach was investigated in the prostate. Ultrasound imaging was used to guide the injection of an adenoviral vector containing a transgene encoding firefly luciferase under the control of the human *hsp70B* promoter into both lobes of the prostates of three beagles. After injection, the left lobe of the prostate was heated using an ultrasound transducer and employing an MRI guidance system. The *hsp* promoter allows induction of the associated transgene only in areas that are subsequently heated after infection. High levels of luciferase expression were observed only in areas exposed to ultrasonic heating (Solcox et al. 2005).

The feasibility of using focused ultrasound to induce hyperthermia in the liver of a rat model to focally induce GFP under the control of an *hsp70B* promoter was examined in a preliminary study. Temperature was non-invasively monitored by temperature-sensitive MRI. This study demonstrated localised gene induction within the liver parenchyma, in good correlation with MRI and histology. Thus, it was shown that the introduced parameters could spatially control gene induction within a parenchymal organ, such as the liver in rats, using focused ultrasound under the control of MRI (Plathow et al. 2005).

5.2.1 MR Temperature Mapping During Ultrasound Exposure

During the thermal procedure, continuous temperature imaging can be performed with MRI using specific pulse sequences and data processing. The excellent linearity and near-independence with respect to tissue type, together with good temperature sensitivity, make the proton resonance frequency (PRF)-based temperature MRI method the preferred choice for many applications at mid to high field strength ($\geq 1\,T$). The PRF methods employ RF-spoiled gradient echo imaging methods. A standard deviation of less than $1°C$ for a temporal resolution below 1 s and a spatial resolution of about 2 mm is feasible for a single slice for immobile tissues. Corrections are necessary for temperature-induced susceptibility effects in the PRF method. Motion artefacts can severely degrade the accuracy of MR temperature maps and must be carefully corrected. The principles and performance of these methods have been reviewed recently. Also, it has been shown that ultrasound imaging may allow temperature mapping. However, the latter method still requires further developments, in particular for in-vivo applications (Pernot et al. 2004; Amini et al. 2005).

Optimal control of the temperature-based treatment requires regulation of the temperature. Recent developments have shown that rapid MR imaging, followed by on-line data processing, and real-time feedback to the focused ultrasound output, combined with new temperature regulation algorithms, may provide such control. The regulation of temperature evolution of the focal point was described based on temperature mapping and a physical model of local energy deposition and heat conduction. The following expression was used for automatic modification of the ultrasound output power $P(t)$ in order to follow a pre-described time evolution of the temperature $\Theta(t)$:

$$P(t) = \frac{1}{\alpha_2(T_{\max})} \left[\frac{d\Theta(t)}{dt} - \alpha_1(T_{\max}) \cdot \nabla^2 T_{\max}(t) + a \cdot [\Theta(t) - T_{\max}(t)] + \frac{a^2}{4} \cdot \Delta(t) \right]$$

(3)

where α_1 and α_2 are the heat diffusivity in the tissue and the HIFU absorption coefficient, respectively. The maximum temperature is indicated as $T_{\max}(t)$, and ∇^2 represents the Laplacian operator. Equation 4 resembles a classical PID (proportional, integral and derivative) type of temperature control, in which the term $\Theta(t)$-$T_{max}(t)$ is the difference between the measured and the planned temperature at time t, and $\Delta(t)$ the integral of the difference between the measured and the planned time evolution. The parameter a is related to the characteristic response time t_r of the regulation loop ($a = 2/t_r$). The objectives are that the temperature in the focal point should quickly reach the target value without overshooting or oscillating, and then remain constant for a user-defined period. It was demonstrated that the regulation system is insensitive to errors in estimates of ultrasound absorption and heat diffusion so long as the ratio of the two parameters is within a fairly large range. Therefore, the temperature trajectory of the focal point can be automatically regulated with a precision that is close to that of the precision of the temperature measurements at the focal point.

6 Conclusion

Ultrasound offers several advantages in local gene delivery and control of expression via radiation forces, local heating, and cavitation effects. Target-specific and non-specific ultrasound contrast agents may further enhance the potential of ultrasound in this emerging field. The combination with MRI appears especially promising since MR contrast agents can be used for pharmacodistribution and nanocarrier tracking. In particular, when using cell-based gene carriers, such as stem cells or immune system cells, this allows tracking during their homing to the target site. In addition, MRI allows non-invasive monitoring of tissue temperature during ultrasound heating, allowing visualisation and control of the heating process. Such methods may be associated with the use of heat-sensitive promoters, since these would allow spatio-temporal control of transgene expression.

References

Amabile PG, Waugh JM, Lewis TN, Elkins CJ, Janas W, Dake MD (2001) High-efficiency endovascular gene delivery via therapeutic ultrasound. J Am Coll Cardiol 37(7):1975–1980

Amini AN, Ebbini ES, Georgiou TT (2005) Noninvasive estimation of tissue temperature via high-resolution spectral analysis techniques. IEEE Trans Biomed Eng 52(2):221–228

Arai Y, Kubo T, Kobayashi K, Ikeda T, Takahashi K, Takigawa M, Imanishi J, Hirasawa Y (1999) Control of delivered gene expression in chondrocytes using heat shock protein 70B promoter. J Rheumatol 26(8):1769–1774

Baek S, March KL (1998) Gene therapy for restenosis: getting nearer the heart of the matter. Circ Res 82(3):295–305

Bao S, Thrall BD, Miller DL (1997) Transfection of a reporter plasmid into cultured cells by sonoporation in vitro. Ultrasound Med Biol 23(6):953–959

Bao S, Thrall BD, Gies RA, Miller DL (1998) In vivo transfection of melanoma cells by lithotripter shock waves. Cancer Res 58(2):219–221

Bekeredjian R, Grayburn PA, Shohet RV (2005) Use of ultrasound contrast agents for gene or drug delivery in cardiovascular medicine. J Am Coll Cardiol 45(3):329–335

Blackburn RV, Galoforo SS, Corry PM, Lee YJ (1998) Adenoviral-mediated transfer of a heat-inducible double suicide gene into prostate carcinoma cells. Cancer Res 58(7):1358–1362

Blake JR, Gibson DC (1987) Cavitation bubbles near boundaries. Ann Rev Fluid Mech 19:99–123

Bos C, Lepetit-Coiffe M, Quesson B, Moonen CT (2005) Simultaneous monitoring of temperature and T1: methods and preliminary results of application to drug delivery using thermosensitive liposomes. Magn Reson Med 54(4):1020–1024

Braiden V, Ohtsuru A, Kawashita Y, Miki F, Sawada T, Ito M, Cao Y, Kaneda Y, Koji T, Yamashita S (2000) Eradication of breast cancer xenografts by hyperthermic suicide gene therapy under the control of the heat shock protein promoter. Hum Gene Ther 11(18):2453–2463

Brennen CE (1995) Cavitation and bubble dynamics. Oxford University Press, New York

Bulte JW, Arbab AS, Douglas T, Frank JA (2004) Preparation of magnetically labeled cells for cell tracking by magnetic resonance imaging. Methods Enzymol 386:275–299

Cao YA, Wagers AJ, Beilhack A, Dusich J, Bachmann MH, Negrin RS, Weissman IL, Contag CH (2004) Shifting foci of hematopoiesis during reconstitution from single stem cells. Proc Natl Acad Sci U S A 101(1):221–226

Chen S, Ding JH, Bekeredjian R, Yang BZ, Shohet RV, Johnston SA, Hohmeier HE, Newgard CB, Grayburn PA (2006) Efficient gene delivery to pancreatic islets with ultrasonic microbubble destruction technology. Proc Natl Acad Sci U S A 103(22):8469–8474

Dalecki D, Child SZ, Raeman CH, Cox C, Carstensen EL (1997a) Ultrasonically induced lung hemorrhage in young swine. Ultrasound Med Biol 23(5):777–781

Dalecki D, Raeman CH, Child SZ, Cox C, Francis CW, Meltzer RS, Carstensen EL (1997b) Hemolysis in vivo from exposure to pulsed ultrasound. Ultrasound Med Biol 23(2):307–313

de Vries IJ, Lesterhuis WJ, Barentsz JO, Verdijk P, van Krieken JH, Boerman OC, Oyen WJ, Bonenkamp JJ, Boezeman JB, Adema GJ, Bulte JW, Scheenen TW, Punt CJ, Heerschap A, Figdor CG (2005) Magnetic resonance tracking of dendritic cells in melanoma patients for monitoring of cellular therapy. Nat Biotechnol 23(11):1407–1413

Dreano M, Brochot J, Myers A, Cheng-Meyer C, Rungger D, Voellmy R, Bromley P (1986) High-level, heat-regulated synthesis of proteins in eukaryotic cells. Gene 49(1):1–8

Dunn F, D. O'Brien W (eds) (1976) Ultrasonic Biophysics. Hutchinson and Ross, Dowden

Evans EA, Waugh R, Melnik L (1976) Elastic area compressibility modulus of red cell membrane. Biophys J 16(6):585–595

Everbach EC, Makin IR, Azadniv M, Meltzer RS (1997) Correlation of ultrasound-induced hemolysis with cavitation detector output in vitro. Ultrasound Med Biol 23(4):619–624

Fechheimer M, Boylan JF, Parker S, Sisken JE, Patel GL, Zimmer SG (1987) Transfection of mammalian cells with plasmid DNA by scrape loading and sonication loading. Proc Natl Acad Sci U S A 84(23):8463–8467

Fossheim SL, Il'yasov KA, Hennig J, Bjornerud A (2000) Thermosensitive paramagnetic liposomes for temperature control during MR imaging-guided hyperthermia: in vitro feasibility studies. Acad Radiol 7(12):1107–1115

Frenkel PA, Chen S, Thai T, Shohet RV, Grayburn PA (2002) DNA-loaded albumin microbubbles enhance ultrasound-mediated transfection in vitro. Ultrasound Med Biol 28(6):817–822

Frenkel V, Li KC. Potential role of pulsed-high intensity focused ultrasound in gene therapy. Future Oncol 2006;2(1):111–119

Frenkel V, Deng C, O'Neill BE et al (2005) Pulsed-high intensity focused ultrasound (HIFU) exposures for enhanced delivery of therapeutics: mechanisms and applications. The 5th International Symposium on Therapeutic Ultrasound, October 27–29, Boston

Frenkel V, Etherington A, Greene M, Quijano J, Xie J, Hunter F, Dromi S, Li KC (2006) Delivery of liposomal doxorubicin (Doxil) in a breast cancer tumor model: investigation of potential enhancement by pulsed-high intensity focused ultrasound exposure. Acad Radiol 13(4):469–479

Gao ZG, Fain HD, Rapoport N (2005) Controlled and targeted tumor chemotherapy by micellar-encapsulated drug and ultrasound. J Control Release 102(1):203–222

Grayburn PA (2002) Current and future contrast agents. Echocardiography 19(3):259–265

Greenleaf WJ, Bolander ME, Sarkar G, Goldring MB, Greenleaf JF (1998) Artificial cavitation nuclei significantly enhance acoustically induced cell transfection. Ultrasound Med Biol 24(4):587–595

Guilhon E, Quesson B, Moraud-Gaudry F, de Verneuil H, Canioni P, Salomir R, Voisin P, Moonen CT (2003a) Image-guided control of transgene expression based on local hyperthermia. Mol Imaging 2(1):11–17

Guilhon E, Voisin P, de Zwart JA, Quesson B, Salomir R, Maurange C, Bouchaud V, Smirnov P, de Verneuil H, Vekris A, Canioni P, Moonen CT (2003b) Spatial and temporal control of transgene expression in vivo using a heat-sensitive promoter and MRI-guided focused ultrasound. J Gene Med 5(4):333–342

Hauger O, Frost EE, van Heeswijk R, Deminiere C, Xue R, Delmas Y, Combe C, Moonen CT, Grenier N, Bulte JW (2006) MR evaluation of the glomerular homing of magnetically labeled mesenchymal stem cells in a rat model of nephropathy. Radiology 238(1):200–210

Hoehn M, Kustermann E, Blunk J, Wiedermann D, Trapp T, Wecker S, Focking M, Arnold H, Hescheler J, Fleischmann BK, Schwindt W, Buhrle C (2002) Monitoring of implanted stem cell migration in vivo: a highly resolved in vivo magnetic resonance imaging investigation of experimental stroke in rat. Proc Natl Acad Sci U S A 99(25):16267–16272

Hou CC, Wang W, Huang XR, Fu P, Chen TH, Sheikh-Hamad D, Lan HY (2005) Ultrasound-microbubble-mediated gene transfer of inducible Smad7 blocks transforming growth factor-beta signaling and fibrosis in rat remnant kidney. Am J Pathol 166(3):761–771

Huang Q, Hu JK, Lohr F, Zhang L, Braun R, Lanzen J, Little JB, Dewhirst MW, Li CY (2000) Heat-induced gene expression as a novel targeted cancer gene therapy strategy. Cancer Res 60(13):3435–3439

Huber PE, Pfisterer P (2000) In vitro and in vivo transfection of plasmid DNA in the Dunning prostate tumor R3327-AT1 is enhanced by focused ultrasound. Gene Ther 7(17):1516–1525

Hueter TF, Bolt RH (1955) Sonics. Wiley, New York

Husseini GA, Myrup GD, Pitt WG, Christensen DA, Rapoport NY (2000) Factors affecting acoustically triggered release of drugs from polymeric micelles. J Control Release 69(1):43–52

Kim HJ, Greenleaf JF, Kinnick RR, Bronk JT, Bolander ME (1996) Ultrasound-mediated transfection of mammalian cells. Hum Gene Ther 7(11):1339–1346

Lawrie A, Brisken AF, Francis SE, Tayler DI, Chamberlain J, Crossman DC, Cumberland DC, Newman CM (1999) Ultrasound enhances reporter gene expression after transfection of vascular cells in vitro. Circulation 99(20):2617–2620

Lawrie A, Brisken AF, Francis SE, Cumberland DC, Crossman DC, Newman CM (2000) Microbubble-enhanced ultrasound for vascular gene delivery. Gene Ther 7(23):2023–2027

Lawrie A, Brisken AF, Francis SE, Wyllie D, Kiss-Toth E, Qwarnstrom EE, Dower SK, Crossman DC, Newman CM (2003) Ultrasound-enhanced transgene expression in vascular cells is not dependent upon cavitation-induced free radicals. Ultrasound Med Biol 29(10): 1453–1461

Lee JM, Takahashi M, Mon H, Koga K, Kawaguchi Y, Kusakabe T (2005) Efficient gene transfer into silkworm larval tissues by a combination of sonoporation and lipofection. Cell Biol Int 29(11):976–979

Lee YH, Peng CA (2005) Enhanced retroviral gene delivery in ultrasonic standing wave fields. Gene Ther 12(7):625–633

Leighton TG (1994) The acoustic bubble. Academic Press, London

Letavernier B, Salomir R, Delmas Y, Rome C, Couillaud F, Desmoulière A, Dubus I, Moreau-Gaudry F, Grosset C, Hauger O, Rosenbaum J, Grenier N, Combe C, Ripoche J, Moonen CT (2008) Ultrasound induced expression of a heat shock promoter-driven transgene delivered in the kidney by genetically modified mesenchymal stem cells. A feasibility study. In: Hynynen K, Jolesz F (eds) Taylor & Francis (in press)

Liu J, Lewis TN, Prausnitz MR (1998) Non-invasive assessment and control of ultrasound-mediated membrane permeabilization. Pharm Res 15(6):918–924

Lokhandwalla M, McAteer JA, Williams JC, Sturtevant B (2001) Mechanical hemolysis in shock wave lithotripsy (SWL): II. In vitro cell lysis due to shear. Phys Med Biol 46:1245–1264

Lu QL, Liang HD, Partridge T, Blomley MJ (2003) Microbubble ultrasound improves the efficiency of gene transduction in skeletal muscle in vivo with reduced tissue damage. Gene Ther 10(5):396–405

Lum AF, Borden MA, Dayton PA, Kruse DE, Simon SI, Ferrara KW (2006) Ultrasound radiation force enables targeted deposition of model drug carriers loaded on microbubbles. J Control Release 111(1–2):128–134

Madio DP, van Gelderen P, DesPres D, Olson AW, de Zwart JA, Fawcett TW, Holbrook NJ, Mandel M, Moonen CT (1998) On the feasibility of MRI-guided focused ultrasound for local induction of gene expression. J Magn Reson Imaging 8(1):101–104

Manome Y, Nakamura M, Ohno T, Furuhata H (2000) Ultrasound facilitates transduction of naked plasmid DNA into colon carcinoma cells in vitro and in vivo. Hum Gene Ther 11(11):1521–1528

Marmottant P, Hilgenfeldt S (2003) Controlled vesicle deformation and lysis by single oscillating bubbles. Nature 423(6936):153–156

May DJ, Allen JS, Ferrara KW (2002) Dynamics and fragmentation of thick-shelled microbubbles. IEEE Trans Ultrason Ferroelectr Freq Control 49(10):1400–1410

Miller DL, Song J (2002) Lithotripter shock waves with cavitation nucleation agents produce tumor growth reduction and gene transfer in vivo. Ultrasound Med Biol 28(10):1343–1348

Miller MW, Miller DL, Brayman AA (1996) A review of in vitro bioeffects of inertial ultrasonic cavitation from a mechanistic perspective. Ultrasound Med Biol 22(9):1131–1154

Mukherjee D, Wong J, Griffin B, Ellis SG, Porter T, Sen S, Thomas JD (2000) Ten-fold augmentation of endothelial uptake of vascular endothelial growth factor with ultrasound after systemic administration. J Am Coll Cardiol 35(6):1678–1686

Nakashima M, Tachibana K, Iohara K, Ito M, Ishikawa M, Akamine A (2003) Induction of reparative dentin formation by ultrasound-mediated gene delivery of growth/differentiation factor 11. Hum Gene Ther 14(6):591–597

Newman CM, Lawrie A, Brisken AF, Cumberland DC (2001) Ultrasound gene therapy: on the road from concept to reality. Echocardiography 18(4):339–347

Newman KD, Dunn PF, Owens JW, Schulick AH, Virmani R, Sukhova G, Libby P, Dichek DA (1995) Adenovirus-mediated gene transfer into normal rabbit arteries results in prolonged vascular cell activation, inflammation, and neointimal hyperplasia. J Clin Invest 96(6):2955–2965

Ng YY, Hou CC, Wang W, Huang XR, Lan HY (2005) Blockade of NFkappaB activation and renal inflammation by ultrasound-mediated gene transfer of Smad7 in rat remnant kidney. Kidney Int Suppl (94):S83–S91

Nishida K, Doita M, Takada T, Kakutani K, Miyamoto H, Shimomura T, Maeno K, Kurosaka M (2006) Sustained transgene expression in intervertebral disc cells in vivo mediated by microbubble-enhanced ultrasound gene therapy. Spine 31(13):1415–1419

Nyborg WL (1996) Basic physics of low frequency therapeutic ultrasound. Kluwer, Boston

Pernot M, Tanter M, Bercoff J, Waters KR, Fink M (2004) Temperature estimation using ultrasonic spatial compound imaging. IEEE Trans Ultrason Ferroelectr Freq Control 51(5):606–615

Pislaru SV, Pislaru C, Kinnick RR, Singh R, Gulati R, Greenleaf JF, Simari RD (2003) Optimization of ultrasound-mediated gene transfer: comparison of contrast agents and ultrasound modalities. Eur Heart J 24(18):1690–1698

Plathow C, Lohr F, Divkovic G, Rademaker G, Farhan N, Peschke P, Zuna I, Debus J, Claussen CD, Kauczor HU, Li CY, Jenne J, Huber P (2005) Focal gene induction in the liver of rats by a heat-inducible promoter using focused ultrasound hyperthermia: preliminary results. Invest Radiol 40(11):729–735

Porter TR, Xie F. Therapeutic ultrasound for gene delivery. Echocardiography18(4):349–353

Rome C, Couillaud F, Moonen CT (2005) Spatial and temporal control of expression of therapeutic genes using heat shock protein promoters. Methods 35(2):188–198

Rooney JA (1970) Hemolysis near an ultrasonically pulsating gas bubble. Science 169(948): 869–871

Schachinger V, Assmus B, Britten MB, Honold J, Lehmann R, Teupe C, Abolmaali ND, Vogl TJ, Hofmann WK, Martin H, Dimmeler S, Zeiher AM (2004) Transplantation of progenitor cells and regeneration enhancement in acute myocardial infarction: final one-year results of the TOPCARE-AMI Trial. J Am Coll Cardiol 44(8):1690–1699

Schratzberger P, Krainin JG, Schratzberger G, Silver M, Ma H, Kearney M, Zuk RF, Brisken AF, Losordo DW, Isner JM (2002) Transcutaneous ultrasound augments naked DNA transfection of skeletal muscle. Mol Ther 6(5):576–583

Shohet RV, Chen S, Zhou YT, Wang Z, Meidell RS, Unger RH, Grayburn PA (2000) Echocardiographic destruction of albumin microbubbles directs gene delivery to the myocardium. Circulation 101(22):2554–2556

Shortencarier MJ, Dayton PA, Bloch SH, Schumann PA, Matsunaga TO, Ferrara KW (2004) A method for radiation-force localized drug delivery using gas-filled liposheres. IEEE Trans Ultrason Ferroelectr Freq Control 51(7):822–831

Silcox CE, Smith RC, King R, McDannold N, Bromley P, Walsh K, Hynynen K (2005) MRI-guided ultrasonic heating allows spatial control of exogenous luciferase in canine prostate. Ultrasound Med Biol 31(7):965–970

Smith RC, Machluf M, Bromley P, Atala A, Walsh K (2002) Spatial and temporal control of transgene expression through ultrasound-mediated induction of the heat shock protein 70B promoter in vivo. Hum Gene Ther 13(6):697–706

Strauer BE, Brehm M, Zeus T, Kostering M, Hernandez A, Sorg RV, Kogler G, Wernet P (2002) Repair of infarcted myocardium by autologous intracoronary mononuclear bone marrow cell transplantation in humans. Circulation 106(15):1913–1918

Suslick KS (1989) Ultrasound: its chemical, physical and biological effects. VCH, London

Taniyama Y, Tachibana K, Hiraoka K, Aoki M, Yamamoto S, Matsumoto K, Nakamura T, Ogihara T, Kaneda Y, Morishita R (2002) Development of safe and efficient novel nonviral gene transfer using ultrasound: enhancement of transfection efficiency of naked plasmid DNA in skeletal muscle. Gene Ther 9(6):372–380

Tata DB, Dunn F, Tindall DJ (1997) Selective clinical ultrasound signals mediate differential gene transfer and expression in two human prostate cancer cell lines: LnCap and PC-3. Biochem Biophys Res Commun 234(1):64–67

Teupe C, Richter S, Fisslthaler B, Randriamboavonjy V, Ihling C, Fleming I, Busse R, Zeiher AM, Dimmeler S (2002) Vascular gene transfer of phosphomimetic endothelial nitric oxide synthase (S1177D) using ultrasound-enhanced destruction of plasmid-loaded microbubbles improves vasoreactivity. Circulation 105(9):1104–1109

Unger EC, McCreery TP, Sweitzer RH (1997) Ultrasound enhances gene expression of liposomal transfection. Invest Radiol 32(12):723–727

Unger EC, Matsunaga TO, McCreery T, Schumann P, Sweitzer R, Quigley R (2002) Therapeutic applications of microbubbles. Eur J Radiol 42(2):160–168

Weinstein JN, Magin RL, Yatvin MB, Zaharko DS (1979) Liposomes and local hyperthermia: selective delivery of methotrexate to heated tumors. Science 204(4389):188–191

Xu L, Zhao Y, Zhang Q, Li Y, Xu Y (2004) Regulation of transgene expression in muscles by ultrasound-mediated hyperthermia. Gene Ther 11(11):894–900

Magnetic Resonance of Mouse Models of Cardiac Disease

Karl-Heinz Hiller(✉), Christiane Waller, Axel Haase, and Peter M. Jakob

Abstract In recent years magnetic resonance imaging (MRI) has become the non-invasive standard for the quantitative evaluation of cardiac function, masses, and infarct size. Wall motion analysis is used to display myocardial dysfunction and microcirculatory deficits can be displayed by perfusion imaging and quantification of the myocardial regional blood volume. Magnetic resonance spectroscopy (MRS) also provides quantitative information on cardiac energetics and, in combination with MRI, insights into cardiac structure and function. The use of both techniques permits complementary data collection within the same experimental setup.

Nevertheless, it should be mentioned that MR does not directly visualize genes or gene product expression but morphological or bioenergetical outcomes of gene expression instead.

In conclusion, cardiac MR is a valuable tool applicable to mouse phenotyping and, also, can be applied to assess the effects of therapeutic agents. Thus, MR of mouse models of cardiac disease has great potential to substantially contribute to the understanding of the underlying pathomechanisms and can help to evaluate new therapy options.

Karl-Heinz Hiller
Physikalisches Institut, Universität Würzburg, 97074 Würzburg, Germany;
MRB Research Center of Magnetic Resonance Bavaria, 97074 Würzburg, Germany
hiller@mr-bavaria.de

W. Semmler and M. Schwaiger (eds.), *Molecular Imaging II.*
Handbook of Experimental Pharmacology 185/II.
© Springer-Verlag Berlin Heidelberg 2008

1 Introduction

In recent years magnetic resonance imaging (MRI) has become an attractive non-invasive imaging modality for experimental animal research. Animal models offer the opportunity to investigate both pathophysiological questions and drug development. The understanding of the mammalian genome allows for the increased generation of animal models for studying cardiovascular development, changes and function.

Because of technical and economic considerations, the transgenic mouse model has become a key tool in experimental animal research. Disease models become an important role of transgenic modeling of the murine heart and it is essential to analyze the phenotypes of the whole organ and whole intact animal level over time with non-invasive imaging modalities. To this end, MRI is used to characterize the phenotype of such models by examining the functional effects of gene expression or gene knock-out directly or to analyze the morphological consequences. One advantage that MRI offers for the characterization of animal models is the repetition of measurements in the same animal at different time points. This is important since the number of animals required to fulfill statistical significance is reduced because the interindividual variance is omitted. Another advantage is the noninvasive nature of MRI in monitoring the progression of a chronic disease and regression during therapy.

MRI allows highly accurate three-dimensional characterization of cardiac structure and function within a single examination. This imaging technique provides high spatial resolution ($<100\,\mu m$), which yields detailed morphological information and allows the quantification of volumetric and functional changes in hearts, especially when underlying ventricular remodeling after myocardial infarction or in dilated cardiomyopathy (Shapiro et al. 1989), but also in vascular disorders such as chronic occlusive arterial disease and restenosis.

The focus of this article is to give an overview of the current methods used in high-resolution MRI in mice and to demonstrate some potential applications for murine cardiac phenotyping. The functional examples discussed here include the analysis of heart function, wall motion, perfusion and vascular imaging. In the future, the use of target-specific contrast agents will also become an important tool in MRI applications.

2 Technical Requirements

The use of murine animals with small size and short cardiac cycle for the determination of normal and abnormal cardiovascular function is challenging. In small animals, typical heart rates are between 300 and 600 beats/min in rats and mice and, therefore, significantly higher than in clinical heart studies. The typical length of the cardiac cycle for a mouse is a tenth of the rate for a human. To minimize motion artifacts, ECG and respiratory gating or navigation is mandatory to obtain high-quality time-resolved cardiac images, especially using magnets with high static field strength (Wood and Henkelman 1986). Different gating strategies have been reported using direct or indirect detection methods. Direct detection methods sense heart and respiratory motion, such as using the ECG signal (Rommel et al. 2000) as a double-trigger unit with optimized gating strategies (Cassidy et al. 2004), or pneumatic (Minard et al. 1998), fiberoptic (Brau et al. 2002), piezoelectric (McKibben and Reo 1992), infrared (Lemieux and Glover 1996) or inductive sensors (Fishbein et al. 2001). Indirect detection methods use the information gathered in an additional navigator MR signal as criteria for accepting or acquiring data (Wang et al. 1996). The detection of an accurate ECG signal without disturbances by interference of RF pulses or gradient switching is also important for the exact quantification of the T_1-dependent perfusion and regional blood-volume values, where knowledge of the exact timing of each image acquisition is necessary.

A comparison of the typical heart weight of mice ($\sim$300 mg) and of humans ($\sim$300 g) demonstrates that the imaging of small-sized animals requires high spatial resolution. The obtainable resolution of a useful animal MR system is limited by the maximum possible gradient strength and by the signal-to-noise ratio (SNR). The acquisition of high-resolution images involves a compromise between imaging time, which reflects the time of data sampling, and technical factors like magnetic field strength, receiver coil design and pulse sequence employed. Increasing the spatial resolution always results in a reduced SNR. To compensate for this loss of sensitivity, higher magnetic field strength ($>$4 Tesla) and optimally designed small receiver coils with high filling factors and sensitivities have been used. Another possibility to increase the SNR is to employ signal averaging, which results in a prolonged measurement time. Additionally, improved gradient systems allow rapid data collection techniques to reduce image acquisition time. The use of fast imaging sequences, such as FLASH (Haase et al. 1986), Turbo FLASH, FISP (Oppelt et al. 1986) or RARE (Hennig et al. 1984), makes it possible to image rapid, time-dependent physiological and pharmacological events. For example, the principle of the FLASH sequence is the excitation of the spin system with small flip angles, which permits very short repetition times and, therefore, a reduction in the acquisition or recording time.

To avoid negative chronotropic and inotropic effects, inhalative anesthetics such as isoflurane or i.v. anesthetics such as propofol are commonly used and given via nose cone or tail vein catheter and allow for short induction and recovery times (Ruff et al. 1998; Waller et al. 2001). In most studies, the temperature of the animals was kept at 37°C, using either circulating water pads or electrical heating pads. In general, the vital functions of the animals during anesthesia have to be carefully controlled.

3 Cine MRI – Volumes and Mass

High-resolution MRI has been successfully applied to a number of transgenic mouse models. Using a well-established cine technique allows for the investigation and accurate determination of morphologic and functional consequences in the cardiovascular system, such as changes in compartment volumes, wall thickness and mass (Manning et al. 1990; Rudin et al. 1991). For example (Ruff et al. 1998; Wiesmann et al. 2000), cine MRI was performed on high-field magnets (7.05 Tesla) using an ECG and respiratory triggered fast gradient echo (FLASH) sequence (Haase et al. 1986) with the following typical imaging parameters: flip angle 30–40°; echo time 1.5 ms; repetition time 4.3 ms (depending on heart rate and number of frames per heart cycle); field of view 30 mm²; image matrix 128–256 × 128–256; in-plane resolution 120–230 μm and slice thickness 0.5–1.0 mm. Typically, 12–16 frames per heart cycle were obtained. A birdcage probe head with an inner diameter of 35 mm was used for transmission and reception of the MR signal. The sizes of the myocardial and ventricular compartments were determined by semi-automated segmentation in the short axis with slice images covering the entire heart. Therefore, for all slices, endocardial borders in both the end-diastolic and end-systolic frames were delineated. These could be clearly distinguished due to the high MRI-derived intrinsic contrast between the blood-filled ventricular cavity and the myocardial tissue caused by nonsaturated spins. The obtained compartment areas were multiplied by the slice thickness to determine the myocardial and ventricular slice volumes. Ventricular volumes were calculated as follows: stroke volume (SV) = end-diastolic volume (EDV) – end-systolic volume (ESV); ejection fraction (EF) = SV/EDV; cardiac output (CO) = SV × heart rate. Myocardial masses were calculated from the multiplication of the total volumes with the specific gravity of the myocardium ($1.05\,\text{g}/\text{cm}^3$). Volumes and masses were calculated with similar reproducibility and accuracy as known from human MR studies. Compared with autopsy data, MRI-determined cardiac masses and volumes were in excellent agreement. Applying this technique (Fig. 1), LV morphology and function can be accurately assessed (Franco et al. 1998; Ruff et al. 1998; Nahrendorf et al. 2003) and hypertrophic changes can be quantified (Siri et al. 1997; Slawson et al. 1998). Kubota et al. (1997) demonstrated significant dilatation and reduction of the

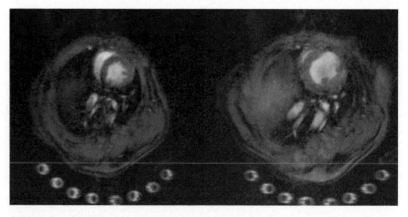

Fig. 1 Diastolic midventricular short-axis cine images of a healthy mouse (*left*) and of a mouse 8 weeks after anterolateral myocardial infarction. (From Nahrendorf et al. 2003)

left ventricular ejection fraction in mice overexpressing TNF-α. Other hypertrophic changes in the left ventricle were also found in other transgenic mouse models, such as guanylyl cyclase. Double-knockout mice developed a significant increase in LV mass without changes in volumes and ejection fraction caused by the lack of the ability to transduce the signal from the atrial natruretic peptide (Franco et al. 1998). Another example is a transgenic mouse model with a heart-specific overexpression of the β_1-adrenergic receptor (Engelhardt et al. 1999). These mice underwent a progressive reduction of left ventricular function, demonstrated by a significant reduction of the LV ejection fraction. In younger mice, the only difference detected was a significantly increased LV mass, whereas ejection fraction and cardiac output were identical in mice with myocardial overexpression of the β_1-adrenergic receptor and wild-type mice. Under dobutamine stress, a lower maximal LV filling rate (dV/dt) was observed, which might be caused by a loss of relaxation reserve during inotropic stimulation. For the assessment of these LV systolic and diastolic dynamics (Fig. 2), Engelhardt et al. (1999) and Wiesmann et al. (2001) used a cine sequence with a higher number of frames and an acquisition window of 4.3 ms per cine frame to visualize the filling processes. This technique requires a microimaging system with rapid gradient performance (maximum gradient strength 870 mT/m and 280 μs rise time).

Cine MRI also allows the quantification of right ventricular (RV) volumes and function (Wiesmann et al. 2002). This is important because gene-targeted mouse models of cardiomyopathy may also develop remodeling in the right heart. The assessment of RV function is more difficult than it is for the LV, due to the complex geometry. Consistent with human physiology, Wiesmann et al. (2002) showed higher RV end-diastolic and end-systolic volumes compared with LV volumes in wild-type mice. In mice with LV heart failure due to myocardial infarction significant structural and functional changes of the RV could be demonstrated. These mice developed a RV dysfunction caused by ligation of the left anterior ascending aorta.

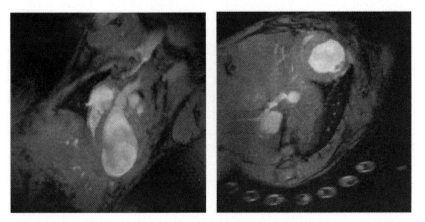

Fig. 2 Coronal (*left*) and short-axis (*right*) end-diastolic cine frame image of a mouse 2 weeks after myocardial infarction. (Courtesy of K.H. Hiller and F. Wiesmann)

Using the cine MRI technique serial assessment of LV cardiac structure and function was reliable and accurate also in neonatal, juvenile and adult growth stages (Wiesmann et al. 2000). Considering the fact, that transgenic mice may develop an early phenotype or even may die within the first days of life, cine MRI may give new insights into the underlying pathophysiology in these models and also allow to follow-up changes during growth by serial measurements in the same animal. Cine MRI also allows serial measurements of cardiac output (Franco et al. 1999) and Nahrendorf et al. (2003) also demonstrated the feasibility of the in-vivo determination of myocardial infarct size. In this study, myocardial infarct size was calculated for each slice by dividing the sum of the endocardial and epicardial circumferences occupied by the infarct with significant thinning and akinesia or dyskinesia during systole by the sum of the total epicardial and endocardial circumferences of the LV.

4 Wall Motion

Besides the quantification of volume and mass, cine MRI is also a valuable tool for obtaining detailed information about left ventricular wall motion. Tagged cine MRI has been used to calculate torsion angles in the left ventricular myocardium of the mouse (Henson et al. 2000). Placing a "tag" mark of saturated spins on the myocardium using distinct prepulses, the variation of this "stamped" pattern or grid in shape and orientation can be followed over the heart cycle (Axel and Dougherty 1989). This allows the quantification of the radial and circumferential motion, as well as the torsion of the ventricle, and reflects abnormalities in the regional wall motion. Another approach to analyze wall motion is the phase contrast MRI method using a segmented FLASH imaging sequence (Streif et al. 2003). This method measures a velocity vector in each voxel with high spatial resolution and is based on the phase contrast flow velocity technique, which belongs to the use of bipolar gradient pulses to induce velocity encoding. Streif et al. (2003) recently showed quantitative velocity maps of myocardial wall motion in the in vivo mouse heart. In infarcted mouse hearts disturbed wall motion was visualized, as well as areas with scar tissue and regions in the remote myocardium (Fig. 3). This phase-contrast method was recently used to determine abnormalities of the murine heart in creatine kinase double-knockout mice, $CK^{-/-}$ (Nahrendorf et al. 2006). The deletion of the creatine kinase enzyme system leads to left ventricular hypertrophy and dilatation of the left ventricle. A marked increase in LV mass was found, and the maximal systolic myocardial contraction velocity was significantly reduced in the $CK^{-/-}$ mice versus wild type, although ejection fraction was preserved. These findings suggest that indices of myocardial function, such as ejection fraction, do not detect all abnormalities in myocardial function in these mice. Therefore, further phenotypic characterization of transgenic mice should include MRI techniques such as motion velocity mapping and myocardial perfusion imaging.

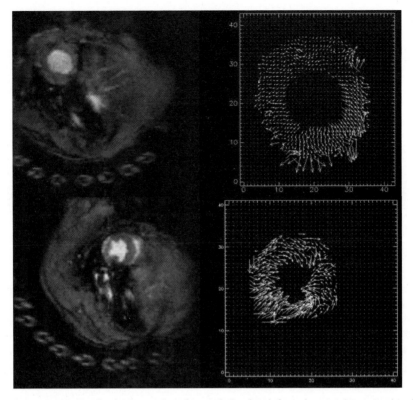

Fig. 3 Representative cine images and motion analysis of an infarcted mouse (*upper row*) and a healthy mouse. The vector plot of the infarcted mouse shows a significant reduction of motion velocity. (Courtesy of J.U.G. Streif)

5 Perfusion MRI

For complete phenotyping of transgenic mice and the full characterization of the viability of the myocardium, the quantification of myocardial microcirculatory parameters such as perfusion or regional blood volume is important. The detection of a reduced myocardial perfusion in hypertrophied hearts might be a significant marker for possible development of systolic dysfunction (Waller et al. 2001; Maestri et al. 2003).

Only a few MRI methods which assess the myocardial perfusion in mice have been presented to date. One possible approach is contrast-enhanced first-pass perfusion MRI (Wilke et al. 1993). The basic principle of this method is tracking the change of signal intensity after administration of a contrast agent. The analysis of the first pass of the contrast agent through the myocardium provides information about the perfusion and regional blood volume in the heart. Although this technique allows absolute quantification in principle (Jerosch-Herold and Wilke 1998), only relative perfusion changes were reported in mice myocardium (Bashir et al. 2000).

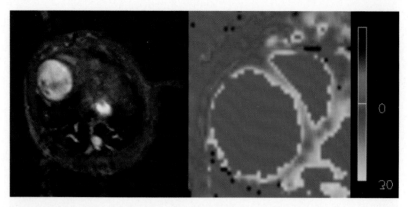

Fig. 4 Representative source image (*left*) of a T_1 dataset of a mouse after myocardial infarction and the corresponding perfusion map (*right*). (Courtesy of J.U.G. Streif)

One reason is that when conventional extracellular contrast agents are applied, only qualitative information on perfusion is provided, since extravascular distribution of these agents implies that the dynamics of signal intensity in tissue are a result of a complex superposition of perfusion and transvascular penetration. In addition, repetitive first-pass measurements are hampered by the residual contrast agent.

Recently, another approach for the assessment of myocardial perfusion in murine hearts was reported (Streif et al. 2005) (Fig. 4). This method is based on magnetic spin-labeling of endogenous water protons within the imaging plane (Schwarzbauer et al. 1996) and also allows the quantification of regional blood volume by application of an intravascular contrast agent like Gd-DTPA-albumin (Kahler et al. 1999). Two different inversion recovery T_1 measurements with global and slice-selective spin inversion using an adiabatic hyperbolic secant inversion pulse were combined for the assessment of perfusion. After initial spin inversion the relaxation of the magnetization was tracked by a series of FLASH images. The beginning of each image acquisition was synchronized with the heart cycle using an ECG trigger unit. The global inversion measurement gives the intrinsic relaxation of the tissue. In case of the slice selective inversion, only spins within the detection slice are affected by the inversion pulse. If spins outside the detection slice, which were in thermal equilibrium, enter the detection slice due to perfusion, they cause an apparent acceleration of the relaxation and reflect information about the perfusion in this area. Perfusion (P) can be calculated by the following equation: $P/\lambda[\text{blood-tissue partition coefficient}] = 1/T_1[\text{slice selective}] - 1/T_1[\text{global}]$, first described by Detre et al. (1992). One major difficulty in this technique is related to the small differences between the T_1 values of the global and the slice selective measurement. To solve this problem, a high SNR and accuracy in determination of the T_1 maps are required.

However, this technique was successfully validated against microspheres (Waller et al. 2000). In the $CK^{-/-}$ mice study already mentioned above, Nahrendorf et al. (2006) used a segmented inversion recovery snapshot FLASH sequence on a Bruker

7-Tesla scanner with a proton resonance frequency of 300.3 MHz, a TE of 1.5 ms, a TR of 2.6 ms, a field of view of 30×30 mm, an in-plane resolution of 230μm and a slice thickness of 2 mm. A significantly diminished myocardial perfusion in these CK-deficient mice was found, which was inversely correlated to their left ventricular mass. This finding might be caused by the reduced capillary density which was described in hypertrophied hearts.

6 Vascular Imaging

Due to the increasing importance of transgenic mouse models in cardiovascular research, MRI has also become a powerful tool for investigating the progression of atherosclerosis in noninvasive long-term experiments. High-resolution MRI was used to visualize atherosclerotic plaques in the aortic wall of apolipoprotein-E-deficient mice, which develop fibroinflammatory atheromatous lesions similar to those observed in humans (Seo et al. 1997; Nakashima et al. 1994). Fayad et al. (1998) first showed morphological changes in wall thickening and diameter of the abdominal aorta in vivo using a spin-echo sequence in a 9.4-T magnet (spatial resolution $100 \times 100 \mu$m, slice thickness 500μm). A subsequent study quantified aortic atherosclerosis over a broad range of lesion severity (Choudhury et al. 2002). Wiesmann et al. (2003) demonstrated the feasibility of MRI to reveal a detailed view of lumen and vessel wall in the aortic root, the ascending and descending aorta as well as in the aortic arch. The data showed an excellent agreement with corresponding cross-sectional histopathology. A "black blood" spin-echo sequence was used with an optimized time delay between the excitation and refocusing pulses to suppress the signal from flowing blood in the cardiac chambers and vessels (spatial resolution $50 \times 100 \mu$m, slice thickness 300μm, TR $\sim 1,000$ ms, TE 10 ms). This method allows a clear definition of cardiac compartments, thoracic vessels and shape of atherosclerotic plaques. To avoid motion artifacts, a reliable ECG- and respiratory-gating system was used on a 7-T experimental MR system. Mean and maximal aortic wall thicknesses were significantly increased in the adult apoE$^{-/-}$ mice compared with wild type. The use of this noninvasive MRI technique might facilitate a systematic investigation of the underlying pathological mechanisms of atherosclerotic disease, and possibly offer new insights.

7 Magnetic Resonance Spectroscopy (MRS)

MRS is the ideal technique to study metabolism and metabolic disorders. In-vivo MRS offers the noninvasive and continuous observation of cardiac energetics and cellular metabolic processes at the molecular level. In recent years, several examples of cardiac MRS applications in mice have been reported. The use of transgenic animals might offer new insights into the regulatory processes of cardiac metabolism.

Chacko et al. (2000) described a one-dimensional chemical-shift imaging (CSI) method to assess spatially resolved cardiac ^{31}P-MRS at physiological heart rates in anaesthetized adult mice. Depending on the functional state a number of different phosphorus-containing metabolites, such as ATP, inorganic phosphate or phosphocreatine (PCr), can be detected. The ratio of these metabolites reflects the state of energy consumption and the enzymatic activities in the heart muscle. Because of the rapid ATP consumption, in an intact heart muscle during increased muscle contraction, the signal of phosphocreatine decreases and the signal of inorganic phosphate increases, because ATP is regenerated from phosphocreatine. Therefore, the ATP signal remains unchanged. It is known that the cardiac PCr/ATP ratio is decreased in several pathologies, such as heart failure and ischemia. Therefore, the "creation" of different creatine kinase knockout mice (CK single or double knockout) permits the investigation of the role of creatine kinase in cardiac metabolic processes (Saupe et al. 2000). This mouse heart showed a reduced concentration of phosphocreatine while heart function remained unchanged. In adult transgenic mice lacking expression of the GLUT4 protein, which is the predominantly insulin-sensitive transporter in the heart muscle, the cardiac PCr level showed a significant increase (Weiss et al. 2002). Unexpectedly, the ATP level remained unchanged. These mice showed a severe left ventricular hypertrophy and a depressed systolic function. Despite hypertrophy, diastolic function was not significantly altered. The investigation of the cardiac bioenergetic status and the metabolic processes of phosphorus-containing metabolites in transgenic mouse models provide new information on reaction mechanisms and might be helpful for the development of therapies.

Recently, proton (^{1}H) spectroscopy was used to study the role of myoglobin in the heart of myoglobin-knockout mice (Merx et al. 2001). These mice showed a benign phenotype, although no myoglobin ^{1}H-MRS signal could be detected. Therefore, the chronic lack of myoglobin might be compensated by other mechanisms.

References

Axel L, Dougherty L (1989) Heart wall motion: improved method of spatial modulation of magnetization for MR imaging. Radiology 172:349–350

Bashir A, Bao J, Simons M, Post M, Burstein D (2000) MR imaging of perfusion defects in mice. Proc Intl Soc Magn Reson Med 8:726

Brau AC, Wheeler CT, Hedlund LW, Johnson GA (2002) Fiber-optic stethoscope: a cardiac monitoring and gating system for magnetic resonance microscopy. Magn Reson Med 47:314–321

Cassidy PJ, Schneider JE, Grieve SM, Lygate C, Neubauer S, Clarke K (2004) Assessment of motion gating strategies for mouse magnetic resonance at high magnetic fields. J Magn Reson Imaging 19:229–237

Chacko VP, Aresta F, Chacko SM, Weiss RG (2000) MRI/MRS assessment of in vivo murine cardiac metabolism, morphology, and function at physiological heart rates. Am J Physiol Heart Circ Physiol 279:H2218–H2224

Choudhury RP, Aguinaldo JG, Rong JX, Kulak JL, Kulak AR, Reis ED, Fallon JT, Fuster V, Fisher EA, Fayad ZA (2002) Atherosclerotic lesions in genetically modified mice quantified in vivo by non-invasive high-resolution magnetic resonance microscopy. Atherosclerosis 162:315–321

Detre J, Leigh JS, Williams DS, Koretsky AP. Perfusion Imaging (1992) Magn Reson Med 23: 37–45

Engelhardt S, Hein L, Wiesmann F, Lohse MJ (1999) Progressive hypertrophy and heart failure in beta1-adrenergic receptor transgenic mice. Proc Natl Acad Sci U S A 96:7059–7064

Fayad ZA, Fallon JT, Shinnar M, Whrli S, Dansky HM, Poon M, Badimon JJ, Charlton SA, Fisher EA, Breslow JL, Fuster V (1998) Noninvasive in vivo high-resolution magnetic resonance imaging of atherosclerotic lesions in genetically engineered mice. Circulation 98: 1541–1547

Fishbein KW, McConville P, Spencer RG (2001) The lever-coil: a simple, inexpensive sensor for respiratory and cardiac motion in MRI experiments. Magn Reson Imaging 19:881–889

Franco F, Dubois SK, Peshock RM, Shohet RV (1998) Megnetic resonance imaging accurately estimates LV mass in a transgenic mouse model of cardiac hypertrophy. Am J Physiol 274: H679–H683

Franco F, Thomas GD, GiroirB, Bryant D, Bullock MC, Chwialkowski MC, Victor RG, Peshock RM (1999) Magnetic resonance imaging and invasive evaluation of development of heart failure in transgenic mice with myocardial expression of tumor necrosis factor-α. Circulation 99: 448–454

Haase A, Frahm J, Matthaei M, Hänicke W, Merboldt KD (1986) FLASH imaging: rapid NMR imaging using low flip angle pulses. J Magn Reson 67:258–266

Hennig J, Nauerth A, Friedburg H, Ratzel D (1984) New rapid imaging procedure for nuclear spin tomography. Radiologe 24:579–580

Henson RE, Song SK, Pastorek JS, Lorenz CH (2000) Left ventricular torsion is equal in mice and humans. Am J Physiol 278:H1117–H1123

Jerosch-Herold M, Wilke N (1998) Magnetic resonance qunatification of the myocardial perfusion reserve with a fermi function model for constrained deconvolution. Med Phys 25:73–84

Kahler E, Waller C, Rommel E, Belle V, Hiller KH, Voll S, Bauer WR, Haase A (1999) Perfusion-corrected mapping of cardiac regional blood volume in rats in vivo. Magn Reson Med 42: 500–506

Kubota T, McTierman CF, Frye CS, Slawson SE, Lemster HB, Koretsky AP, Demetris AJ, Feldman AM (1997) Dilated cardiomyopathy in transgenic mice with cardiac-specific over-expression of tumor necrosis factor-alpha. Circ Res 81:627–635

Lemieux SK, Glover GH (1996) An infrared device for monitoring the respiration of small rodents during magnetic resonance imaging. J Magn Reson Imaging 6:561–564

Maestri R, Milia AF, Salis MB, Graiani G, Lagrasta C, Monica M, Corradi D, Emanueli C, Madeddu P (2003) Cardiac hypertrophy and microvascular deficit in kinin B2 receptor knock-out mice. Hypertension 41:1151–1155

Manning WJ, Wei JY, Fossel ET, Burstein D (1990) Measurement of left ventricular mass in rats using electrocardiogram-gated magnetic resonance imaging. Am J Physiol 258:H1181–H1186

McKibben CK, Reo NV (1992) A piezoelectric respiratory monitor for in vivo NMR. Magn Reson Med 27:338–342

Merx MW, Flogel U, Stumpe T, Godecke A, Decking UK, Schrader J (2001) Myoglobin facilitates oxygen diffusion. FASEB J 15:1077–1079

Minard KR, Wind RA, Phelps RL (1998) A compact respiratory-triggering device for routine microimaging of laboratory mice. J Magn Reson Imaging 8:1343–1348

Nahrendorf M, Hu K, Fraccarollo D, Hiller KH, Haase A, Bauer WR, Ertl G (2003) Time course of right ventricular remodeling in rats with experimental myocardial infarction. Am J Physiol Heart Circ Physiol 284:H241–H248

Nahrendorf M, Hiller KH, Hu K, Ertl G, Haase A, Bauer WR (2003) Cardiac magnetic resonance imaging in small animal models of human heart failure. Med Image Anal 7:369–375

Nahrendorf M, Streif JUG, Hiller KH, Hu K, Nordbeck P, Ritter O, Sosnovik D, Bauer L, Neubauer S, Jakob PM, Ertl G, Spindler M, Bauer WR (2006) Multimodal functional cardiac MRI in creatine kinase-deficient mice reveals subtle abnormalities in myocardial perfusion and mechanics. Am J Physiol Heart Circ Physiol 290:H2516–H2521

Nakashima Y, Plump AS, Raines EW, Breslow JL, Ross R (1994) ApoE-deficient mice develop lesions of all phases of atherosclerosis throughout the arterial tree. Arterioscler Thromb 14: 133–140

Oppelt A, Graumann R, Barfuss H, Fischer H, Hartl W, Schajor W (1986) FISP – a new fast MRI sequence. Electromedica 54:15–18

Rommel E, Kuhstrebe J, Wiesmann F, Szimtenings M, Streif J, Haase A (2000) A double trigger unit for ECG and breath triggered mouse heart imaging. MAGMA 11:250

Rudin M, Pedersen B, Umemura K, Zierhut W (1991) Determination of rat heart morphology and function in vivo in two models of cardiac hypertrophy by means of magnetic resonance imaging. Basic Res Cardiol 86:165–174

Ruff J, Wiesmann F, Hiller KH, Neubauer S, Rommel E, Haase A (1998) Influence of isoflurane anesthesia on contractility of mouse heart in vivo. An NMR imaging study. MAGMA 6:169

Ruff J, Wiesmann F, Hiller KH, Voll S, von Kienlin M, Bauer WR, Rommel E, Neubauer S, Haase A (1998) Magnetic resonance microimaging for noninvasive quantification of myocardial function and mass in the mouse. Magn Reson Med 40:43–48

Saupe KW, Spindler M, Hopkins JC, Shen W, Ingwall JS (2000) Kinetic, thermodynamic, and developmental consequences of deleting creatine kinase isoenzymes from the heart. Reaction kinetics of the creatine kinase isoenzymes in the intact heart. J Biol Chem 275:19742–19746

Schwarzbauer C, Morissey S, Haase A (1996) Quantitative magnetic resonance imaging of perfusion using magnetic labeling of water protons within the detection slice. Magn Reson Med 35: 540-546

Seo HS, Lombardi DM, Polinsky P, Powell-Braxton L, Bunting S, Schwartz SM, Rosenfeld ME (1997) Peripheral vascular stenosis in apolipoprotein E-deficient mice. Potential roles of lipid deposition, medial atrophy, and adventitial inflammation. Arterioscler Thromb Vasc Biol 17:3593–601

Shapiro EP, Rogers WJ, Beyar, R, Soulen RL, Zerhouni EA, Lima JA, Weiss JL (1989) Determination of left ventricular mass by magnetic resonance imaging in hearts deformed by acute infarction. Circulation 79:706–711

Siri FM, Jelicks LA, Leinwand LA, Gardin JM (1997) Gated magnetic resonance imaging of normal and hypertrophied murine hearts. Am J Physiol 272:H2394–H2402

Slawson SE, Roman BB, Williams DS, Koretsky AP (1998) Cardiac MRI of the normal and hypertrophied mouse heart. Magn Reson Med 39:980–987

Streif JUG, Herold V, Szimtenings M, Lanz TE, Nahrendorf M, Wiesmann F, Bauer WR, Rommel E, Haase A (2003) In vivo time-resolved quantitative motion mapping of the murine myocardium with phase contrast MRI. Magn Reson Med 49:315–321

Streif JUG, Nahrendorf M, Hiller KH, Waller C, Wiesmann F, Rommel E, Haase A, Bauer WR (2005) In vivo assessment of absolute perfusion and intracapillary blood volume in the murine myocardium by spin labeling magnetic resonance imaging. Magn Res Med 53:584–592

Waller C, Kahler E, Hiller KH, Hu K, Nahrendorf M, Voll S, Haase A, Ertl G, Bauer WR (2000) Myocardial perfusion and intracapillary blood volume in rats at rest and with coronary dilatation: MR imaging in vivo with use of a spin-labeling technique. Radiology 215:189–197

Waller C, Hiller KH, Kahler E, Hu K, Nahrendorf M, Voll S, Haase A, Ertl G, Bauer WR (2001) Serial magnetic resonance imaging of microvascular remodeling in the infarcted rat heart. Circulation 103:1564–1569

Wang Y, Rossman PJ, Grimm RC, Riederer SJ, Ehmann RL (1996). Navigator-echo-based real-time respiratory gating and triggering for reduction of respiration effects in three-dimensional coronary MR angiography. Radiology 198:55–60

Weiss RG, Chatham JC, Georgakopolous D, Charron MJ, Walliman T, Kay L, Walzel B, Wang Y, Kass DA, Gerstenblith G, Chacko VP (2002) An increase in the myocardial PCr/ATP ratio in GLUT4 null mice. FASEB J 15:1077–1079

Wiesmann F, Ruff J, Hiller KH, Rommel E, Haase A, Neubauer S (2000) Developmental changes of cardiac function and mass assessed with MRI in neonatal, juvenil, and adult mice. Am J Physiol Heart Circ Physiol 278:H652–H657

Wiesmann F, Ruff J, Dienesch C, Laupold A, Illinger R, Frydrychowicz A, Hiller KH, Rommel E, Haase A, Neubauer S (2001) Dobutamine stress magnetic resonance microimaging in mice: acute changes of cardiac geometry and function in normal and failing murine hearts. Circ Res 88:563–569

Wiesmann F, Frydrychowicz A, Rautenberg J, Illinger R, Rommel E, Haase A, Neubauer S (2002) Analysis of right ventricular function in healthy mice and a murine model of heart failure by in vivo MRI. Am J Physiol Heart Circ Physiol 283:H1065–H1071

Wiesmann F, Szimtenings M, Frydrychowicz A, Illinger R, Hunecke A, RommelE, Neubauer S, Haase A (2003) High-resolution MRI with cardiac and respiratory gating allows for accurate in vivo atherosclerotic plaque visualization in the murine aortic arch. Magn Reson Med 50:69–74

Wilke N, Simm C, Zhang J, Ellermann J, Ya X, Merkle H, Path G, Ludemann H, Bache R, Urgurbil K (1993) Contrast-enhanced first pass myocardial perfusion imaging: correlation between myocardial blood flow in dogs at rest and during hyperemia. Magn Res Med 29:485–497

Wood ML, Henkelman RM (1986) The magnetic field dependence of the breathing artifact. Magn Reson Imaging 4:387–392

Translational Imaging: Imaging of Apoptosis

H. William Strauss(✉), Francis Blankenberg, Jean-Luc Vanderheyden, and Jonathan Tait

Abstract Since its original description in 1972, apoptosis or programmed cell death has been recognized as the major pathway by which the body precisely regulates the number and type of its cells as part of normal embryogenesis, development, and homeostasis. Later it was found that apoptosis was also involved in the pathogenesis of a number of human diseases, cell immunity, and the action of cytotoxotic drugs and radiation therapy in cancer treatment. As such, the imaging of apoptosis with noninvasive techniques such as with radiotracers, including annexin V and lipid proton magnetic resonance spectroscopy, may have a wide range of clinical utility in both the diagnosis and monitoring therapy of a wide range of human disorders. In this chapter we review the basic biochemical and morphologic features of apoptosis and the methods developed thus far to image this complex process in humans.

1 History

Over four decades ago John Kerr described an unusual form of cell death. Evaluating the liver following acute ligation of the portal vein in rats (O'Rourke and Ellem 2000), Kerr observed that some cells appeared to shrink and disappear without

H. William Strauss
Memorial Sloan Kettering Hospital, 1275 York Ave., Room S-212, Nuclear Medicine, New York, NY 10021
straussh@mskcc.org

W. Semmler and M. Schwaiger (eds.), *Molecular Imaging II.*
Handbook of Experimental Pharmacology 185/II.
© Springer-Verlag Berlin Heidelberg 2008

producing any inflammation. This observation contrasted with the findings of typical necrosis, where cells lose membrane integrity, spill their contents into surrounding tissues, and cause inflammation. Since the cells decreased in size as they died, this type of cell death was initially named shrinkage necrosis. John Kerr, in conjunction with his collaborators, Andrew Wyllie, Alistair Currie and other colleagues, observed this type of noninflammatory cell death was in embryogenesis, effective tumor therapy, and the withdrawal of hormonal support in endocrine organs such as the adrenal gland (Kerr et al. 1972).

According to his personal account, Kerr's observation of this type of cell death began with his Ph.D. thesis, where he was challenged to identify the cause of rapid shrinkage of liver tissue that followed interruption of the portal venous blood supply. In the ischemic lobes, scattered sites in the surviving parenchyma converted into small round masses of cytoplasm that often contained specks of condensed nuclear chromatin. These masses were taken up and digested by other hepatic cells as well as by specialized mononuclear phagocytes. Although it was clear that these cells were dying, the process was different from necrosis, since it was not associated with inflammation, the mitochondria and ribosomes remained intact, and extracellular bodies, occasionally occurring in clusters, suggested budding from the surface of the cells (Kerr 2002). Working with Jeffrey Searle, similar observations were made in histologic specimens of basal cell carcinoma (Kerr and Searle 1972). The incidence of 'shrinkage necrosis' was increased by treatment with radiotherapy. Professor Curry, while a visiting professor working with Kerr in Brisbane, described a similar observation made by his colleague Dr. Wyllie in the adrenal cortex of rats treated with prednisolone (to suppress ACTH) (Wylie et al. 1973). Dr. Curry demonstrated a similar type of cell death associated with regression of experimental rat breast carcinoma following removal of the ovaries. In a seminal article, Kerr, Wyllie and Curry coined the term apoptosis, derived from two Greek words, 'apo' which means *from* and 'ptosis' which means *falling*, to describe this type of cell death.

Since the original description, many investigators have defined specific intracellular processes that allow the apoptotic cell to undergo an organized shut-down and dissolution process that allows the cell to disappear without a trace. Major components of the biochemical modifications of apoptotic cells include: (1) Activation of a series of cysteine protease enzymes (i.e., caspases), to crosslink and cleave specific intracellular proteins. Each of the caspases is associated with a specific inhibitor, allowing the system to be strictly regulated by a number of positive and negative feedback mechanisms. (2) DNA molecules are degraded into 50- to 300-kb-sized pieces. (3) Leakage of potassium and chloride from the intracellular environment, which results in loss of intercellular water and an associated decrease in cell size. Pieces of the cell undergoing apoptosis are packaged in small vesicles derived from the cell membrane. These cell pieces are called "apoptosomes." (4) Cells undergoing apoptosis signal their neighbors by expressing phosphatidylserine (PS) on the external leaflet of the cell membrane (Gottlieb 2005) (as well as apoptosomes). PS is one of the four major phospholipids that make up the cell membrane (the other three are phosphatidylethanolamine, sphingomyelin, and phosphatidylcholine). Normal cell polarization confines PS to the inner leaflet of the cell membrane. Cells undergoing apoptosis lose this polarization, resulting in the expression of PS on the outer leaflet of the cell membrane. The expression of PS on the outer leaflet of the membrane signals neighboring cells that the expressing cell is undergoing apoptosis. A combination of macrophages and adjacent normal cells then phagocytize the remaining components of the cell carcass.

There are several approaches to specifically stain histologic specimens to detect apoptosis. One approach looks for DNA degradation based on nick end-labeling of DNA in the cell (TUNEL stain), another utilizes fluorescein or rhodamine labeled annexin, a protein with nanomolar affinity for cell membrane-bound phosphatidylserine. An alternative approach employs radiolabeled forms of annexin for in-vivo imaging of apoptosis (with either single-photon or positron imaging). In this chapter, we initially focus on the most recent history of radiolabeled annexin V imaging in both animals and humans, followed by a discussion of other imaging modalities, such as lipid proton MR spectroscopy, that have been used to study apoptosis.

2 Physiology of Annexin V Binding and Internalization

Annexin V (MW $\approx 36,000$) is an endogenous human protein that is widely distributed intracellularly, with very high concentrations in the placenta and lower concentrations in endothelial cells, kidney, myocardium, skeletal muscle, skin, red cells, platelets and monocytes. Although the precise physiologic function of annexin is uncertain, the protein has several well-studied functions, including: inhibition of coagulation [annexin was originally discovered because of its ability to trap calcium (annex calcium) and prevent clotting]; inhibition of phospholipase A2, an enzyme responsible for the release of arachidonic acid from the cell membrane – a component of the inflammatory process; and inhibition of protein kinase C, a system responsible for intracellular signaling (Boersma et al. 2005). Annexin levels in normal subjects is about 7 ng per ml of plasma. During pregnancy, circulating levels of annexin increase, often to 30 ng per ml of plasma. The physiologic reason for this increase is unclear, but may relate to prevention of clotting in the placenta (Wu et al. 2006).

The binding of annexin V to sites of PS expression in vivo has been found to be extremely complex and difficult to model. While annexin V is a relatively large protein (about half the molecular weight of albumin), it was shown early on that the protein can be internalized at sites of ischemic injury both in the heart and brain and cross the intact blood brain barrier (Fig. 1) (D'Arceuil et al. 2000). The transport of exogenously administered annexin V, a protein normally found almost exclusively within cells, also must occur across a protein gradient, suggesting the existence of an energy-dependent pump mechanism.

Annexin V binding to rafts of PS exposed on a cell's surface with internalization via a newly discovered unique pathway of pinocytosis (Kenis et al. 2004). This pathway consists of, first, the disassembly of the cortical actin network underlying

Controls

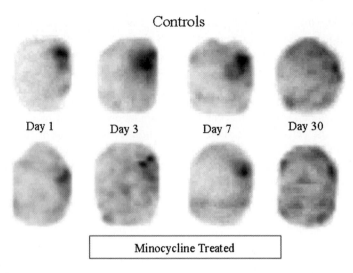

Fig. 1 Minocycline treatment reduces infarct volume. Horizontal tomographic images through the cerebral hemispheres of mice with focal distal middle cerebral artery occlusion and infarction treated with minocycline [an inhibitor of casapse-3 (apoptotic cascade)] (22.5 mg/kg i.p. bid × 7 days) or saline (*controls*). Images were obtained using a LumaGEM small animal SPECT system (Gamma Medica Instruments; Los Angeles, Calif.) with a single-headed detector and a 1-mm pinhole collimator (64 × 64 imaging matrix, 3 degrees per step, 30 s per step for a 360-degree rotation with a radius of rotation of 2.0 cm. Animals were administered 5–10 mCi of 99mTc-HYNIC-annexin V (20–50 μg/kg of protein) 1 h prior to imaging by penile vein injection. Note the marked decrease in annexin V uptake in the left MCA infarct in minocycline treated mice compared with control at all time points

the PS-exposing membrane patch. Annexin A5 then binds to PS, crystallizes on the cell surface as closely packed trimers that cause the underlying membrane to bend inward. The invaginated membrane patch then closes on itself and is transported into the cytosol in a microtubule-dependent manner. This pathway, apparently, is not related to clathrin- or caveolin-mediated endocytosis as it is neither actin-driven nor preceded by membrane ruffling.

Other investigations of annexin V binding have found that PS can be expressed at low levels in a reversible fashion under condition of cell stress that does not necessarily commit a cell to apoptotic cell death (Lejeune et al. 1998; Hammill et al. 1999; Furukawa et al. 2000; Lin et al. 2000; Maiese et al. 2000; Martin et al. 2000; Strauss et al. 2000; Geske et al. 2001; Yang et al. 2002). These studies showed that intermediate levels of PS exposure were noted in cells with no other morphologic features of apoptosis which could be readily reversed upon removal of physiologic stressors such as nitric-oxide, p53 activation, allergic mediators and growth factor deprivation. If these observations play out in vivo, then PS expression may define tissues at risk for cell death that may recover or be amendable to therapeutic intervention. Radiolabeled annexin V imaging may, therefore, be vastly more sensitive to regions of cellular injury as both stressed and dying cells can bind the tracer.

Annexin imaging can, therefore, define territory at risk and potentially salvageable with prompt intervention.

Better understanding of PS expression in vivo along with the mechanisms of exogenous annexin localization may lead to use of the annexin V pinocytic pathway to introduce drugs and other molecules into cells expressing PS that could halt or even reverse a wide variety of cellular injuries and stress.

3 PET and SPECT Imaging with Radiolabeled Annexin V

Annexin has been radiolabeled with iodine-125, iodine-124, fluorine-18, technetium-99m and gallium-68. The half-lives of the tracers limit the choices of imaging time. Typically, the tracer clears from the blood rapidly. When labeled with ^{123}I, there was <4% residual in the blood 40 min after injection (Lahorte et al. 2003). However there is significant nonspecific distribution in soft tissue, which has much slower clearance. Based on sequential imaging studies, once annexin binds to sites expressing PS, it appears that the signal persists, suggesting that imaging should be performed several hours after injection to maximize contrast while maintaining a reasonable count rate.

An array of human imaging studies have been performed with recombinant human annexin V. Initial studies utilized ^{99m}Tc-labeled annexin to detect thrombi in the atria of patients with atrial fibrillation. This work was a direct extension of the experimental studies in rabbits with atrial thrombi (Tait et al. 1994). Although excellent imaging results were seen in pigs (Stratton et al. 1995), the human results were disappointing, and the use of annexin for atrial thrombus detection was abandoned. However, the initial promising results in experimental animals with apoptosis suggested the ^{99m}Tc-rh-annexin V could be clinically useful to detect apoptosis in vivo. Two clinical trials were performed with ^{99m}Tc-N$_2$S$_2$-rh-annexin, the same formulation used in the clot detection trial. The first study was designed to detect graft rejection in heart transplant recipients. Detection of transplant rejection was based on the work of Vriens et al. (1998), which clearly delineated uptake in experimental heart transplant graft rejection (Fig. 2). Narula et al. (2001) studied 18 cardiac allograft recipients. Thirteen patients had negative and five had positive myocardial uptake of annexin V as seen by ECG-gated SPECT imaging. Endocardial biopsies obtained within 2 days of the scan demonstrated histologic evidence of at least moderate transplant rejection.

In the second trial, Belhocine et al. (2002) studied 15 cancer patients in late stage small-cell and non-small-cell lung cancers (SCLC and NSCLC), Hodgkins, non-Hodgkins lymphomas (HL and NHL), and metastatic breast cancers (BC). Two sets of images were recorded: the first immediately prior to starting chemotherapy and the second immediately after the first course of treatment. In eight patients with no increase in annexin V uptake post therapy there was no response to chemotherapy.

To reduce the complexity of preparing the radiolabeled material, alternative labeling approaches were sought and hydrazino nicotinamide (HYNIC) was

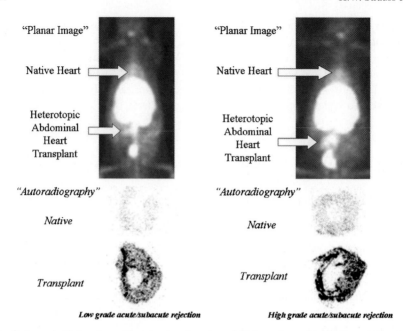

Fig. 2 Annexin V imaging of low-grade subacute and high-grade acute rejection. ACI rats received PVG heterotopic cardiac allografts sewn into the abdominal aorta and vena cava. Following transplant animals were treated with either subtherapeutic doses of cyclosporine (5 mg/kg p.o. qd, subacute low grade rejection) or saline control (high grade acute rejection) for 4 days. Planar images were obtained 1 h after injection of 2–3 mCi of ^{99m}Tc-HYNIC-annexin V (64 × 64 matrix, parallel hole collimator). Immediately after imaging, animals were euthanized and the native and allograft hearts were removed and 60-µm histologic sections were obtained and placed on a digital phosphor storage screen overnight and then readout. Note that on both the planar and autoradiographic images there is little uptake of tracer in the native hearts compared with the abdominal heterotopic allografts. Also note the marked reduction in tracer uptake in low grade/subacute versus the untreated control

selected as the coupling molecule (Kemerink et al. 2003). HYNIC [succinimidyl (6-hydrazinopyridine-3-carboxylic acid)], also known as [succinimidyl (6-hydrazinonicotinic acid)], is covalently attached to rh-annexin V and the resultant compound is lyophilized and stored for labeling with ^{99m}Tc as needed. Labeling with ^{99m}Tc is performed by simply reacting the conjugate with ^{99m}Tc pertechnetate in the presence of stannous tricine for 5–10 min at room temperature. The whole procedure has been reduced to a standardized two-vial kit that can be ready for patient use within 30 min of receiving 20–30 mCi of sterile ^{99m}Tc-pertechnetate from a local radiopharmacy or generator.

Unfortunately, although ^{99m}Tc-HYNIC-annexin V is not concentrated in the liver or excreted in the bowel; it concentrates in the cortex of the kidney, limiting visualization of any structures in this region (Boersma et al. 2003).

In spite of this shortcoming, clinical trials are testing the clinical utility of HYNIC-annexin V in determining the efficacy of chemotherapy in oncology patients

(Blankenberg 2003; Haas et al. 2004; Kartachova et al. 2004; Vermeersch et al. 2004; Rottey et al. 2006), detection of apoptosis in areas of acute myocardial infarction (Narula et al. 2003; Thimister et al. 2003), defining the activity of rheumatoid arthritis (personal communication: R. Hustinx and C. Beckers, Liege, Belgium), ischemic preconditioning (Riksen et al. 2005, 2006; Rongen et al. 2005), detecting vulnerable plaque (Kiestelaer et al. 2004), acute stroke (Blankenberg et al. 2006; Lorberboym et al. 2006), and Alzheimer's dementia (Lampl et al. 2006).

In patients with late-stage (IIIB and IV) small-cell and non-small-cell lung cancer (Belhocine et al. 2004), imaging at 24 and 48 h post injection may not be required to get an optimal signal. At 24 h after the start of treatment, in the subset of patients with a partial response to platinum-based chemotherapy ($n = 5$), only one patient had increase tumor uptake of ^{99m}Tc-HYNIC-annexin V, while the four remaining patients showed an unexpected decrease in tracer uptake, suggesting that the therapy may have had an effect on tumor vasculature, limiting the delivery of the tracer to the lesion (Ran et al. 2002).

Another observation was the presence of a low level of Tc-99m annexin V uptake in the lesions *immediately prior* to chemotherapy correlated with tumor response. This observation suggested that the lesions had ongoing apoptosis, raising the likelihood of an apoptotic response to chemotherapy. An alternative explanation is increased expression of PS on vascular endothelial cells during neoangiogenesis (van de Wiele et al. 2003).

The timing of injection and imaging is also important in imaging apoptosis following acute myocardial infarction (Flotats and Carrio 2003; Taki et al. 2004). Thimister's clinical study of patients with acute infarction (Thimister et al. 2003) demonstrated the highest annexin V localization the first day after infarction. The lesions were reduced in size and intensity when the patients were restudied with ^{99m}Tc-annexin V days to months after the acute event.

There are alternative methods to radiolabel annexin V, including the use of self-chelating annexin V mutants that have lower concentrations in the kidneys of rodents compared with HYNIC-annexin V (Tait et al. 2000). The best-studied annexin V mutant with an endogenous site for ^{99m}Tc chelation is known as V117. The protein contains six amino acids added at the N-terminus, followed by amino acids 1-320 of wild-type annexin V. Amino acid Cys-316 is also mutated to serine in this molecule. Technetium-99m chelation is thought to occur via formation of an N_3S structure involving the N-terminal cysteine and the immediately adjacent amino acids. The purified protein is then reduced and can be stored for later labeling with ^{99m}Tc using glucoheptonate as the exchange reagent.

Another self-chelating annexin V mutant, V128, is a fusion protein with an endogenous Tc chelation site (Ala-Gly-Gly-Cys-Gly-His) added to the N-terminus of annexin V (Jin et al. 2004; Tait et al. 2005). Both V117 and V128 have major advantages over the HYNIC chelator with regard to renal retention of ^{99m}Tc, with attendant decreased abdominal background and renal radiation dose.

It would be helpful to quantify radiolabeled annexin concentration at lesions sites. Since PET has major advantages for quantitative imaging, several approaches to label annexin V with ^{18}F have been developed. Two laboratories have used

N-succinimidyl 4-fluorobenzoate (Grierson et al. 2004; Murakami et al. 2004) to synthesize ^{18}F-annexin V. The fluorine-labeled agent has lower uptake in the liver, spleen, and kidney compared with HYNIC-annexin V.

4 Recent Developments in the Assay of Modified Forms of Annexin V

Most imaging investigations have used annexin V that has been randomly modified with bifunctional agents attached to the protein's accessible amino groups, as outlined above. In addition, researchers have tested chemically modified annexin V with a variety of different in-vitro assays and have generally concluded that the protein can withstand up to average derivatization stoichiometry of 2 mol/mol without a loss in PS binding affinity (Blankenberg et al. 1998; Zijlstra et al. 2003; Boersma et al. 2004; Schellenberger et al. 2004a, 2004b; Dekker et al. 2005). However, these results have been called into question by the work of Bazzi and Nelsestuen (1991), who found that the binding of annexins to membranes is negatively cooperative (i.e., a negative Hill Effect) with respect to protein. This means that binding measurements made by titrating PS expressing cells with labeled annexin V until full saturation will overestimate the binding affinity measured at higher protein concentrations. To make matters worse, many in-vitro binding measurements have been made with calcium at 1.8 or 2.5 mmol/l rather than 1.25 mmol/l. Because the affinity of annexin V binding to cells declines greatly over a calcium range of 2.5–1.25 mmol/l (Tait et al. 2004) these results also may not accurately predict in-vitro and in-vivo binding of modified protein.

Tait et al. (2004) have recently developed a newer method of measuring the membrane-binding affinity of annexin V, titrating with calcium (an ion necessary for PS binding) instead of protein. In addition, site-specific labeled forms of fluorescent or radioactive labels (as opposed to the standard random amino group labeling approach) are used for the competition with modified annexin. Finally, the assay is performed under conditions of very low occupancy ($\leq$1% of membrane-binding sites occupied at saturation), thus avoiding the confounding effects seen as the membrane becomes more crowded (i.e., the negative Hill Effect). These conditions best simulate the situation in vivo in which annexin V binding occurs at a calcium concentration of 1.25 mmol/l (the typical value for ionized calcium in vivo) and very low membrane occupancy with respect to the protein.

In related work, Tait et al. (2005) have constructed and systematically tested a set of self-chelating mutants of annexin V, including annexin V-128, that have varying numbers of calcium binding sites both in vitro with the new assay system and in vivo in mice undergoing cycloheximide-induced liver apoptosis (Tait et al. 2005). It was found that all four calcium binding sites are needed for full in-vitro and in-vivo binding of annexin V. Mutation (loss of function) of any one the four calcium binding sites decreased in-vivo location of tracer by 25% and any two site mutations resulted in a 50% decline. These results indicate that mini-forms of annexin with only one calcium ion binding site are unlikely to be useful as imaging agents (Mukherjee et al. 2006). Comparison of HYNIC, mercaptoacetyltriglycine (MAG_3), fluorescein isothiocyanate, and biotin-labeled annexin V with annexin V-128 showed a 50% decrease in liver uptake of tracer when randomly modified with respect to self-chelating (site-specific) protein (Tait et al. 2005). Furthermore, modification of annexin V with as little as 0.5 mol HYNIC/mol protein is sufficient to lower in-vitro and in-vivo bioactivity substantially.

In summary, it appears that the self-chelating mutant annexin V-128 with site-specific modification is the best approach to development of annexin V-based SPECT, PET and fluorescent probes in the near future.

5 Other Potential Tracers

Several types of annexin V derivatives have been developed for the in-vivo imaging of apoptosis, including AnxCLIO-Cy5.5, a magneto-optical (iron) nanoparticle that can be used as a bifunctional tracer in MR and fluorescence imaging (Sosnovik et al. 2005), another annexin V-indocyanine fluorophore (a bisfunctional succinimidyl ester of Cy5.5) (Yang et al. 2006), annexin V-conjugated quantum dots with a parmagnetic lipidic coating (DTPA) for MR and fluorescent imaging (van Tilborg et al. 2006), ^{64}Cu-labeled streptavidin imaging following pretargeting of PS with biotinylated annexin V (Cauchon et al. 2007), and another self-chelating (with ^{99m}Tc) annexin subfamily of proteins called annexin B1 (Luo et al. 2005). All these tracers with the exception of the self-chelating annexin B1, however, rely on the random modification of annexin V with bifunctional molecules, which necessarily results in a dramatic loss of in-vivo PS binding affinity compared with the wild-type protein as mentioned previously. As for annexin B1, it appears to have a high renal retention (50% I.D.) similar to HYNIC modified forms of the protein for reasons that are still unclear. Furthermore, in-vitro assays to validate each tracer rely on the use of fluorescent forms of annexin V that also have been randomly modified and, typically, are done at relatively high protein concentrations that can greatly over-estimate the measured binding affinities.

Another class of possible alternative tracers for the imaging of apoptosis selectively or nonselectively target the early loss of membrane asymmetry and exposure of anionic phospholipids on the cell surface. These include mimics of annexin V such as those peptidic vectors found by phage display technologies (Laumonier et al. 2006), nonselective cationic liposomes (Bose et al. 2004), sensing of the phosphate moiety on PS with Zn(II)-di-picolylamine (DPA) complexes (Hanshaw and Smith 2005; Quinti et al. 2006), and the development of radiolabeled and iron-labeled forms of the C2A domain of synaptotagmin I, a neural protein with a relatively weak PS binding capacity (10- to 100-fold less than wild-type annexin V) (Zhao et al. 2006). A disadvantage of the nonselective anionic phospholipid and phosphate binding tracers is the potential for hemolysis and other forms of cytotoxicity found with other types of nonselective agents such as Ro09-0198, a tetracyclic

19-amino-acid polypeptide that recognizes and forms a tight equimolar complex with phosphatidylethanolamine (PE) on biological membranes (Emoto et al. 1996).

The last class of possible new tracers for apoptosis focus on the development of caspase-3-specific binding peptides that rely not on membrane changes but on the activation of the caspase cascade of mitochondrial and cytoplasmic enzymes believed to occur prior to the exposure of PS on the cell surface. These agents include a small membrane permeant, caspase-activable far-red fluorescent peptide composed of a Tat-based permeation peptide fused to an L-amino acid effector caspase recognition sequence DEVD (Bullok and Piwnica-Worms 2005), and WC-II-89 (a non-peptide-based isatin sulfonamide caspase inhibiting analogue), labeled with ^{18}F for PET imaging (Zhao et al. 2006). While caspase-based agents hold promise they have as yet not been tested in vivo and previous attempts yielded relatively low target-to-background activities (Haberkom et al. 2001).

6 Lipid Proton MR Spectroscopy

The first MR technique applied to the detection of apoptosis was lipid proton MR spectroscopy (Blankenberg et al. 1996, 1997; Engelmann et al. 1996). These studies described apoptosis-specific changes, including a selective increase in CH_2 (methylene) relative to CH_3 (methyl) mobile lipid proton signal intensities (1.3 and 0.9 ppm, respectively). The rise in CH_2 resonance occurred with a wide range of apoptotic drugs as well as apoptosis associated with serum (growth factor) deprivation. The ratio of CH_2/CH_3 also had a strong linear correlation with other markers of programmed cell death, including fluorescent annexin V cytometry and DNA ladder formation. While there was a rise in the methylene resonance there was no detectable change in total lipid composition or new lipid synthesis, suggesting an increase in membrane mobility as opposed to increased amounts of lipid within cells.

These observations have largely been confirmed by subsequent investigations though the source of the increased methylene signal intensity seen with apoptosis has been determined to arise from the formation of osmophilic lipid ($0.2–2.0 \mu m$) droplets with the cytoplasm (Hakumaki et al. 1998). These droplets contain variable amounts of polyunsaturated fatty acids associated largely with 18:1 and 18:2 lipid moieties and an accumulation of TAGs (triacylglycerides). The accumulation of TAGs are believed to be related to phospholipase-A_2 activation and the formation of ceramide, (a regulatory molecule in mediating membrane related apoptotic events) with a long -CH_2-chain.

Despite the differences in the drugs used and their mechanisms of action, and the different types of cells studied, the increase in the lipid signal, as evidenced by the increase in the 1.3 p.p.m. intensity, seems to hold in all situations. Therefore, a selective increase in CH_2 and CH_3 mobile lipid protons, principally of CH_2, permits the calculation of a ratio of CH_2 to CH_3 signal as a measure of the presence and degree of apoptosis within a sample or voxel in most situations. Decreases in other chemical species, such as glutamine and glutamate, choline-containing metabolites, taurine and reduced glutathione, can also be seen with apoptotic cell death. By contrast, necrosis in general is characterized by a completely different profile of ^{1}H-NMR in which there is a significant increase in all the metabolites examined, with the exception of CH_2 mobile lipids that remain unchanged coupled to a decrease in reduced glutathione.

This early spectroscopic work, however, was severely limited by the lack of a method that could permit high spectral resolution of excised whole tissue. Therefore, investigations were conducted with treated cell suspensions in deuteriated (D_2O) phosphate-buffered saline or lipid extracts of tissue, a process that necessarily introduces artifacts. These problems arise as tissues are semi-solid in nature and contain highly heterogeneous microenvironments that lead to marked restriction of molecular motion and high magnetic susceptibility (i.e., dipole couplings and chemical shift anisotropy). The result is strong interactions between the spins of each proton leading to severe dephasing with T2 shorting (signal intensity loss) and relatively broad spectral lines. Additionally, spin-spin interactions have an angular dependence with respect to the main magnetic field. In liquids (and lipid extracts of tissue) molecules can freely move at rates faster than these dipole interactions and are effectively averaged, giving sharp well defined spectral lines and long T2 relaxation times.

With the advent of magic angle spinning (MAS) proton spectroscopy in the early 1990s, the problems with obtaining high-resolution spectra from whole-tissue samples have largely been overcome (Cheng et al. 1998; Moka et al. 1998; Adebodun et al. 1992). It is known that if a sample is spun mechanically, at a rate faster than the spectral broadening originating from these interactions (about 2.5 kHz), and at the 'magic angle' of 54°44' with respect to the main magnetic field, the contribution from these interactions to the MR spectral broadening can be significantly reduced.

Ex-vivo MAS and conventional in-vivo MR spectroscopy of patients with cervical carcinomas pre and post radiation therapy showed that the apoptotic activity could be well predicted from the lipid metabolites in HR MAS MR spectra, whereas tumor cell fraction and density were predicted from cholines, creatine, taurine, glucose, and lactate (Mahon et al. 2004; Lyng et al. 2007). Clinical studies using lipid proton MR spectroscopy, however, will be at least in the near term be limited to those organs that are accessible to surface (or endovaginal, endorectal) coils that are needed to detect the relative small changes in lipid signal with scattered regions of apoptosis typically found within a voxel of tissue, or in organs such as the brain that are mostly free of motion artifacts and subcutaneous fat that can bleed as noise into the desired lipid signal.

7 Diffusion-weighted MR Imaging (DWI)

DWI is an alternative measure of apoptosis in response to radiation and chemotherapy (Lidar et al. 2004; Valonen et al. 2004; Charles-Edwards and deSouza 2006; Deng et al. 2006). DWI generates image contrast by using the diffusion properties of water within tissues. Diffusion can be predominantly unidirectional (anisotropic) or not (isotropic) and can be restricted or free depending on the amount of water in the extracellular (relatively unrestricted) or intracellular (restricted) compartments. Diffusion sensitized (weighted) images can be acquired with magnetic gradients of different magnitudes generating an apparent diffusion coefficient (ADC) map. As increases in cellularity are reflected as restricted motion DWI has been used in n cancer imaging to distinguish between tumor and peri-tumoral edema (unrestricted). DWI may also be valuable in monitoring treatment where changes due to cell swelling and apoptosis are measurable as changes in ADC. The magnitude of changes however are small (i.e., less than 50% of control) and maybe difficult to separate tumor shrinkage, necrosis, etc. that can occur with therapy. Therefore, more studies are needed to confirm the validity of DWI as a marker of therapeutic efficacy in the clinic.

References

Adebodun F, Chung J, Montez B, Oldfield E, Shan X (1992) Spectroscopic studies of lipids and biological membranes: carbon-13 and proton magic-angle sample-spinning nuclear magnetic resonance study of glycolipid-water systems.Biochemistry 31:4502–4509
Bazzi MD, Nelsestuen GL (1991) Highly sequential binding of protein kinase C and related proteins to membranes. Biochemistry. 30:7970–7977
Belhocine T, Steinmetz N, Hustinx R, Bartsch P, Jerusalem G, Seidel L, Rigo P, Green A (2002) Increased uptake of the apoptosis-imaging agent (99m)Tc recombinant human Annexin V in human tumors after one course of chemotherapy as a predictor of tumor response and patient prognosis. Clin Cancer Res 8:2766–2774
Belhocine T, Steinmetz N, Li C, Green A, Blankenberg FG (2004) The imaging of apoptosis with the radiolabeled annexin V: optimal timing for clinical feasibility. Technol Cancer Res Treat 3:23–32
Blankenberg FG (2003) Molecular imaging: The latest generation of contrast agents and tissue characterization techniques. J Cell Biochem 90:443–453
Blankenberg FG, Storrs RW, Naumovski L, Goralski T, Spielman D (1996) Detection of apoptotic cell death by proton nuclear magnetic resonance spectroscopy. Blood 87:1951–1956
Blankenberg FG, Katsikis PD, Storrs RW, Beaulieu C, Spielman D, Chen JY, Naumovski L, Tait JF (1997) Quantitative analysis of apoptotic cell death using proton nuclear magnetic resonance spectroscopy. Blood 89:3778–3786
Blankenberg FG, Katsikis PD, Tait JF et al (1998) In vivo detection and imaging of phosphatidylserine expression during programmed cell death. Proc Natl Acad Sci USA 95: 6349–6354
Blankenberg FG, Kalinyak J, Liu L, Koike M, Cheng D, Goris ML, Green A, Vanderheyden JL, Tong DC, Yenari MA (2006) 99mTc-HYNIC-annexin V SPECT imaging of acute stroke and its response to neuroprotective therapy with anti-Fas ligand antibody
Eur J Nucl Med Mol Imaging 33:566–574
Boersma HH, Liem IH, Kemerink GJ, Thimister PW, Hofstra L, Stolk LM, van Heerde WL, Pakbiers MT, Janssen D, Beysens AJ, Reutelingsperger CP, Heidendal GA (2003) Comparison between human pharmacokinetics and imaging properties of two conjugation methods for 99mTc-annexin A5. Br J Radiol 76:553–560

Boersma HH, Stolk LM, Kenis H et al (2004) The ApoCorrect assay: a novel, rapid method to determine the biological functionality of radiolabeled and fluorescent Annexin A5. Anal Biochem 327:126–134

Boersma HH, Kietselaer BL, Stolk LM, Bennaghmouch A, Hofstra L, Narula J, Heidendal GA, Reutelingsperger CP (2005) Past, present, and future of annexin A5: from protein discovery to clinical applications. J Nucl Med 46:2035–2050

Bose S, Tuunainen I, Parry M, Medina OP, Mancini G, Kinnunena PKJ (2004) Binding of cationic liposomes to apoptotic cells. Anal Biochem 331:385–394

Bullok K, Piwnica-Worms D (2005) Synthesis and characterization of a small, membrane-permeant, caspase-activatable far-red fluorescent peptide for imaging apoptosis. J Med Chem 48:5404–5407

Cauchon N, Langlois R, Rousseau JA, Tessier G, Cadorette J, Lecomte R, Hunting DJ, Pavan RA, Zeisler SK, van Lier JE (2007) PET imaging of apoptosis with ^{64}Cu-labeled streptavidin following pretargeting of phosphatidylserine with biotinylated annexin-V. Eur J Nucl Med Mol Imaging 34:247–258

Charles-Edwards EM, deSouza NM (2006) Diffusion-weighted magnetic resonance imaging and its application to cancer. Cancer Imaging 6:135–143

Cheng LL, Chang IW, Louis DN, Gonzalez RG (1998) Correlation of high-resolution magic angle spinning proton magnetic resonance spectroscopy with histopathology of intact human brain tumor specimens. Cancer Res 58:1825–1832

D'Arceuil H, Rhine W, de Crespigny A, Yenari M, Tait JF, Strauss WH, Engelhorn T, Kastrup A, Moseley M, Blankenberg FG (2000) 99mTc annexin V imaging of neonatal hypoxic brain injury. Stroke 31:2692–2700

Dekker B, Keen H, Shaw D et al (2005) Functional comparison of annexin V analogues labeled indirectly and directly with iodine-124. Nucl Med Biol 32:403–413

Deng J, Miller FH, Rhee TK, Sato KT, Mulcahy MF, Kulik LM, Salem R, Omary RA, Larson AC (2006) Diffusion-weighted MR imaging for determination of hepatocellular carcinoma response to ttrium-90 radioembolization. J Vasc Interv Radiol 17:1195–200

Emoto K, Kobayashi T, Yamaji A, Aizawa H, Yahara I, Inoue K, Umeda M (1996) Redistribution of phosphatidylethanolamine at the cleavage furrow of dividing cells during cytokinesis. Proc Natl Acad Sci U S A 93:12867–12872

Engelmann J, Henke J, Willker W, Kutscher B, Nossner G, Engel J, Leibfritz D (1996) Early stage monitoring of miltefosine induced apoptosis in KB cells by multinuclear NMR spectroscopy. Anticancer Res 16(3B):1429–1439

Flotats A, Carrio I (2003) Non-invasive in vivo imaging of myocardial apoptosis and necrosis. Eur J Nucl Med Mol Imaging 30:615–630

Furukawa Y, Bangham CRM, Taylor GP, Weber JN, Osame M (2000) Frequent reversible membrane damage in peripheral blood B cells in human T cell lymphotrophic virus type I (HTLV-I)-associated myelopathy/tropical spastic paraparesis (HAM/TSP). Clin Exp Immunol 120: 307–316

Geske FJ, Lieberman R, Strange R, Gerschenson LE (2001) Early stages of p53-induced apoptosis are reversible. Cell Death Differ 8:182–191

Gottlieb RA (2005) Apoptosis. In: Lichtman MA, Beutler E, Kipps TJ, Seligsohn U, Kaushansky K, Prcha JT (eds) Williams Hematology, Part III: Molecular and cellular hematology, 7th edn. McGraw-Hill, pp 125–130

Grierson JR, Yagle KJ, Eary JF, Tait JF, Gibson DF, Lewellen B, Link JM, Krohn KA (2004) Production of [F-18]fluoroannexin for imaging apoptosis with PET. Bioconjug Chem 15: 373–379

Haas RL, de Jong D, Valdes Olmos RA, Hoefnagel CA, van den Heuvel I, Zerp SF, Bartelink H, Verheij M (2004) In vivo imaging of radiation-induced apoptosis in follicular lymphoma patients. Int J Radiat Oncol Biol Phys 59:782–787

Haberkom U, Kinscherf R, Krammer PH, Mier W, Eisenhut M (2001) Investigation of a potential scintigraphic marker of apoptosis: radioiodinated Z-Val-Ala-DL-Asp(O-methyl)-fluoromethyl ketone. Nucl Med Biol 28:793–798

Hakumaki JM, Poptani H, Puumalainen AM, Loimas S, Paljarvi LA, Yla-Herttuala S, Kauppinen RA (1998) Quantitative 1H nuclear magnetic resonance diffusion spectroscopy of BT4C rat glioma during thymidine kinase-mediated gene therapy in vivo: identification of apoptotic response. Cancer Res 58:3791–3799

Hammill AK, Uhr JW, Scheuermann RH (1999) Annexin V staining due to loss of membrane asymmetry can be reversible and precede commitment to apoptotic death. Exp Cell Res 251: 16–21

Hanshaw RG, Smith BD (2005) New reagents for phosphatidylserine recognition and detection of apoptosis. BioorgMed Chem 13:5035–5042

Jin M, Smith C, Hsieh HY, Gibson DF, Tait JF (2004) Essential role of B-helix calcium binding sites in annexin V-membrane binding. J Biol Chem 279:40351–40357

Kartachova M, Haas RL, Olmos RA, Hoebers FJ, van Zandwijk N, Verheij M (2004) In vivo imaging of apoptosis by 99mTc-annexin V scintigraphy: visual analysis in relation to treatment response. Radiother Oncol 72:333–339

Kemerink GJ, Liu X, Kieffer D, Ceyssens S, Mortelmans L, Verbruggen AM, Steinmetz ND, Vanderheyden J-L, Green A, Verbeke K (2003) Safety, biodistribution, and dosimetry of 99mTc-HYNIC-annexin V, a novel human recombinant annexin V for human application. J Nucl Med 44:947–952

Kenis H, van Genderen H, Bennaghmouch A, Rinia HA, Frederik P, Narula J, Hofstra L, Reutelingsperger CP (2004) Cell surface-expressed phosphatidylserine and annexin A5 open a novel portal of cell entry. J Biol Chem 279:52623–52629

Kerr JF (2002) History of the events leading to the formulation of the apoptosis concept. Toxicology 181–182:471–474

Kerr JFR, Searle JA (1972) A suggested explanation for the paradoxically slow growth of basal cell carcinomas that contain numerous mitotic figures. J Pathology 107:41–44

Kerr JF, Wylie AH, Currie AR (1972) Apoptosis: the basic biological phenomenon with wide-ranging implications in tissue kinetics. Brit J of Cancer 26:239–257

Kiestelaer BLJH, Reutelingsperger CPM, Heidendal GAK, Daemen MJAP, Mess WH, Hofstra L (2004) Noninvasive detection of plaque instability with use of radiolabeled annexin A5 in patients with carotid-artery atherosclerosis. New Engl J Med 350:1472–1473

Lahorte CM, van de Wiele C, Bacher K, van den Bossche B, Thierens H, van Belle S, Slegers G, Dierckx RA (2003) Biodistribution and dosimetry study of 123I-rh-annexin V in mice and humans. Nucl Med Commun 24:871–880

Lampl Y, Lorberboym M, Blankenberg FG, Sadeh M, Gilad R (2006) Annexin V SPECT imaging of phosphatidylserine expression in patients with dementia. Neurology 66:1253–1254

Laumonier C, Segers J, Laurent S, Michel A, Coppee F, Belayew A, Elst LV, Muller RN (2006) A New Peptidic Vector for Molecular Imaging of Apoptosis, Identified by Phage Display Technology. J Biomol Screen 11:537–545

Lejeune M, Ferster A, Cantinieaux B, Sariban E (1998) Prolonged but reversible neutrophil dysfunctions differentially sensitive to granulocyte colony-stimulating factor in children with acute lymphoblastic leukemia. Br J Haematol 102:1284–1291

Lidar Z, Mardor Y, Jonas T, Pfeffer R, Faibel M, Nass D, Hadani M, Ram Z (2004) Convection-enhanced delivery of paclitaxel for the treatment of recurrent malignant glioma: a phase I/II clinical study. J Neurosurg 100:472–479

Lin SH, Vincent A, Shaw T, Maynard KI, Maiese K (2000) Prevention of nitric oxide-induced neuronal injury through the modulation of independent pathways of programmed cell death. J Cereb Blood Flow Metab 20:1380–1391

Lorberboym M, Blankenberg FG, Sadeh M, Lampl Y (2006) In vivo imaging of apoptosis in patients with acute stroke: correlation with blood-brain barrier permeability. Brain Res 1103: 13–19

Luo Q-Y, Zhang Z-Y, Wang F, Lu H-K, Guo Y-Z, Zhu R-S (2005) Preparation, in vitro and in vivo evaluation of 99mTc-Annexin B1: A novel radioligand for apoptosis imaging. Biochemical and Biophysical Research Communications 335:1102–1106

Lyng H, Sitter B, Bathen TF, Jensen LR, Sundfør K, Kristensen GB, Gribbestad IS (2007) Metabolic mapping by use of high-resolution magic angle spinning 1H MR spectroscopy predicts apoptosis in cervical carcinomas. BMC Cancer 7:11

Mahon MM, Williams AD, Soutter WP, Cox IJ, McIndoe GA, Coutts GA, Dina R, deSouza NM (2004) ^{1}H magnetic resonance spectroscopy of invasive cervical cancer: an in vivo study with ex vivo corroboration. NMR Biomed 17:1–9

Maiese K, Vincent AM (2000) Membrane asymmetry and DNA degradation: functionally distinct determinants of neuronal programmed cell death. J Neurosci Res 59:568–580

Martin S, Pombo I, Poncet P, David B, Arock M, Blank U (2000) Immunologic stimulation of mast cells leads to the reversible exposure of phosphatidylserine in the absence of apoptosis. Int Arch Allergy Immunol 123(3):249–258

Moka D, Vorreuther R, Schicha H, Spraul M, Humpfer E, Lipinski M, Foxall PJ, Nicholson JK, Lindon JC (1998) Biochemical classification of kidney carcinoma biopsy samples using magic-angle-spinning 1H nuclear magnetic resonance spectroscopy. J Pharm Biomed Anal 17: 125–132

Mukherjee A, Kothari K, Toth G, Szemenyei E, Sarma HD, Kornyei J, Venkatesh M (2006) 99mTc-labeled annexin V fragments: a potential SPECT radiopharmaceutical for imaging cell death.Nucl Med Biol 33(5):635–643

Murakami Y, Takamatsu H, Taki J, Tatsumi M, Noda A, Ichise R, Tait JF, Nishimura S (2004) 18F-labelled annexin V: a PET tracer for apoptosis imaging. Eur J Nucl Med Mol Imaging 31:469–474

Narula J, Strauss HW (2003) Invited commentary: P.S.* I love you: implications of phosphatidyl serine (PS) reversal in acute ischemic syndromes. J Nucl Med 44:397–399

Narula J, Acio ER, Narula N, Samuels LE, Fyfe B, Wood D, Fitzpatrick JM, Raghunath PN, Tomaszewski JE, Kelly C, Steinmetz N, Green A, Tait JF, Leppo J, Blankenberg FG, Jain D, Strauss HW (2001) Annexin-V imaging for noninvasive detection of cardiac allograft rejection. Nat Med 7:1347–1352

O'Rourke MGE, Ellem KAO (2000) John Kerr and apoptosis. Med J Australia 173:616–617

Quinti L, Weissleder R, Tung C-H (2006) A fluorescent nanosensor for apoptotic cells. Nano Lett 6:488–490

Ran S, Downes A, Thorpe PE (2002) Increased exposure of anionic phospholipids on the surface of tumor blood vessels. Cancer Res 62:6132–6140

Riksen NP, Oyen WJ, Ramakers BP, Van den Broek PH, Engbersen R, Boerman OC, Smits P, Rongen GA (2005) Oral therapy with dipyridamole limits ischemia-reperfusion injury in humans. Clin Pharmacol Ther 78:52–59

Riksen NP, Zhou Z, Oyen WJ, Jaspers R, Ramakers BP, Brouwer RM, Boerman OC, Steinmetz N, Smits P, Rongen GA (2006) Caffeine prevents protection in two human models of ischemic preconditioning. J Am Coll Cardiol 48:700–707

Rongen GA, Oyen WJ, Ramakers BP, Riksen NP, Boerman OC, Steinmetz N, Smits P (2005) Annexin A5 scintigraphy of forearm as a novel in vivo model of skeletal muscle preconditioning in humans. Circulation 111:173–178

Rottey S, Slegers G, Van Belle S, Goethals I, Van de Wiele C (2006) Sequential 99mTc-hydrazinonicotinamide-annexin V imaging for predicting response to chemotherapy. J Nucl Med 47:1813–1818

Schellenberger EA, Weissleder R, Josephson L (2004a) Optimal modification of annexin V with fluorescent dyes. Chembiochem 5:271–274

Schellenberger EA, Sosnovik D, Weissleder R, Josephson L (2004b) Magneto/optical annexin V, a multimodal protein. Bioconjug Chem 15:1062–1067

Sosnovik DE, Schellenberger EA, Nahrendorf M, Novikov MS, Matsui T, Dai G, Reynolds F, Grazette L, Rosenzweig A, Weissleder R, Josephson L (2005) magnetic resonance imaging of cardiomyocyte apoptosis with a novel magneto-optical nanoparticle. Magn Reson Med 54: 718–724

Stratton JR, Dewhurst TA, Kasina S, Reno JM, Cerqueira MD, Baskin DG, Tait JF (1995) Selective uptake of radiolabeled annexin V on acute porcine left atrial thrombi. Circulation 92:
3113–3121

Strauss HW, Narula J, Blankenberg FG (2000) Radioimaging to identify myocardial cell death and
probably injury. Lancet 356:180–181

Tait JF, Cerqueira MD, Dewhurst TA, Fujikawa K, Ritchie JL, Stratton JR (1994) Evaluation of
annexin V as a platelet-directed thrombus targeting agent. Thromb Res 75:491–501

Tait JF, Brown DS, Gibson DF, Blankenberg FG, Strauss HW (2000) Development and characterization of annexin V mutants with endogenous chelation sites for (99m)Tc. Bioconjug Chem
11:918–925

Tait JF, Gibson DF, Smith C (2004) Measurement of the affinity and cooperativity of annexin
V-membrane binding under conditions of low membrane occupancy. Anal Biochem 329:
112–119

Tait JF, Smith C, Blankenberg FG (2005) Structural requirements for in vivo detection of cell death
with 99mTc-annexin V. J Nucl Med 46:807–815

Taki J, Higuchi T, Kawashima A, Tait JF, Kinuya S, Muramori A, Matsunari I, Nakajima K,
Tonami N, Strauss HW (2004) Detection of cardiomyocyte death in a rat model of ischemia
and reperfusion using 99mTc-labeled annexin V. J Nucl Med 45:1536–1541

Thimister PW, Hofstra L, Liem IH, Boersma HH, Kemerink G, Reutelingsperger CP,
Heidendal GA (2003) In vivo detection of cell death in the area at risk in acute myocardial
infarction. J Nucl Med 44:391–396

Valonen PK, Lehtimaki KK, Vaisanen TH, Kettunen MI, Grohn OH, Yla-Herttuala S,
Kauppinen RA (2004) Water diffusion in a rat glioma during ganciclovir-thymidine kinase
gene therapy-induced programmed cell death in vivo: correlation with cell density. J Magn
Reson Imaging 19:389–396

van de Wiele C, Lahorte C, Vermeersch H, Loose D, Mervillie K, Steinmetz ND, Vanderheyden JL,
Cuvelier CA, Slegers G, Dierck RA (2003) Quantitative tumor apoptosis imaging using
technetium-99m-HYNIC annexin V single photon emission computed tomography. J Clin Oncol 21:3483–3487

van Tilborg GAF, Mulder WJM, Chin PTK, Storm G, Reutelingsperger CP, Nicolay K, Strijkers GJ
(2006) Annexin A5-conjugated quantum dots with a paramagnetic lipidic coating for the multimodal detection of apoptotic cells. Bioconjugate Chem 17:865–868

Vermeersch H, Ham H, Rottey S, Lahorte C, Corsetti F, Dierckx R, Steinmetz N, Van de Wiele C
(2004) Intraobserver, interobserver, and day-to-day reproducibility of quantitative 99mTc-
HYNIC annexin-V imaging in head and neck carcinoma. Cancer Biother Radiopharm 19:
205–210

Vriens PW, Blankenberg FG, Stoot JH, Ohtsuki K, Berry GJ, Tait JF, Strauss HW, Robbins RC
(1998) The use of technetium Tc 99m annexin V for in vivo imaging of apoptosis during cardiac
allograft rejection. J Thorac Cardiovasc Surg 116:844–853

Wu XX, Arslan AA, Wein R, Reutlingsperger CP, Lockwood CJ, Kuczynski E, Rand JH (2006)
Analysis of circulating Annexin A5 parameters during pregnancy: absence of differences between women with recurrent spontaneous pregnancy losses and controls. Am J Obstet Gyn
195:971–978

Wylie AH, Kerr JFR, Curry JR (1973) Cell death in the normal neonatal rat adrenal cortex. J Path
111:255–261

Yang MY, Chuang H, Chen RF, Yang KD (2002) Reversible phosphatidylserine expression on
blood granulocytes related to membrane perturbation but not DNA strand breaks. J Leukoc
Biol 71:231–237

Yang SK, Attipoe S, Klausner AP, Tian R, Pan D, Rich TA, Turner TT, Steers WD, Lysiak JJ
(2006) In vivo detection of apoptotic cells in the testis using fluorescence labeled annexin V in
a mouse model of testicular torsion. J Urol 176:830–835

Zhao M, Zhu X, Ji S, Zhou J, Ozker KS, Fang W, Molthen RC, Hellman RS (2006) ^{99m}Tc-Labeled
C2A Domain of synaptotagmin I as a target-specific molecular probe for noninvasive imaging
of acute myocardial infarction. J Nucl Med 47:1367–1374

Zhou D, Chu W, Rothfuss J, Zeng C, Xu J, Jones L, Welch MJ, Mach RH (2006) Synthesis, radiolabeling, and in vivo evaluation of an 18F-labeled isatin analog for imaging caspase-3 activation in apoptosis. Bioorg Med Chem Lett 16:5041–5046.

Zijlstra S, Gunawan J, Burchert W (2003) Synthesis and evaluation of a 18F-labelled recombinant annexin-V derivative, for identification and quantification of apoptotic cells with PET. Appl Radiat Isot 58:201–207

Molecular Imaging of PET Reporter Gene Expression

Jung-Joon Min and Sanjiv S. Gambhir(✉)

Abstract Multimodality molecular imaging continues to rapidly expand and is impacting many areas of biomedical research as well as patient management. Reporter-gene assays have emerged as a very general strategy for indirectly monitoring various intracellular events. Furthermore, reporter genes are being used to monitor gene/cell therapies, including the location(s), time variation, and magnitude of gene expression. This chapter reviews reporter gene technology and its major preclinical and clinical applications to date. The future appears quite promising for the continued expansion of the use of reporter genes in many evolving biomedically related arenas.

1 Introduction

Present imaging technologies rely mostly on nonspecific morphological, physiological, or metabolic changes that differentiate pathological from normal tissue rather than identifying specific molecular events (e.g., gene expression) responsible for disease. Molecular imaging usually exploits specific molecular probes as

Sanjiv S. Gambhir
Molecular Imaging Program at Stanford, The James H Clark Center, 318 Campus Drive, East Wing, 1st Floor, Stanford, CA 94305-5427
sgambhir@stanford.edu

W. Semmler and M. Schwaiger (eds.), *Molecular Imaging II.*
Handbook of Experimental Pharmacology 185/II.
© Springer-Verlag Berlin Heidelberg 2008

the source of image signal. This change in emphasis from a non-specific to a specific approach represents a significant paradigm shift, the impact of which is that imaging can now provide the potential for understanding integrative biology, earlier detection and characterization of disease, and evaluation of treatment. We have previously suggested several important goals in molecular imaging research (Massoud and Gambhir 2003), namely: (1) to develop non-invasive in vivo imaging methods that reflect specific molecular processes, such as gene expression, or more complex molecular interactions, such as protein-protein interactions; (2) to monitor multiple molecular events near-simultaneously; (3) to follow trafficking and targeting of cells; (4) to optimize drug and gene therapy; (5) to image drug effects at a molecular and cellular level; (6) to assess disease progression at a molecular pathological level; and (7) to create the possibility of achieving all of the above goals of imaging in a rapid, reproducible, and quantitative manner, so as to be able to monitor time-dependent experimental, developmental, environmental, and therapeutic influences on gene products in the same animal or patient.

Molecular imaging has its roots in the field of nuclear medicine. Nuclear medicine is focused on characterizing enzyme activity, receptor/transporter levels and the biodistribution of various radiolabeled substrates (tracers). Positron emission tomography (PET) imaging is attractive because it provides high spatial resolution and is more sensitive than single-photon emission computed tomography (SPECT) imaging (by at least one log order). Thus, it provides quantitative information about the distribution of the tracer that is immediately translated into concentration of the tracer in the tissue(s) of interest. This latter feature is important because it allows quantitative determination of levels of molecular target in a tissue region of interest. In addition to dramatic advances in new high-resolution PET scanners for small animal imaging, related progress in molecular and cell biology techniques, and in the development of specific imaging probes have all contributed to the rapid expansion of nuclear medicine techniques to study diseases. These advances are now being explored to characterize molecular events and disease processes such as molecular interactions, gene expression, cell trafficking, and apoptosis. In this chapter, we focus on the use of PET molecular imaging to study reporter-gene expression. The concept of a reporter gene is first introduced followed by types and then applications.

2 Imaging Reporter Genes

For over a decade, molecular biologists have used reporter genes both in cell culture and in vivo to monitor gene expression. Imaging of gene expression in living subjects can be directed either at genes externally transferred into cells of organ systems (transgenes) or at endogenous genes. Most current applications of reporter-gene imaging are of the former variety. By adopting state-of-the-art molecular biology techniques, it is now possible to better image cellular/molecular events in living subjects. One can also engineer cells that will accumulate imaging probes of choice, either to act as generic gene 'markers' for localizing and tracking these cells, or to target a specific biological process or pathway. In the last few years there has been a veritable explosion of activity in the field of reporter-gene imaging, with the aim of determining the location(s), time-variation, and magnitude of reporter-gene expression within living subjects (Gambhir et al. 2000b; Phelps 2000; Massoud and Gambhir 2003).

Reporter genes are used in various ways to study promoter/enhancer elements involved in gene expression, induction of gene expression using inducible promoters, and endogenous gene expression through the use of transgenes containing endogenous promoters fused to the reporter gene of choice. In all these cases, transcription of the reporter gene can be tracked and, therefore, gene expression can be studied. Conventional reporter genes typically include the bacterial gene *chloramphenicol acetyl transferase (CAT)*, *lacZ* gene (with the protein product β-galactosidase), *alkaline phosphatase (ALP)*, or *β-lactamase (BLA)*. Autoradiography of a chromatogram (when using *CAT*), enzyme assay (when using *lacZ*) or immunohistochemistry (when using *CAT* or *lacZ*) can then be used to assay cell extracts for the product of the reporter gene (Lewin 2000). A reporter gene such as *ALP*, which can lead to a protein product secreted into the blood stream, can also be used, thereby allowing monitoring in living animals. However, the location(s) of reporter gene expression is not able to be determined in this case, because only the blood can be easily sampled.

Other conventional reporter genes, such as *green fluorescent protein (GFP)* (Hoffman 2005) and *luciferase* (Bhaumik and Gambhir 2002; Contag and Bachmann 2002), whose protein products are used for light production, allow for localization in some small living animals. Although small animals or animals transparent to light can be imaged with a cooled charged coupled device (CCD) camera, these imaging techniques are somewhat limited because of their lack of generalizability and detailed tomographic resolution (Biswal and Gambhir 2003). In contrast, PET imaging techniques offer the possibility of monitoring the location(s), magnitude, and time-variation of reporter-gene expression with a very high sensitivity and tomographic detail for use in living small and large animals, including humans.

2.1 Characteristics of the Ideal Reporter Gene/Probe

In theory, the ideal reporter gene/probe would have the following characteristics (Gambhir and Massoud 2004):

- The reporter gene should be present (but not expressed) in mammalian cells in order to prevent an immune response.
- The specific reporter probe should accumulate only where the reporter gene is expressed.
- No reporter probe should accumulate when the reporter gene is not being expressed.
- The product of the reporter gene should also be non-immunogenic.

- The reporter probe should be stable in vivo and not be metabolized before reaching its target.
- The reporter probe should clear rapidly from the circulation and not interfere with detection of specific signal. Neither the reporter probe nor its metabolites should be cytotoxic.
- The size of the reporter gene with its driving promoter should be small enough to fit into a delivery vehicle (e.g., plasmids, viruses), except that this is not required for transgenic applications.
- The reporter probe should not be prevented from reaching its destination(s) by natural biological barriers.
- The image signal should correlate well with levels of both reporter-gene mRNA and protein in living subjects.

At present, no single reporter gene/probe system satisfies all of these criteria. The availability of multiple systems, each satisfying some of the criteria, provides a choice based on the application areas of interest. Additionally, the availability of multiple reporter gene/reporter probes facilitates monitoring the expression of more than one reporter gene in the same living subject.

2.2 Classification of Imaging Reporter Gene Systems

A broad classification of reporter systems consists of those where the gene product is intracellular (Fig. 1a), or is associated with the cell membrane (Fig. 1a, b). Examples of intracellular reporters include herpes simplex virus type 1 thymidine kinase (HSV1-tk) (Gambhir et al. 2000b; Serganova and Blasberg 2005), cytosine deaminase (Haberkorn et al. 1996; Haberkorn and Altmann 2001), to name a few. Examples of reporters on or in the cell surface in the form of receptors include the dopamine 2 receptor (D2R) (Gambhir et al. 2000b; Herschman et al. 2000), and receptors for somatostatin (Zinn and Chaudhuri 2002), or the sodium iodide symporter (NIS) (Chung 2002; Dingli et al. 2003). The major advantages of intracellular protein expression are the relatively uncomplicated expression strategy and

---

Fig. 1 a–c Three different types of PET imaging reporter gene/probe strategies. a Enzyme-based reporter-gene imaging system: a radiotracer, such as ^{18}F-FHBG, acts as a substrate, which is phosphorylated by the imaging reporter enzyme, such as HSV1-tk, to result in intracellular trapping of the probe in cells expressing the imaging reporter gene. b Receptor-based reporter-gene imaging system: radiotracers, such as ^{18}F-FESP or radiolabeled somatostatin analogues, are ligand molecular probes interacting with the expressed receptor, such as dopamine-2-receptor (D2R) or somatostatin receptor (SSTR2), to result in trapping of the probe on/in cells expressing the D2R gene or SSTR2 gene. c Transporter-based reporter gene imaging system: expression of a transporter, such as sodium iodide symporter (NIS), results in cell uptake of the reporter probe, such as radioiodide, than would not otherwise occur. Note in this approach nothing traps the reporter probe so there is a window of opportunity for imaging before the reporter probe may leak back out of the cell. (Adapted from Massoud and Gambhir 2003)

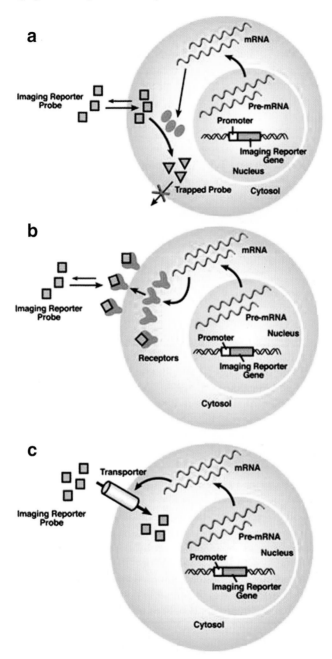

lack of recognition of the expression product by the immune system. An additional advantage is the potential for signal amplification if the reporter protein can act on a reporter probe and is then free to continue to act on other reporter probes. Differently, the major advantages of surface-expressed receptors and acceptors are favorable kinetics (sometimes avoiding the need for the tracer to penetrate into a cell) and the fact that synthetic reporters can be engineered to recognize FDA approved imaging probes.

2.2.1 Herpes Simplex Virus Type 1 Thymidine Kinase (HSV1-tk)

Wild-type herpes simplex virus type 1 thymidine kinase *(HSV1-tk)* and a mutant HSV1-tk gene, *HSV1-sr39tk,* are the most common reporter genes used in current molecular imaging studies using radiolabeled substrate and PET imaging. Products of the *HSV1-tk* and *HSV1-sr39tk* genes are enzymes that have less substrate specificity than mammalian thymidine kinase 1 (TK1) and can phosphorylate a wider range of substrate analogues. Substrates that have been studied to date as PET reporter probes for HSV1-tk can be classified into two main categories (Fig. 2): pyrimidine nucleoside derivatives, such as FIAU (5-iodo-2′-fluoro-2′deoxy-1-β-D-arabino-furanosyl-uracil) (Tjuvajev et al. 1995, 1996, 1998, 1999, 2002) and FEAU (2′-fluoro-2′-deoxyarabinofuranosyl-5-ethyluracil) (Kang et al. 2005), and acycloguanosine derivatives (e.g., FPCV; fluoropenciclovir, FHBG; 9-[4-fluoro-3-(hydrommethyl) butyl] guanine) (Alauddin et al. 1996; Alauddin and Conti 1998; Gambhir et al. 1998; Alauddin et al. 1999; Gambhir et al. 1999, 2000a; Iyer et al. 2001a; Min et al. 2003; Alauddin et al. 2004; Kang et al. 2005), and have been investigated in terms of sensitivity and specificity. These radiolabeled reporter probes are transported into cells, and are trapped as a result of phosphorylation by HSV1-tk. When used in non-pharmacological tracer doses, these substrates can serve as PET- or SPECT-targeted reporter probes by their accumulation in only cells expressing the *HSV1-tk* gene. In order to improve sensitivity, a mutant version of this gene, *HSV1-sr39tk,* was derived using site-directed mutagenesis to obtain an enzyme more effective at phosphorylating ganciclovir (GCV) (and also less efficient at phosphorylating the endogenous competitor thymidine) with consequent gain in imaging signal (Gambhir et al. 2000a). Recently, it has been reported that the *HSV1-sr39tk* reporter gene system with ^{18}F-PCV or ^{18}F-FHBG is a better combination over the *HSV1-tk* reporter gene system with FIAU in C6 cell mouse xenografts (Iyer et al. 2001a; Min et al. 2003). It is important to note that since endogenous levels of thymidine can change, an important benefit of the mutant HSV1-sr39tk over HSV1-tk is the reduced sensitivity to any such changes, since HSV1-sr39tk was specifically selected as its protein product is less able to phosphorylate thymidine (Green 2000). The combination of [124]I-FEAU/HSV1-tk compared with ^{18}F-FHBG/HSV1-sr39tk needs further investigation to determine which is more optimal. FEAU has the advantage of primarily renal excretion and thus low background signal in the gastrointestinal tract compared with the other imaging probes.

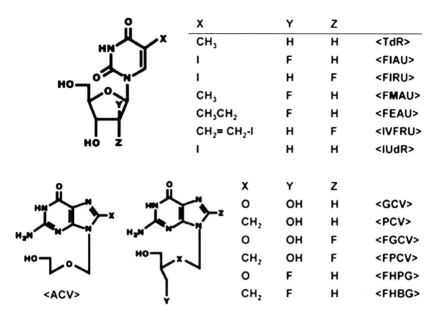

X	Y	Z	
CH₃	H	H	\<TdR\>
I	F	H	\<FIAU\>
I	H	F	\<FIRU\>
CH₃	F	H	\<FMAU\>
CH₃CH₂	F	H	\<FEAU\>
CH₂=CH₂-I	H	F	\<IVFRU\>
I	H	H	\<IUdR\>

X	Y	Z	
O	OH	H	\<GCV\>
CH₂	OH	H	\<PCV\>
O	OH	F	\<FGCV\>
CH₂	OH	F	\<FPCV\>
O	F	H	\<FHPG\>
CH₂	F	H	\<FHBG\>

\<ACV\>

Fig. 2 Structures of thymidine and HSV1-tk reporter gene substrates. *TdR* (thymidine), 5-methyluracil-2′-deoxyribose; *FIAU* 2′-fluoro-2′-deoxy-b-D-arabinofuranosyl-5-iodouracil; *FIRU* 2′-fluoro-2′-deoxy-5-iodo-1-b-D-ribofuranosyl-uracil; *FMAU* 2′-fluoro-2′-deoxy-5-methyl-1-b-D-arabinofuranosyl-uracil; *FEAU* 2′-fluoro-2′-deoxyarabinofuranosyl-5-ethyluracil; *IVFRU* 2′-fluoro-2′-deoxy-5-iodovinyl-1-b-ribofuranosyl-uracil; *IUdR* 2′-deoxy-5-iodo-1-b-D-ribofuranosyl-uracil; *ACV* 9-[(2-hydroxy-1-ethoxy)methyl]guanine (acyclovir); *GCV* 9-[(2-hydroxy-1-(hydroxymethyl)ethoxy)methyl]guanine (ganciclovir); *PCV* 9-[4-hydroxy-3-(hydroxymethyl)butyl]guanine (penciclovir); *FGCV* 8-fluoro-9-[(2-hydroxy-1-(hydroxymethyl)ethoxy)methyl]guanine (fluoroganciclovir); *FPCV* 8-fluoro-9-[4-hydroxy-3-(hydroxymethyl)butyl]guanine (fluoropenciclovir); *FHPG* 9-[(3-fluoro-1-hydroxy-2-propoxy)methyl]guanine; *FHBG* 9-(4-fluoro-3-hydroxymethylbutyl) guanine. (Adapted from Kang et al. 2005)

HSV1-tk and *HSV1-sr39tk* are nonhuman genes and pose a small risk of generating an immune response against cells and tissue transduced with these genes, although in some cancer applications an immune response may be desirable. One potential approach to reduce this risk is to use the human thymidine kinase 2 (*hTK2*) gene. The *hTK2* gene is minimally expressed in the mitochondria of most human tissues and can be used as a human reporter gene. The hTK2 enzyme has a spectrum of substrate specificity similar to that of viral thymidine kinase. The substrate specificity is broader and less restricted in comparison with that of human thymidine kinase 1 (hTK1), and hTK2 has been shown to phosphorylate radiolabeled FIAU and FEAU. Therefore, radiolabeled FIAU or FEAU can be administered to patients, and hTK2 may provide an alternative human thymidine kinase reporter system for use in human subjects (Serganova and Blasberg 2005), although this requires further research. Further reviews of the *HSV1-tk* reporter gene are to be found in previous publications (Gambhir et al. 2000b; Iyer et al. 2005).

2.2.2 Dopamine 2 Receptor (hD2R)

The dopamine 2 receptor *(hD2R)* reporter gene has also been validated as a PET reporter on the cell surface in the form of receptors while using ^{18}F-labeled fluoroethylspiperone (FESP) as the reporter probe ligand (MacLaren et al. 1999). The advantages of this system are that the expression of hD2R is largely limited to the striatal-nigral system of the brain, and that an established radiolabeled probe, FESP, has been extensively used to image striatal-nigral D2 receptors in human subjects (Barrio et al. 1989). The potential problem with this approach is the possibility that circulating endogenous ligands binding to ectopically expressed *D2R* might constitute a chronic stimulus, provoking undesired biological responses. A mutant *D2R* (e.g., *D2R80A*, mutation of Asp80) that uncouples signal transduction while maintaining affinity for FESP has also been reported (Liang et al. 2001).

The disadvantage of this system is that the clinically available D2 receptor ligands are highly lipophilic and are extensively accumulated and excreted by the liver. Therefore, the abdomen will be difficult to evaluate with these tracers (Herzog et al. 1990). Further reviews of the D2R reporter gene are to be found in previous publications (Herschman 2004a, 2004b).

2.2.3 Somatostatin Receptor Subtype-2 (hSSTR2)

Somatostatin receptor imaging has been developed to demonstrate efficacy for detection of naturally SSTR-positive neuroendocrine and lung cancers (van Eijck et al. 1999). Similar to the D2R system, the *hSSTR2* gene has been suggested as a potential reporter gene for human studies (Rogers et al. 1999, 2000), because the expression of *hSSTR2* gene is largely limited to carcinoid tumors. Octreotide, P829, and P2045 are synthetic somatostatin analogues that preferentially bind with high affinity to somatostatin receptor subtypes 2, 3, and 5 of human, mouse, or rat origin (Kundra et al. 2002; Zinn and Chaudhuri 2002). Of further significance, somatostatin analogue PET tracers are available with potential for imaging applications using the *hSSTR2* reporter gene (Anderson et al. 2001; Henze et al. 2001; Hofmann et al. 2001).

Similar to D2R, expression of hSSTR2 can provoke biological activity by endogenous ligands. In order to have reporter receptor without biological activity, a model epitope-tagged receptor was constructed by fusing the hemagglutinin (HA) sequence on the extracellular N-terminus of the hSSTR2 gene. The HA tag was chosen owing to availability of anti-HA antibodies or antibody fragments, which can be radiolabeled. The next step in the evolution of the HA-hSSTR2 fusion reporter will be to ablate binding of somatostatin or its analogues by introducing an amino acid mutation in the transmembrane region of hSSTR2 (Kundra et al. 2002; Zinn and Chaudhuri 2002). Further reviews of *hSSTR2* reporter gene are to be found in previous publications (Zinn and Chaudhuri 2002; Buchsbaum et al. 2004, 2005).

2.2.4 Sodium Iodide Symporter (NIS)

The sodium iodide symporter (NIS) is expressed primarily on the basolateral membrane of thyroid epithelial cells. It is responsible for active iodide uptake in thyrocytes, the first essential step in a series of biochemical changes culminating in the incorporation of the ion within tyrosine residues in thyroglobulin, the precursor for thyroid hormone biosynthesis (Dingli et al. 2003). NIS is also expressed at lower levels in many other organs, such as the salivary and lacrimal glands, stomach, choroid plexus, lactating mammary gland, kidney epithelial cells and placenta. Ion binding to NIS is nonrandom; two sodium ions bind first, followed by an iodide ion. NIS can transport into cells many other anions coupled with sodium transport. These include ClO_3^-, SCN^-, $SeCN^-$, NO_3^-, Br^-, TcO_4^-, RhO_4^- and ^{211}At (Eskandari et al. 1997; Carlin et al. 2002; Van Sande et al. 2003).

NIS has been utilized in combination with ^{124}I to monitor reporter-gene expression using PET (Groot-Wassink et al. 2002; Dingli et al. 2006). ^{124}I is not an ideal radiotracer due to its low positron yield (23%) and the concomitant emission of high-energy gamma photons that make accurate dosimetric calculations difficult (Pentlow et al. 1991). However, its long half-life (4.12 days) allows tracking of slow biochemical processes and a cyclotron need not be on site for production of the isotope. In spite of intrinsic limitation of spatial resolution compared with PET, gamma camera imaging has provided adequate data for monitoring and quantification of in-vivo gene expression as well as dosimetric calculations (Vadysirisack et al. 2006). NIS has been extensively investigated to image gene expression in the myocardium, tumors, metastasis, and to image cell trafficking (Marsee et al. 2004; Lee et al. 2005, 2006; Vadysirisack et al. 2006; Lim et al. 2007).

NIS has several potential advantages over the other reporter systems: (1) NIS is a physiologically expressed protein that only rarely induces an immune reaction. (2) The radiotracers used in combination with NIS are readily commercially available at a low cost and are already approved by the US Food and Drug Administration for clinical applications. However, intracellular retention has generally been found to be low, with a half-life of approximately 30 min (Chung 2002). A large percentage of radioiodide will be accumulated in the thyroid (up to 25% of the injected dose in euthyroid patients) (Anton et al. 2004). Further reviews of the NIS reporter gene are to be found in previous publications (Chung 2002; Dingli et al. 2003; Baker and Morris 2004)

2.2.5 Multimodality Reporters

An important recent development in multimodality reporter systems is the fusion reporter system, which facilitates study using both optical and PET imaging (Ray et al. 2003; Ray et al. 2004). This fusion reporter gene expresses a bi- or tri-fusion of coding elements for enzymes involved in different modalities. Bi-fusion contains coding regions for *Renilla* luciferase and HSV1-sr39tk enzyme, while tri-fusion contains those for monomeric red fluorescent protein (mRFP), synthetic *Renilla* luciferase and HSV1-sr39tk enzyme. Cellular fluorescence expression can be monitored using microscopic techniques, while in-vivo monitoring can be performed using both optical and PET imaging. This fusion reporter offers the possibility of using the particular imaging technique that best suits the application and also doing all three applications with the one reporter gene; fluorescence for monitoring individual cells, bioluminescence for highly sensitive in-vivo imaging with small animals, and PET for accurate quantitation and for the translation to humans (Massoud and Gambhir 2003; Acton and Zhou 2005).

2.2.6 Miscellaneous Reporter Genes

The reporter genes discussed above have not only their advantages but also their own intrinsic disadvantages. Therefore, there is still the need for other types of imaging reporter genes. In a limited publication, human norepinephrine transporter (hNET) has been investigated as a reporter gene (Anton et al. 2004; Buursma et al. 2005). Using both radioiodine labeled meta-iodobenzylguanidine (MIBG) or ^{11}C-m-hydroxyephedrine (mHED), transduction of tumor cells with *NET* gene showed highly specific uptake and significant retention in vitro and in vivo.

Another new reporter-gene imaging system is one that uses the estrogen receptor ligand-binding domain (ERL) as a reporter gene and ^{18}F-labeled estradiol (FES) for reporter probe (Takamatsu et al. 2005; Furukawa et al. 2006). By performing PET imaging, ERL-expressing teratoma of calf muscle was successfully visualized using FES.

Four categories of applications of PET reporter-gene technology are reviewed next: imaging of cell trafficking, imaging of immunotherapies, imaging of gene therapies, and imaging of molecular interactions such as protein-protein interactions.

3 Applications of Reporter Gene Imaging

3.1 *Imaging Cell Trafficking*

3.1.1 Immune Cells/Cancer Cells

An important application of PET reporter-gene technology is to noninvasively monitor cell transplantation and trafficking. Imaging can be used to look at different properties of cellular trafficking, including metastasis, stem cell transplantation, and lymphocyte response to inflammation. PET radiotracers and reporter genes have been used to study cell migration and antitumor responses. ^{18}F-FDG, a common PET tracer used to look at the cellular metabolism of glucose as a good indicator of neoplasia, is highly retained in lymphocytes. This aspect of FDG has been exploited to follow monocyte trafficking (Paik et al. 2002). Botti et al. (1997) compared

FDG, as well as ^{99m}Tc-hexamethazine and ^{111}In-oxine labeling in activated lymphocytes to determine which method would be best for tracking adoptively transferred T-lymphocytes in patients. ^{64}Cu-pyruvaldehyde-bis(N^4-methylthiosemicarbazone) (Cu-PTSM), has also been assessed in a glioma cell line and in splenocytes by our group (Adonai et al. 2002). The cells were labeled ex vivo with tracer and subsequently injected and monitored in the living animal with microPET. Le et al. (2002) assessed the role of the BCR-ABL oncogene and G2A [G protein-coupled receptor (GPCR) predominantly expressed in lymphocytes] in lymphoid leukemogenesis using bone marrow cells marked with HSV1-tk. By adapting murine transplantation models of BCR-ABL-induced leukemia for micro PET imaging, they revealed that G2A functions as a negative modifier of BCR-ABL-induced leukemogenesis, and have developed a system with the potential to study preleukemic events and candidate cellular/biological processes. Utilizing *HSV1-sr39tk* as a reporter gene in adoptively transferred lymphocytes, Dubey et al. (2003) were able to show that T-cell anti-tumor responses could be quantified using microPET. Similarly, Koehne et al. (2003) showed that Epstein-Barr virus (EBV)-specific T-lymphocytes, marked with HSV1-tk, can be shown to traffic and accumulate in EBV$^+$ tumors in mice using microPET. More recently, Shu et al. (2005) kinetically measured the induction and therapeutic modulations of cell-mediated immune responses in bone marrow chimeric mice generated by engraftment of hematopoietic stem cells transduced by a triple reporter gene encoding hRluc, EGFP, and HSV1-sr39tk. These approaches can be used to assess the effects of immunomodulatory agents intended to potentiate the immune response to cancer, and can also be useful for the study of other cell-mediated immune responses, including autoimmunity. Monitoring cell trafficking is feasible in many disease conditions, although careful consideration must be taken in choosing the labeling agent (possible toxicity) and/or the reporter gene (possible immunogenicity). These types of studies would allow for better understanding of the disease process, and the response of neoplastic and immune cells to therapeutics. We are currently also imaging patients being treated with their own engineered T-cells for recurrent gliobastoma. The cells are marked with the *HSV1-tk* reporter gene and the patients imaged with FHBG and PET. Initial results are encouraging, but many more patients will have to be imaged before any definitive conclusions can be made.

Further reviews are to be found in previous publications (Hildebrandt and Gambhir 2004; Ottobrini et al. 2005; Lucignani et al. 2006).

3.1.2 Stem Cells

Because of the capacity for indefinite reproduction, together with the ability to produce differentiated progeny, stem-cell transplantation holds potential promise for treating a wide variety of human diseases, including Parkinson's disease, Alzheimer's disease, stroke, heart disease and rheumatological diseases. The mechanisms may be related to stem cells secreting multiple arteriogenic cytokines, providing a mechanical scaffold, or recruiting other beneficial cells to the diseased territory. However, most techniques used for the analysis of stem-cell survival in animal models have relied on postmortem histology to determine the fate and migratory behavior of the stem cells. This approach, however, precludes any sort of noninvasive longitudinal monitoring. An approach which would allow for the monitoring of stem cell activities within the context of the intact whole-body system, rather than with histological slides, would allow us to gain further insight into the underlying biological and physiological properties of stem cells.

Several imaging strategies are currently under active investigation, including direct radionuclide or ferromagnetic labeling, and reporter-gene labeling (Wu et al. 2004; Chang et al. 2006). In a study of radionuclide labeling, Aicher et al. (2003) injected indium-111 oxine-labeled endothelial progenitor cells into the infarcted myocardia of nude rats, and imaged them at 24–96 h, using a gamma camera. Hofmann et al. (2005) isolated bone marrow cells (BMCs) by bone marrow aspiration from patients after percutaneous coronary intervention 5–10 days after their first acute myocardial infarctions. BMCs were radiolabeled with ^{18}F-FDG and were reintroduced directly into the infracted area via intracoronary artery infusion. By use of PET imaging, only 1.3–2.6% of BMCs were found to be localizing around the infracted area, whereas the majority congregated in the liver and spleen within 1–1.5 h after intracoronary infusion. In a separate study, Kraitchman et al. (2005) compared the sensitivity of SPECT with that of MRI in tracking the mobilization of MSCs (mesenchymal stem cells) after intravenous injections into a dog with myocardial infarction. By double-labeling MSCs with ^{111}In-oxine and ferumoxides-poly-L-lysine, SPECT was able to detect MSCs in the infarcted myocardium within the first 24 h until 7 days after injection, whereas MRI was unable to detect the small numbers of cells homing in to the site. However, the main limitation associated with radionuclide-labeling approaches is that radionuclides have physical half-lives, making it possible to monitor cell distribution only for a limited number of days.

Reporter-gene imaging provides several unique advantages over other imaging techniques. First, in contrast to radionuclide-labeling techniques, only viable cells can be detected because accumulation of reporter probe requires expression of the reporter-gene product. Second, the reporter gene can be integrated into the cellular chromosomes and passed on from parent to daughter cells, thereby permitting tracking of cell proliferation. Finally, multiple reporter genes can be combined for multimodality visualization or can be combined with specific promoters for analyses of molecular pathways or differentiation processes in a precise manner (Barbash et al. 2003; Hofmann et al. 2005).

During the process of reporter-gene labeling, the cells are transfected with reporter genes before being implanted into the myocardium (Wu et al. 2003a). In cases in which the cells remain alive, the reporter gene will be expressed. In cases in which the cells are dead, the reporter gene will not be expressed. Employing this approach, Wu et al. (2003a) recently used embryonic cardiomyoblasts which express HSV1-tk or firefly luciferase (Fluc) reporter genes, which they then noninvasively tracked using either micro-PET or bioluminescence optical imaging. Drastic reductions were noted in signal intensity within the first 1–4 days, and this was tentatively attributed

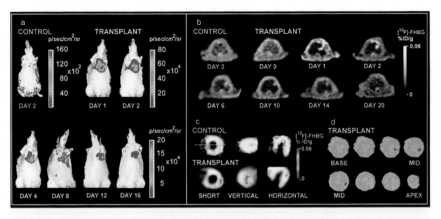

Fig. 3 a–d Reporter-gene imaging of cardiac cell transplantation in living animals. **a** Optical imaging showing a representative rat transplanted with embryonic cardiomyoblasts expressing the firefly luciferase reporter gene (*Fluc*) that emits significant cardiac bioluminescence activity on days 1, 2, 4, 8, 12, and 16 ($P < 0.05$ vs control). The control rat (injected with cardiomyoblasts transfected with *HSV1-sr39tk*, which served as a negative control) has background signal only. **b** MicroPET imaging shows longitudinal imaging of ^{18}F-FHBG reporter activity in a representative rat transplanted with cardiomyoblasts expressing the *HSV1-sr39tk* reporter gene (*gray scale*). **c** Detailed tomographic views of cardiac microPET images are shown in the short, vertical, and horizontal axis. On day 2, a representative transplant rat has significant activity at the lateral wall, as shown by the ^{18}F-FHBG reporter activity image (*color scale*) overlaid on the ^{13}N-ammonia perfusion image (*gray scale*). In contrast, the control rat (injected with cardiomyoblasts transfected with *Fluc*, which served as a negative control) has homogeneous ^{13}N-ammonia perfusion but background ^{18}F-FHBG reporter activity. **d** Autoradiography of the same study rat confirms trapping of ^{18}F radioactivity by transplanted cells at the lateral wall at a finer spatial resolution (approximately 50 μm). (*p/sec*/cm^2/*sr* photons/second/centimeter squared/steridian; *ID/g* injected dose/gram) (Adapted from Wu et al. 2003a)

to acute donor cell death as the result of inflammation, adenoviral toxicity, ischemia, or apoptosis (Fig. 3).

In a recent study Cao et al. (2006) conducted the first investigation to study the kinetics of embryonic stem (ES) cell survival, proliferation, and migration after intramyocardial transplantation by using a multimodality imaging strategy. In this study, mouse ES cells carrying a novel triple-fusion (TF) reporter gene consisting of Fluc, monomeric red fluorescent protein (mRFP), and herpes simplex virus type-1 truncated sr39 thymidine kinase (HSV1-ttk) were injected into the myocardium of adult nude rats. By use of bioluminescence and PET imaging system, the survival and proliferation of injected ES cells were followed in vivo for 4 weeks (Fig. 4). Postmortem analysis revealed teratoma formation by week 4. Interestingly, *HSV1-ttk*, besides being a PET reporter gene, can also be used as a suicide gene by administering pharmacologic dosages of ganciclovir, which can terminate deoxyribonucleic acid synthesis in cells that carry the viral *HSV-ttk*. Intraperitoneal injection of ganciclovir (50 mg/kg twice daily), starting at week 3 after cell transplantation, successfully ablated teratomas in the treated group, as demonstrated by the disappearance of PET and bioluminescence signals.

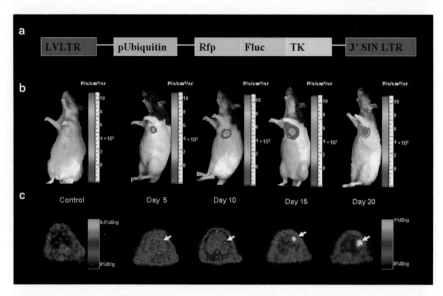

Fig. 4 a–c Multimodality molecular imaging of embryonic stem cells in living animals. **a** Schema of the *TF* reporter gene containing fusion of *Fluc*, monomeric red fluorescence protein (*Rfp*), and truncated HSV1-ttk (*TK*). **b** Optical bioluminescence imaging showing mouse ES cells expressing the *Fluc* gene on day 4 and at week 1, week 2, week 3, and week 4 after intramyocardial transplantation. **c** Detailed tomographic view of cardiac PET imaging of ^{18}F-FHBG activity showing mouse ES cells expressing the HSV1-ttk reporter gene at corresponding time points. *LVLTR* lentivirus long terminal repeats, *pUbiquitin* ubiquitin promoter, *SIN* self-inactivating. (Adapted from Cao et al. 2006)

More recently, Kim et al. (2006) successfully imaged pancreatic islet graft survival using PET imaging. They generated HSV1-sr39tk-expressing recombinant adenovirus rAD-TK and dual gene-expressing recombinant adenovirus rAD-vID10-ITK, by placing the Epstein Barr viral open reading frame, bcrf-1, which encodes viral interleukin-10 (vIL-10) as the first cistron and HSV1-sr39tk as the second, the genes being co-expressed with the aid of the encephalomyocarditis virus (EMCV) internal ribosomal entry site (IRES). They chose *bcrf-1* as a potential therapeutic gene because its product, vIL-10, protects transplanted islets from immunological attack by regulating autoimmune activity. The expression level of vIL-10 protein paralleled the expression of HSV1-SR39tk protein. After infecting islets from C57BL/6 mice with rAD-TK, they transplanted them into the liver of recipient C57BL/6 mice, injected ^{18}F-FHBG and performed scanning. With PET scanning, insulin secretory capacity of transplanted islets and expression of the gene encoding vIL-10 was measurable (Fig. 5). According to this study, quantitative in vivo PET imaging is a valid method for facilitating the development of protocols for prolonging islet survival, with the potential for tracking human transplants.

One potential concern regarding the use of reporter genes is that they may exert adverse effects on stem-cell biology and function. To address this issue, Wu et al. (2006) recently compared gene expression profiling in ES cells expressing the

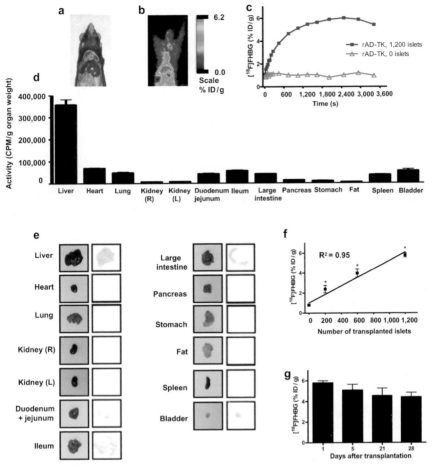

Fig. 5 a–g PET scanning of transplanted islets in the liver. A total of 1,200 islets infected with rAD-TK at a multiplicity of infection (m.o.i.) of 250 were transplanted into the liver. **a** Photographs of C57BL/6 mice indicating the liver position. **b** Representative coronal, MAP-reconstructed slices of PET images in an islet-transplanted C57BL/6 mouse. **c** TACs of the regions of interest (ROIs). **d, e** Determination of radioactivity by γ-spectroscopy and organ autoradiography from the mouse represented in **a–c**. **f** Correlation between the number of transplanted islets and the PET signal. **g** Time-course monitoring of transplanted islets in the liver. All data represent the mean ± SEM. Significance was tested using ANOVA with a Newman-Keuls post-hoc test. *$P < 0.05$ (versus liver with no islet transplants) (Adapted from Kim et al. 2006)

TF reporter gene with normal ES cells. Microarray analysis revealed only a small percentage of genome (1–2%) that underwent transcriptional changes in ES cells with TF. Out of 20,371 genes studied, 173 were down-regulated and 123 were up-regulated. The down-regulated genes were involved with cell-cycle regulation, cell death, and nucleotide metabolism, whereas the up-regulated genes were involved in antiapoptosis and homeostasis pathways. However, despite transcriptional changes resulting from the introduction of exogenous TF reporter genes, there appear to be no significant effects on ES cell viability, proliferation, and differentiation pathways (Cao et al. 2006; Wu et al. 2006). Thus, in light of its unique abilities to image cells longitudinally and noninvasively, multimodality molecular/reporter gene imaging holds tremendous promise as a tool to track the fate of stem cells in stem-cell therapy.

The issue of reporter-gene silencing has been recently evaluated (Krishnan et al. 2006). Reporter gene silencing is due to DNA methylation and histone deacetylation and can affect in-vivo cellular and molecular imaging. Silencing of a reporter gene leads to a lack of mRNA and therefore no imaging signal. This phenomenon could be tackled by using an inhibitor of DNA methyltransferase enzymes (e.g., 5-azacytidine) that removes methyl groups bound to CpG islands or by an inhibitor of histone deacetylase enzymes (e.g., TSA) that converts chromatin to an open structure that is more accessible for gene transcription. Our ongoing efforts focus on using endogenous promoters which have less of a propensity for being silenced, such as β-actin or ubiquitin, to circumvent this issue. Further review of stem-cell imaging is to be found in previous publications (Wu et al. 2004; Chang et al. 2006).

3.2 Imaging Gene Therapies

Monitoring of in-vivo gene expression is critical for the evaluation of the success or failure of the gene therapy approaches. Tissue biopsy might provide some insight into this issue but some organs are not accessible and repeated biopsies are invasive and are rarely clinically feasible. Thus, imaging techniques for noninvasive and longitudinal monitoring of therapeutic gene expression are highly desirable. Previously, to assay the expression of a therapeutic gene, invasive techniques were used, but reporter genes have been validated that can be used in PET imaging, to study gene expression in vivo.

The reporter gene can itself be the therapeutic gene or can be coupled to the therapeutic gene (Gambhir et al. 2000b). In the former approach, the reporter gene and therapeutic gene are one and the same. For example, anticancer gene therapy using HSV1-tk and GCV can be coupled with imaging of the accumulation of radiolabeled probes (^{18}F-FHBG or ^{124}I-FIAU). Yaghoubi et al. (2005) used the PET reporter probe, ^{18}F-FHBG to monitor HSV1-sr39tk expression in C6 glioma tumors (C6sr39) implanted subcutaneously in nude mice that were being treated repetitively with the prodrug GCV. ^{18}F-FHBG and ^{18}F-FDG imaging data indicated that exposure of C6sr39 tumors to GCV causes the elimination of ^{18}F-FHBG-accumulating C6sr39 cells and selects for regrowth of tumors unable to accumulate ^{18}F-FHBG. In a separate clinical pilot study, Jacobs et al. (2001) used ^{124}I-FIAU PET imaging of humans in a prospective gene-therapy trial of intratumorally infused liposome-gene complex (LIPO-HSV1-tk), followed by GCV administration in five recurrent glioblastoma patients. This study showed that [^{124}I]FIAU PET is feasible and that vector-mediated gene expression may predict a therapeutic effect. Another reporter,

NIS, which facilitates the uptake of iodide by thyroid follicular cells, is also being applied in radioiodide gene therapy (Chung 2002). The conventional radioiodide or ^{99m}Tc-pertechnetate scintigraphy has been used to directly monitor NIS expression. Since the iodine is not trapped, the issue of efflux has to be optimized, but initial studies show significant promise. Human somatostatin subtype 2 receptor (hSSTR2) is also being applied in radiotargeted gene therapy in combination with radiolabeled synthetic somatostatin analogues (Buchsbaum et al. 2005).

3.2.1 Transcriptional Targeting

Transcriptional targeting is feasible because a tissue- or disease-specific promoter can be activated in the cells of choice in the presence of the proper subset of activators, while remaining relatively silent in other nontarget cells. A wide range of tissue-specific and tumor-selective promoters (TSPs) has been developed for gene therapy of cancer (Nettelbeck et al. 2000; Wu et al. 2003b). These strategies allow an additional level of control for gene therapy, as even if a vector is delivered to nontarget tissues, transcriptional targeting provides a second level of specificity and primarily activates the gene(s) of interest only in the desired tissues. However, transgene expression involving the use of TSPs is generally lower than constitutive viral promoters (e.g., CMV) due to their weak transcriptional activity.

A two-step transcriptional amplification (TSTA) method for amplifying gene expression using relatively weak promoters has been developed by Iyer et al. (2005). In this approach, a specific promoter of choice directs the potent transcription activator VP16, which in turn is directed to drive the transcription of the gene(s) of interest. This approach can enhance the activity of the prostate specific antigen (PSA) promoter over a range of up to 1,000-fold (Iyer et al. 2001b; Zhang et al. 2002). A follow-up application has been documented with enhancement of the carcinoembryonic antigen (CEA) promoter to boost HSV1-tk expression. Greater tumor cell killing of CEA positive breast cancer cell and accumulation of ^{131}I-FIAU tumor signal recorded by gamma camera were documented in this study (Qiao et al. 2002).

The potency and specificity of the PSA promoter-based TSTA expression system was retained while using an adenoviral delivery vector (Sato et al. 2003; Zhang et al. 2003). In a very recent study (Johnson et al. 2005), combined ^{18}F-FHBG PET and CT were utilized to monitor intratumoral gene transfer and therapy mediated by the prostate-specific AdTSTA-sr39tk or AdCMV-sr39tk adenoviral vectors (Fig. 6). Loss of FHBG PET signal in the tumor was observed, which correlated with destruction of tumor cells. In this study, tissue-specific TSTA suicide gene therapy was demonstrated to be superior to the constitutive approach in minimizing systemic liver toxicity evidenced by no hepatic radioactivity in PET images. A lentivirus carrying the TSTA expression cassette also exhibited regulated, cell-specific and long-term expression (Iyer et al. 2004). In a separate study (Dong et al. 2004), the regulation of the *GRP78* promoter, which regulates the expression of a stress-inducible chaperone protein, GRP78, was examined in human breast tumor by ^{18}F-FHBG. ^{18}F-FHBG PET signals were documented in breast tumors stably

Pre-Rx   **Post-Rx**

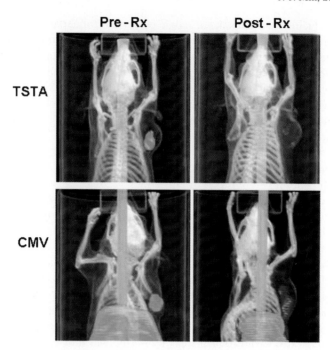

Fig. 6 MicroPET/CT imaging of suicide gene therapy. A total of 1×10^9 infectious units of prostate-targeted AdTSTA-sr39tk (TSTA) or constitutive active AdCMV-sr39tk (CMV) were intratumorally injected into androgen dependent LAPC-4 tumors, human prostate cancer xenografts on mice on day 0. MicroPET/CT imaging performed prior to ganciclovir (GCV) treatment on day 7 showed tumor-limited expression in the TSTA-treated animals, but the CMV-treated animal showed strong expression in the liver as well. After receiving GCV treatment, ^{18}F-FHBG PET signals at day 22 were diminished in the tumors and the liver of the CMV animals. (Adapted from Johnson et al. 2005).

transduced by a retrovirus carrying *HSV1-tk* driven by the *GRP78* promoter. The signal was further induced by photodynamic therapy. All these strategies continue to show the ability to use transcriptional targeting as a method of providing further specificity in gene therapy, while using transcriptional amplification to insure robust gene expression. Further details are provided elsewhere (Iyer et al. 2005)

3.2.2 Linked Gene Expression Strategies

This approach involves *indirect* imaging of therapeutic transgene expression using expression of a reporter gene whose expression is coupled to a therapeutic transgene of choice. This strategy requires proportional and constant coexpression of both the reporter gene and the therapeutic gene over a wide range of transgene expression levels. An advantage of this approach is that it provides for a much wider application of therapeutic transgene imaging, because various imaging reporter genes can be coupled to various therapeutic transgenes while utilizing the same imaging probe each time. Linking the expression of a therapeutic gene to a reporter gene has been validated using PET and optical imaging through a variety of different molecular constructs. Examples include fusion approaches (Ray et al. 2003, 2004), bicistronic approaches using internal ribosomal entry site (IRES) (Yu et al. 2000; Liang et al. 2002), dual-promoter approaches (Hemminki et al. 2002; Zinn et al. 2002), a bi-directional transcriptional approach (Sun et al. 2001), and a two vector administration approach (Yaghoubi et al. 2001b).

A fusion gene approach can be used in which two or more different genes are joined in such a way that their coding sequences are in the same reading frame, and thus a single protein with properties of both the original proteins is produced. An advantage of the fusion gene approach is that the expression of the linked genes is absolutely coupled (unless the spacer between the two proteins is cleaved). However, the fusion protein does not always yield functional activity for both of the individual proteins and/or may not localize in an appropriate subcellular compartment (Min and Gambhir 2004). Another approach is to insert an internal ribosomal entry site (IRES) sequence between the two genes so that they are transcribed into a single mRNA from the same promoter but translated into two separate proteins. Although the IRES sequence leads to proper translation of the downstream cistron from a bicistronic vector, translation from the IRES can be cell-type-specific and the magnitude of expression of the gene placed distal to the IRES is often attenuated (Yu et al. 2000). Two different genes expressed from distinct promoters within a single vector (dual-promoter approach) may avoid some of the attenuation and tissue variation problems of an IRES-based approach (Zinn et al. 2002). The bidirectional transcriptional approach utilizes a vector in which the therapeutic and reporter genes can each be driven by a minimal CMV promoter induced by tetracycline-responsive element (TRE), transcribing separated mRNA from each gene, which would then be translated into separate protein products (Sun et al. 2001). This system also avoids the attenuation and tissue variation problems of the IRES-based approach and may prove to be one of the most robust approaches developed to date. Another way to image both the therapeutic and reporter genes can be through administration of two separate vectors, by cloning of the therapeutic and reporter genes in two different vectors but driven by the same promoter. Further details on imaging gene therapy have been reviewed by Min et al. (2004) and Iyer et al. (2005).

4 Clinical Applications and Future Prospects

One of the key objectives of reporter gene imaging is to be able to translate strategies from small animal models to clinically applicable methods. In this context, some recent clinical studies have incorporated imaging to monitor cancer gene therapy. For example, repetitive PET imaging was performed to assess a cationic liposome-mediated *HSV1-tk* suicide gene transfer into glioblastoma (Jacobs et al. 2001; Reszka et al. 2005). Vector-mediated *HSV1-tk* gene expression was monitored by ^{124}I-FIAU in five patients with recurrent glioblastoma. In one patient, specific ^{124}I-FIAU uptake was detected within the infused tumor. After GCV treatment, signs of necrosis were observed by FDG-PET indicating HSV1-tk-mediated treatment response. This study may have had limited imaging findings because of the relatively poor efficiency of gene transduction when using liposomes. The use of the ^{18}F-FHBG probe was studied in healthy human volunteers to characterize the biodistribution, radiation dosimetry, and routes of clearance of the reporter probe. The results showed that FHBG exhibited good pharmacokinetic properties and rapid clearance suitable for applications in patients (Yaghoubi et al. 2001a). More interestingly, FHBG-PET has been recently used by us to monitor *HSV1-tk* suicide gene expression in patients with hepatocellular carcinoma (Penuelas et al. 2005a, 2005b). Gene expression was evident in all patients who received a viral

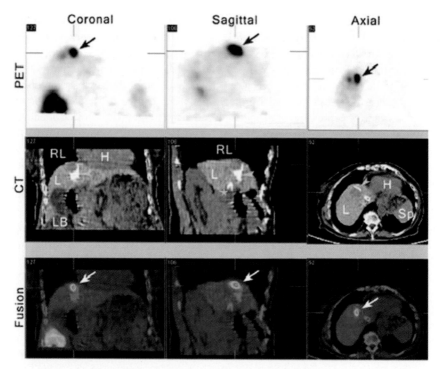

Fig. 7 PET imaging of adenoviral-mediated transgene expression in liver cancer patients. PET-CT imaging of *HSV1-tk* transgene expression in humans. Columns 1 to 3 show the 5-mm-thick coronal, sagittal, and transaxial slices, respectively, from an ^{18}F-FHBG-PET-CT study in patient 5. All sections are centered on the treated tumor lesion (*dotted lines* in the CT images) and show ^{18}F-FHBG accumulation at the tumor site (*arrows*). Anatomic-metabolic correlation can be obtained by fused PET-CT imaging. The white spots on the liver seen on the CT images correspond to lipiodol retention (*arrowheads*) after transarterial embolization of the tumor and a transjugular intrahepatic portosystemic shunt (⋆). Tracer signal can be seen in the treated lesion (*arrows*), whereas no specific accumulation of the tracer can be seen in the necrotic, lipiodol-retaining regions around it. *H* heart, *L* liver, *LB* large bowel, *RL* right lung, *Sp* spleen. (Adapted from Penuelas et al. 2005b)

dose of 7.7×10^9 pfu or more (Fig. 7). These findings help support the use of the FHBG-HSV1-tk system to directly monitor the expression of a therapeutic gene in future gene therapy trials. Currently, human trials with T-cells and dendritic cells expressing the HSV1-tk reporter and consecutive ^{18}F-FHBG PET imaging are underway and should help form the basis for cellular imaging in humans with FHBG-PET.

Molecular imaging strategies will likely expand significantly over the next few years as imaging and molecular genetic technologies continue to evolve. The explosion in genetic engineering is expected to generate more robust gene transfer vectors, both viral and nonviral. Bicistronic/bidirectional vectors, which can be easily modified, and tissue-specific amplification techniques will likely expand. Continued refinements in chemistry of molecular probe development should give rise to a new generation of probes with greater sensitivity and specificity. Advances in detector technology and image reconstruction techniques for PET should help to produce a newer generation of imaging instruments with better spatial resolution, sensitivity, and significantly improved throughput time. Multimodality reporter gene approaches will likely expand so that investigators may readily move between the various imaging technologies The potential power of molecular imaging to see fundamental biological processes in a new light will not only help to enhance our knowledge and understanding but should also accelerate considerably the rate of discovery in the biological sciences.

References

Acton PD, Zhou R (2005) Imaging reporter genes for cell tracking with PET and SPECT. Q J Nucl Med Mol Imaging 49(4):349–360

Adonai N, Nguyen KN, Walsh J, Iyer M, Toyokuni T, Phelps ME, McCarthy T, McCarthy DW, Gambhir SS (2002) Ex vivo cell labeling with 64Cu-pyruvaldehyde-bis(N4-methylthiosemicarbazone) for imaging cell trafficking in mice with positron-emission tomography. Proc Natl Acad Sci U S A 99(5):3030–3035

Aicher A, Brenner W, Zuhayra M, Badorff C, Massoudi S, Assmus B, Eckey T, Henze E, Zeiher AM, Dimmeler S (2003) Assessment of the tissue distribution of transplanted human endothelial progenitor cells by radioactive labeling. Circulation 107(16):2134–2139

Alauddin MM, Conti PS (1998) Synthesis and preliminary evaluation of 9-(4-[18F]-fluoro-3-hydroxymethylbutyl)guanine ([18F]FHBG): a new potential imaging agent for viral infection and gene therapy using PET. Nucl Med Biol 25(3):175–180

Alauddin MM, Conti PS, Mazza SM, Hamzeh FM, Lever JR (1996) 9-[(3-[18F]-fluoro-1-hydroxy-2-propoxy)methyl]guanine ([18F]-FHPG): a potential imaging agent of viral infection and gene therapy using PET. Nucl Med Biol 23(6):787–792

Alauddin MM, Shahinian A, Gordon EM, Conti PS (2004) Direct comparison of radiolabeled probes FMAU, FHBG, and FHPG as PET imaging agents for HSV1-tk expression in a human breast cancer model. Mol Imaging 3(2):76–84

Alauddin MM, Shahinian A, Kundu RK, Gordon EM, Conti PS (1999) Evaluation of 9-[(3-18F-fluoro-1-hydroxy-2-propoxy)methyl]guanine ([18F]-FHPG) in vitro and in vivo as a probe for PET imaging of gene incorporation and expression in tumors. Nucl Med Biol 26(4):371–376

Anderson CJ, Dehdashti F, Cutler PD, Schwarz SW, Laforest R, Bass LA, Lewis JS, McCarthy DW (2001) 64Cu-TETA-octreotide as a PET imaging agent for patients with neuroendocrine tumors. J Nucl Med 42(2):213–221

Anton M, Wagner B, Haubner R, Bodenstein C, Essien BE, Bonisch H, Schwaiger M, Gansbacher B, Weber WA (2004) Use of the norepinephrine transporter as a reporter gene for non-invasive imaging of genetically modified cells. J Gene Med 6(1):119–126

Baker CH, Morris JC (2004) The sodium-iodide symporter. Curr Drug Targets Immune Endocr Metabol Disord 4(3):167–174

Barbash IM, Chouraqui P, Baron J, Feinberg MS, Etzion S, Tessone A, Miller L, Guetta E, Zipori D, Kedes LH, Kloner RA, Leor J (2003) Systemic delivery of bone marrow-derived mesenchymal stem cells to the infarcted myocardium: feasibility, cell migration, body distribution. Circulation 108(7):863–868

Barrio JR, Satyamurthy N, Huang SC, Keen RE, Nissenson CH, Hoffman JM, Ackermann RF, Bahn MM, Mazziotta JC, Phelps ME (1989) 3-(2′-[18F]fluoroethyl)spiperone: in vivo biochemical and kinetic characterization in rodents, nonhuman primates, and humans. J Cereb Blood Flow Metab 9(6):830–839

Bhaumik S, Gambhir SS (2002) Optical imaging of Renilla luciferase reporter gene expression in living mice. Proc Natl Acad Sci U S A 99(1):377–382

Biswal S, Gambhir SS (2003) Monitoring gene therapy using in vivo molecular imaging techniques. In: Smyth Templeton N (ed) Gene therapy: therapeutic mechanisms and strategies, Dekker, New York Basel, pp 447–480

Botti C, Negri DR, Seregni E, Ramakrishna V, Arienti F, Maffioli L, Lombardo C, Bogni A, Pascali C, Crippa F, Massaron S, Remonti F, Nerini-Molteni S, Canevari S, Bombardieri E (1997) Comparison of three different methods for radiolabelling human activated T lymphocytes. Eur J Nucl Med 24(5):497–504

Buchsbaum DJ, Chaudhuri TR, Yamamoto M, Zinn KR (2004) Gene expression imaging with radiolabeled peptides. Ann Nucl Med 18(4):275–283

Buchsbaum DJ, Chaudhuri TR, Zinn KR (2005) Radiotargeted gene therapy. J Nucl Med 46 Suppl 1:179S–186S

Buursma AR, Beerens AM, de Vries EF, van Waarde A, Rots MG, Hospers GA, Vaalburg W, Haisma HJ (2005) The human norepinephrine transporter in combination with 11C-m-hydroxyephedrine as a reporter gene/reporter probe for PET of gene therapy. J Nucl Med 46(12):2068–2075

Cao F, Lin S, Xie X, Ray P, Patel M, Zhang X, Drukker M, Dylla SJ, Connolly AJ, Chen X, Weissman IL, Gambhir SS, Wu JC (2006) In vivo visualization of embryonic stem cell survival, proliferation, and migration after cardiac delivery. Circulation 113(7):1005–1014

Carlin S, Mairs RJ, Welsh P, Zalutsky MR (2002) Sodium-iodide symporter (NIS)-mediated accumulation of [(211)At]astatide in NIS-transfected human cancer cells. Nucl Med Biol 29(7):729–739

Chang GY, Xie X, Wu JC (2006) Overview of stem cells and imaging modalities for cardiovascular diseases. J Nucl Cardiol 13(4):554–569

Chung JK (2002) Sodium iodide symporter: its role in nuclear medicine. J Nucl Med 43(9): 1188–1200

Contag CH, Bachmann MH (2002) Advances in in vivo bioluminescence imaging of gene expression. Annu Rev Biomed Eng 4:235–260

Dingli D, Kemp BJ, O'Connor MK, Morris JC, Russell SJ, Lowe VJ (2006) Combined I-124 positron emission tomography/computed tomography imaging of NIS gene expression in animal models of stably transfected and intravenously transfected tumor. Mol Imaging Biol 8(1):16–23

Dingli D, Russell SJ, Morris JC 3rd (2003) In vivo imaging and tumor therapy with the sodium iodide symporter. J Cell Biochem 90(6):1079–1086

Dong D, Dubeau L, Bading J, Nguyen K, Luna M, Yu H, Gazit-Bornstein G, Gordon EM, Gomer C, Hall FL, Gambhir SS, Lee AS (2004) Spontaneous and controllable activation of suicide gene expression driven by the stress-inducible grp78 promoter resulting in eradication of sizable human tumors. Hum Gene Ther 15(6):553–561

Dubey P, Su H, Adonai N, Du S, Rosato A, Braun J, Gambhir SS, Witte ON (2003) Quantitative imaging of the T cell antitumor response by positron-emission tomography. Proc Natl Acad Sci U S A 100(3):1232–1237

Eskandari S, Loo DD, Dai G, Levy O, Wright EM, Carrasco N (1997) Thyroid Na + /I-symporter mechanism, stoichiometry, and specificity. J Biol Chem 272(43):27230–27238

Furukawa T, Lohith TG, Takamatsu S, Mori T, Tanaka T, Fujibayashi Y (2006) Potential of the FES-hERL PET reporter gene system — basic evaluation for gene therapy monitoring. Nucl Med Biol 33(1):145–151

Gambhir S, Massoud TF (2004) Molecular imaging fundamentals. In: Ell PJ, Gambhir S (eds) Nuclear medicine in clinical diagnosis and treatment, Elsevier, London, pp 1845–1870

Gambhir SS, Barrio JR, Wu L, Iyer M, Namavari M, Satyamurthy N, Bauer E, Parrish C, MacLaren DC, Borghei AR, Green LA, Sharfstein S, Berk AJ, Cherry SR, Phelps ME, Herschman HR (1998) Imaging of adenoviral-directed herpes simplex virus type 1 thymidine kinase reporter gene expression in mice with radiolabeled ganciclovir. J Nucl Med 39(11):2003–2011

Gambhir SS, Barrio JR, Phelps ME, Iyer M, Namavari M, Satyamurthy N, Wu L, Green LA, Bauer E, MacLaren DC, Nguyen K, Berk AJ, Cherry SR, Herschman HR (1999) Imaging adenoviral-directed reporter gene expression in living animals with positron emission tomography. Proc Natl Acad Sci U S A 96(5):2333–2338

Gambhir SS, Bauer E, Black ME, Liang Q, Kokoris MS, Barrio JR, Iyer M, Namavari M, Phelps ME, Herschman HR (2000a) A mutant herpes simplex virus type 1 thymidine kinase reporter gene shows improved sensitivity for imaging reporter gene expression with positron emission tomography. Proc Natl Acad Sci U S A 97(6):2785–2790

Gambhir SS, Herschman HR, Cherry SR, Barrio JR, Satyamurthy N, Toyokuni T, Phelps ME, Larson SM, Balatoni J, Finn R, Sadelain M, Tjuvajev J, Blasberg R (2000b) Imaging transgene expression with radionuclide imaging technologies. Neoplasia 2(1–2):118–138

Green LA (2000) A proposal for quantitating herpes simplex virus type 1 thymidine kinase reporter gene expression in living animals using positron emission tomography and a tracer kinetic model for radiolabeled acyclic guanosine analogues. In: Biomathematics, University of California, Los Angeles, p 170

Groot-Wassink T, Aboagye EO, Glaser M, Lemoine NR, Vassaux G (2002) Adenovirus biodistribution and noninvasive imaging of gene expression in vivo by positron emission tomography using human sodium/iodide symporter as reporter gene. Hum Gene Ther 13(14):1723–1735

Haberkorn U, Altmann A (2001) Imaging methods in gene therapy of cancer. Curr Gene Ther 1(2):163–182

Haberkorn U, Oberdorfer F, Gebert J, Morr I, Haack K, Weber K, Lindauer M, van Kaick G, Schackert HK (1996) Monitoring gene therapy with cytosine deaminase: in vitro studies using tritiated-5-fluorocytosine. J Nucl Med 37(1):87–94

Hemminki A, Zinn KR, Liu B, Chaudhuri TR, Desmond RA, Rogers BE, Barnes MN, Alvarez RD, Curiel DT (2002) In vivo molecular chemotherapy and noninvasive imaging with an infectivity-enhanced adenovirus. J Natl Cancer Inst 94(10):741–749

Henze M, Schuhmacher J, Hipp P, Kowalski J, Becker DW, Doll J, Macke HR, Hofmann M, Debus J, Haberkorn U (2001) PET imaging of somatostatin receptors using [68GA]DOTA-D-Phe1-Tyr3-octreotide: first results in patients with meningiomas. J Nucl Med 42(7):1053–1056

Herschman HR (2004a) Noninvasive imaging of reporter gene expression in living subjects. Adv Cancer Res 92:29–80

Herschman HR (2004b) PET reporter genes for noninvasive imaging of gene therapy, cell tracking and transgenic analysis. Crit Rev Oncol Hematol 51(3):191–204

Herschman HR, MacLaren DC, Iyer M, Namavari M, Bobinski K, Green LA, Wu L, Berk AJ, Toyokuni T, Barrio JR, Cherry SR, Phelps ME, Sandgren EP, Gambhir SS (2000) Seeing is believing: non-invasive, quantitative and repetitive imaging of reporter gene expression in living animals, using positron emission tomography. J Neurosci Res 59(6):699–705

Herzog H, Coenen HH, Kuwert T, Langen KJ, Feinendegen LE (1990) Quantification of the whole-body distribution of PET radiopharmaceuticals, applied to 3-N-([18F]fluoroethyl)spiperone. Eur J Nucl Med 16(2):77–83

Hildebrandt IJ, Gambhir SS (2004) Molecular imaging applications for immunology. Clin Immunol 111(2):210–224

Hoffman RM (2005) The multiple uses of fluorescent proteins to visualize cancer in vivo. Nat Rev Cancer 5(10):796–806

Hofmann M, Maecke H, Borner R, Weckesser E, Schoffski P, Oei L, Schumacher J, Henze M, Heppeler A, Meyer J, Knapp H (2001) Biokinetics and imaging with the somatostatin receptor PET radioligand (68)Ga-DOTATOC: preliminary data. Eur J Nucl Med 28(12):1751–1757

Hofmann M, Wollert KC, Meyer GP, Menke A, Arseniev L, Hertenstein B, Ganser A, Knapp WH, Drexler H (2005) Monitoring of bone marrow cell homing into the infarcted human myocardium. Circulation 111(17):2198–2202

Iyer M, Barrio JR, Namavari M, Bauer E, Satyamurthy N, Nguyen K, Toyokuni T, Phelps ME, Herschman HR, Gambhir SS (2001a) 8-[18F]Fluoropenciclovir: an improved reporter probe for imaging HSV1-tk reporter gene expression in vivo using PET. J Nucl Med 42(1):96–105

Iyer M, Wu L, Carey M, Wang Y, Smallwood A, Gambhir SS (2001b) Two-step transcriptional amplification as a method for imaging reporter gene expression using weak promoters. Proc Natl Acad Sci U S A 98(25):14595–14600

Iyer M, Salazar FB, Lewis X, Zhang L, Carey M, Wu L, Gambhir SS (2004) Noninvasive imaging of enhanced prostate-specific gene expression using a two-step transcriptional amplification-based lentivirus vector. Mol Ther 10(3):545–552

Iyer M, Sato M, Johnson M, Gambhir SS, Wu L (2005) Applications of molecular imaging in cancer gene therapy. Curr Gene Ther 5(6):607–618

Jacobs A, Voges J, Reszka R, Lercher M, Gossmann A, Kracht L, Kaestle C, Wagner R, Wienhard K, Heiss WD (2001) Positron-emission tomography of vector-mediated gene expression in gene therapy for gliomas. Lancet 358(9283):727–729

Johnson M, Sato M, Burton J, Gambhir SS, Carey M, Wu L (2005) Micro-PET/CT monitoring of herpes thymidine kinase suicide gene therapy in a prostate cancer xenograft: the advantage of a cell-specific transcriptional targeting approach. Mol Imaging 4(4):463–472

Kang KW, Min JJ, Chen X, Gambhir SS (2005) Comparison of [14C]FMAU, [3H]FEAU, [14C]FIAU, and [3H]PCV for monitoring reporter gene expression of wild type and mutant herpes simplex virus type 1 thymidine kinase in cell culture. Mol Imaging Biol 7(4):296–303

Kim SJ, Doudet DJ, Studenov AR, Nian C, Ruth TJ, Gambhir SS, McIntosh CH (2006) Quantitative micro positron emission tomography (PET) imaging for the in vivo determination of pancreatic islet graft survival. Nat Med 12(12):1423–1428

Koehne G, Doubrovin M, Doubrovina E, Zanzonico P, Gallardo HF, Ivanova A, Balatoni J, Teruya-Feldstein J, Heller G, May C, Ponomarev V, Ruan S, Finn R, Blasberg RG, Bornmann W, Riviere, I, Sadelain M, O'Reilly RJ, Larson SM, Tjuvajev JG (2003) Serial in vivo imaging of the targeted migration of human HSV-TK-transduced antigen-specific lymphocytes. Nat Biotechnol 21(4):405–413

Kraitchman DL, Tatsumi M, Gilson WD, Ishimori T, Kedziorek D, Walczak P, Segars WP, Chen HH, Fritzges D, Izbudak I, Young RG, Marcelino M, Pittenger MF, Solaiyappan M, Boston RC, Tsui BM, Wahl RL, Bulte JW (2005) Dynamic imaging of allogeneic mesenchymal stem cells trafficking to myocardial infarction. Circulation 112(10):1451–1461

Krishnan M, Park JM, Cao F, Wang D, Paulmurugan R, Tseng JR, Gonzalgo ML, Gambhir SS, Wu JC (2006) Effects of epigenetic modulation on reporter gene expression: implications for stem cell imaging. FASEB J 20(1):106–108

Kundra V, Mannting F, Jones AG, Kassis AI (2002) Noninvasive monitoring of somatostatin receptor type 2 chimeric gene transfer. J Nucl Med 43(3):406–412

Le LQ, Kabarowski JH, Wong S, Nguyen K, Gambhir SS, Witte ON (2002) Positron emission tomography imaging analysis of G2A as a negative modifier of lymphoid leukemogenesis initiated by the BCR-ABL oncogene. Cancer Cell 1(4):381–391

Lee KH, Bae JS, Lee SC, Paik JY, Matsui T, Jung KH, Ko BH, Kim BT (2006) Evidence that myocardial Na/I symporter gene imaging does not perturb cardiac function. J Nucl Med 47(11):1851–1857

Lee KH, Kim HK, Paik JY, Matsui T, Choe YS, Choi Y, Kim BT (2005) Accuracy of myocardial sodium/iodide symporter gene expression imaging with radioiodide: evaluation with a dual-gene adenovirus vector. J Nucl Med 46(4):652–657

Lewin B (2000) Genes VII. Oxford University Press, New York

Liang Q, Gotts J, Satyamurthy N, Barrio J, Phelps ME, Gambhir SS, Herschman HR (2002) Non-invasive, repetitive, quantitative measurement of gene expression from a bicistronic message by positron emission tomography, following gene transfer with adenovirus. Mol Ther 6(1):73–82

Liang Q, Satyamurthy N, Barrio JR, Toyokuni T, Phelps MP, Gambhir SS, Herschman HR (2001) Noninvasive, quantitative imaging in living animals of a mutant dopamine D2 receptor reporter gene in which ligand binding is uncoupled from signal transduction. Gene Ther 8(19): 1490–1498

Lim SJ, Paeng JC, Kim SJ, Kim SY, Lee H, Moon DH (2007) Enhanced expression of adenovirus-mediated sodium iodide symporter gene in MCF-7 breast cancer cells with retinoic acid treatment. J Nucl Med 48(3):398–404

Lucignani G, Ottobrini L, Martelli C, Rescigno M, Clerici M (2006) Molecular imaging of cell-mediated cancer immunotherapy. Trends Biotechnol 24(9):410–418

MacLaren DC, Gambhir SS, Satyamurthy N, Barrio JR, Sharfstein S, Toyokuni T, Wu L, Berk AJ, Cherry SR, Phelps ME, Herschman HR (1999) Repetitive, non-invasive imaging of the dopamine D2 receptor as a reporter gene in living animals. Gene Ther 6(5):785–791

Marsee DK, Shen DH, MacDonald LR, Vadysirisack DD, Lin X, Hinkle G, Kloos RT, Jhiang SM 2004 Imaging of metastatic pulmonary tumors following NIS gene transfer using single photon emission computed tomography. Cancer Gene Ther 11(2):121–127

Massoud TF, Gambhir SS (2003) Molecular imaging in living subjects: seeing fundamental biological processes in a new light. Genes Dev 17(5):545–580

Min JJ, Gambhir SS (2004) Gene therapy progress and prospects: noninvasive imaging of gene therapy in living subjects Gene Ther 11(2):115–125

Min JJ, Iyer M, Gambhir SS (2003) Comparison of [18F]FHBG and [14C]FIAU for imaging of HSV1-tk reporter gene expression: adenoviral infection vs stable transfection. Eur J Nucl Med Mol Imaging 30(11):1547–1560

Nettelbeck DM, Jerome V, Muller R (2000) Gene therapy: designer promoters for tumour targeting. Trends Genet 16(4):174–181

Ottobrini L, Lucignani G, Clerici M, Rescigno M (2005) Assessing cell trafficking by noninvasive imaging techniques: applications in experimental tumor immunology. Q J Nucl Med Mol Imaging 49(4):361–366

Paik JY, Lee KH, Byun SS, Choe YS, Kim BT (2002) Use of insulin to improve [18 F]fluorodeoxyglucose labelling and retention for in vivo positron emission tomography imaging of monocyte trafficking. Nucl Med Commun 23(6):551–557

Pentlow KS, Graham MC, Lambrecht RM, Cheung NK, Larson SM (1991) Quantitative imaging of I-124 using positron emission tomography with applications to radioimmunodiagnosis and radioimmunotherapy. Med Phys 18(3):357–366

Penuelas I, Haberkorn U, Yaghoubi S, Gambhir SS (2005a) Gene therapy imaging in patients for oncological applications. Eur J Nucl Med Mol Imaging 32 Suppl 2:S384–S403

Penuelas I, Mazzolini G, Boan JF, Sangro B, Marti-Climent J, Ruiz M, Ruiz J, Satyamurthy N, Qian C, Barrio JR, Phelps ME, Richter JA, Gambhir SS, Prieto J (2005b) Positron emission tomography imaging of adenoviral-mediated transgene expression in liver cancer patients. Gastroenterology 128(7):1787–1795

Phelps ME (2000) Inaugural article: positron emission tomography provides molecular imaging of biological processes. Proc Natl Acad Sci U S A 97(16):9226–9233

Qiao J, Doubrovin M, Sauter BV, Huang Y, Guo ZS, Balatoni J, Akhurst T, Blasberg RG, Tjuvajev JG, Chen SH, Woo SL (2002) Tumor-specific transcriptional targeting of suicide gene therapy. Gene Ther 9(3):168–175

Ray P, Wu AM, Gambhir SS 2003 Optical bioluminescence and positron emission tomography imaging of a novel fusion reporter gene in tumor xenografts of living mice. Cancer Res 63(6): 1160–1165

Ray P, De A, Min JJ, Tsien RY, Gambhir SS (2004) Imaging tri-fusion multimodality reporter gene expression in living subjects. Cancer Res 64(4):1323–1330

Reszka RC, Jacobs A, Voges J (2005) Liposome-mediated suicide gene therapy in humans. Methods Enzymol 391:200–208

Rogers BE, McLean SF, Kirkman RL, Della Manna D, Bright SJ, Olsen CC, Myracle AD, Mayo MS, Curiel DT, Buchsbaum DJ (1999) In vivo localization of [(111)In]-DTPA-D-Phe1-octreotide to human ovarian tumor xenografts induced to express the somatostatin receptor subtype 2 using an adenoviral vector. Clin Cancer Res 5(2):383–393

Rogers BE, Zinn KR, Buchsbaum DJ (2000) Gene transfer strategies for improving radiolabeled peptide imaging and therapy. Q J Nucl Med 44(3):208–223

Sato M, Johnson M, Zhang L, Zhang B, Le K, Gambhir SS, Carey M, Wu L (2003) Optimization of adenoviral vectors to direct highly amplified prostate-specific expression for imaging and gene therapy. Mol Ther 8(5):726–737

Serganova I, Blasberg R (2005) Reporter gene imaging: potential impact on therapy. Nucl Med Biol 32(7):763–780

Shu CJ, Guo S, Kim YJ, Shelly SM, Nijagal A, Ray P, Gambhir SS, Radu CG, Witte ON (2005) Visualization of a primary anti-tumor immune response by positron emission tomography. Proc Natl Acad Sci U S A 102(48):17412–17417

Sun X, Annala AJ, Yaghoubi SS, Barrio JR, Nguyen KN, Toyokuni T, Satyamurthy N, Namavari M, Phelps ME, Herschman HR, Gambhir SS (2001) Quantitative imaging of gene induction in living animals. Gene Ther 8(20):1572–1579

Takamatsu S, Furukawa T, Mori T, Yonekura Y, Fujibayashi Y (2005) Noninvasive imaging of transplanted living functional cells transfected with a reporter estrogen receptor gene. Nucl Med Biol 32(8):821–829

Tjuvajev JG, Stockhammer G, Desai R, Uehara H, Watanabe K, Gansbacher B, Blasberg RG (1995) Imaging the expression of transfected genes in vivo. Cancer Res 55(24):6126–6132

Tjuvajev JG, Finn R, Watanabe K, Joshi R, Oku T, Kennedy J, Beattie B, Koutcher J, Larson S, Blasberg RG (1996) Noninvasive imaging of herpes virus thymidine kinase gene transfer and expression: a potential method for monitoring clinical gene therapy. Cancer Res 56(18): 4087–4095

Tjuvajev JG, Avril N, Oku T, Sasajima T, Miyagawa T, Joshi R, Safer M, Beattie B, DiResta G, Daghighian F, Augensen F, Koutcher J, Zweit J, Humm J, Larson SM, Finn R, Blasberg R (1998) Imaging herpes virus thymidine kinase gene transfer and expression by positron emission tomography. Cancer Res 58(19):4333–4341

Tjuvajev JG, Chen SH, Joshi A, Joshi R, Guo ZS, Balatoni J, Ballon D, Koutcher J, Finn R, Woo SL, Blasberg RG (1999) Imaging adenoviral-mediated herpes virus thymidine kinase gene transfer and expression in vivo. Cancer Res 59(20):5186–5193

Tjuvajev JG, Doubrovin M, Akhurst T, Cai S, Balatoni J, Alauddin MM, Finn R, Bornmann W, Thaler H, Conti PS, Blasberg RG (2002) Comparison of radiolabeled nucleoside probes (FIAU, FHBG, and FHPG) for PET imaging of HSV1-tk gene expression. J Nucl Med 43(8): 1072–1083

Vadysirisack DD, Shen DH, Jhiang SM (2006) Correlation of Na + /I-symporter expression and activity: implications of Na + /I-symporter as an imaging reporter gene. J Nucl Med 47(1): 182–190

van Eijck CH, de Jong M, Breeman WA, Slooter GD, Marquet RL, Krenning EP (1999) Somatostatin receptor imaging and therapy of pancreatic endocrine tumors. Ann Oncol 10 Suppl 4: 177–181

Van Sande J, Massart C, Beauwens R, Schoutens A, Costagliola S, Dumont JE, Wolff J (2003) Anion selectivity by the sodium iodide symporter. Endocrinology 144(1):247–252

Wu JC, Chen IY, Sundaresan G, Min JJ, De A, Qiao JH, Fishbein MC, Gambhir SS (2003a) Molecular imaging of cardiac cell transplantation in living animals using optical bioluminescence and positron emission tomography. Circulation 108(11):1302–1305

Wu JC, Tseng JR, Gambhir SS (2004) Molecular imaging of cardiovascular gene products. J Nucl Cardiol 11(4):491–505

Wu JC, Spin JM, Cao F, Lin S, Xie X, Gheysens O, Chen IY, Sheikh AY, Robbins RC, Tsalenko A, Gambhir SS, Quertermous T (2006) Transcriptional profiling of reporter genes used for molecular imaging of embryonic stem cell transplantation. Physiol Genomics 25(1):29–38

Wu L, Johnson M, Sato M (2003b) Transcriptionally targeted gene therapy to detect and treat cancer. Trends Mol Med 9(10):421–429

Yaghoubi S, Barrio JR, Dahlbom M, Iyer M, Namavari M, Satyamurthy N, Goldman R, Herschman HR, Phelps ME, Gambhir SS (2001a) Human pharmacokinetic and dosimetry studies of [(18)F]FHBG: a reporter probe for imaging herpes simplex virus type-1 thymidine kinase reporter gene expression. J Nucl Med 42(8):1225–1234

Yaghoubi SS, Barrio JR, Namavari M, Satyamurthy N, Phelps ME, Herschman HR, Gambhir SS (2005) Imaging progress of herpes simplex virus type 1 thymidine kinase suicide gene therapy in living subjects with positron emission tomography. Cancer Gene Ther 12(3):329–339

Yaghoubi SS, Wu L, Liang Q, Toyokuni T, Barrio JR, Namavari M, Satyamurthy N, Phelps ME, Herschman HR, Gambhir SS (2001b) Direct correlation between positron emission tomographic images of two reporter genes delivered by two distinct adenoviral vectors. Gene Ther 8(14):1072–1080

Yu Y, Annala AJ, Barrio JR, Toyokuni T, Satyamurthy N, Namavari M, Cherry SR, Phelps ME, Herschman HR, Gambhir SS (2000) Quantification of target gene expression by imaging reporter gene expression in living animals. Nat Med 6(8):933–937

Zhang L, Adams JY, Billick E, Ilagan R, Iyer M, Le K, Smallwood A, Gambhir SS, Carey M, Wu L (2002) Molecular engineering of a two-step transcription amplification (TSTA) system for transgene delivery in prostate cancer. Mol Ther 5(3):223–232

Zhang L, Johnson M, Le KH, Sato M, Ilagan R, Iyer M, Gambhir SS, Wu L, Carey M (2003) Interrogating androgen receptor function in recurrent prostate cancer. Cancer Res 63(15):4552–4560

Zinn KR, Chaudhuri TR (2002) The type 2 human somatostatin receptor as a platform for reporter gene imaging. Eur J Nucl Med Mol Imaging 29(3):388–399

Zinn KR, Chaudhuri TR, Krasnykh VN, Buchsbaum DJ, Belousova N, Grizzle WE, Curiel DT, Rogers BE (2002) Gamma camera dual imaging with a somatostatin receptor and thymidine kinase after gene transfer with a bicistronic adenovirus in mice. Radiology 223(2):417–425

Noninvasive Cell Tracking

Fabian Kiessling

Abstract Cell-based therapies may gain future importance in defeating different kinds of diseases, including cancer, immunological disorders, neurodegenerative diseases, cardiac infarction and stroke. In this context, the noninvasive localization of the transplanted cells and the monitoring of their migration can facilitate basic research on the underlying mechanism and improve clinical translation.

In this chapter, different ways to label and track cells in vivo are described. The oldest and only clinically established method is leukocyte scintigraphy, which enables a (semi)quantitative assessment of cell assemblies and, thus, the localization of inflammation foci. Noninvasive imaging of fewer or even single cells succeeds with MRI after labeling of the cells with (ultrasmall) superparamagentic iron oxide particles (SPIO and USPIO). However, in order to gain an acceptable signal-to-noise ratio, at a sufficiently high spatial resolution of the MR sequence to visualize a small amount of cells, experimental MR scanners working at high magnetic fields are usually required. Nevertheless, feasibility of clinical translation has been achieved by showing the localization of USPIO-labeled dendritic cells in cervical lymph nodes of patients by clinical MRI.

Cell-tracking approaches using optical methods are important for preclinical research. Here, cells are labeled either with fluorescent dyes or quantum dots, or

Fabian Kiessling
Abteilung Medizinische Physik in der Radiologie, Deutsches Krebsforschungszentrum, Im Neuenheimer Feld 280, 69120 Heidelberg
f.kiessling@dkfz.de

W. Semmler and M. Schwaiger (eds.), *Molecular Imaging II.*
Handbook of Experimental Pharmacology 185/II.
© Springer-Verlag Berlin Heidelberg 2008

transfected with plasmids coding for fluorescent proteins such as green fluorescent protein (GFP) or red fluorescent protein (RFP). The advantage of the latter approach is that the label does not get lost during cell division and, thus, makes imaging of proliferating transplanted cells (e.g., tumor cells) possible.

In summary, there are several promising options for noninvasive cell tracking, which have different strengths and limitations that should be considered when planning cell-tracking experiments.

1 Current Status of Cell-based Therapies

Cell migration plays an important role in the progression and defense of various diseases, including local infections, autoimmunological disorders, graft rejection, tissue repair, and cancer. In this context, the local interplay between migrated lymphocytes, monocytes and granulocytes induces the cellular and humoral immunoresponse and plays also a major role in the removal of necrotic material. Beside their role in the defense of bacterial and viral infections, their responsibility for tumor immunity is the focus of intense research.

In contrast to the cells of the immune system, progenitor cells are more involved in tissue remodelling and repair. For example, the differentiation of progenitor cells to stromal and vascular cells improves revascularization in infarctions and, thus, decreases the duration of hypoxia. This can be supported by the release of transmitters and growth factors from the progenitor cells, which trigger local tissue activation, proliferation and regeneration. In brain and cardiac infarctions, even a differentiation to neurons and cardiomyocytes has been postulated, respectively. This, however, is still discussed controversially.

Two therapeutic options result from these observations. The first is to use cells of the immune system as specific mediators of immune response; the second is to use progenitor cells for the renewal of stable tissues.

While in bacterial infections the use of leucocytes is more restricted to diagnostic procedures, much effort has been taken in cell-based immuno-therapy strategies to defeat cancer.

In this regard, one possible procedure is to load dendritic cells in vitro with tumor antigens and retransfer them into the organism, where they present the antigens at their surface, thus inducing proliferation of $CD4^+$ T-lymphocytes and activation of $CD8^+$ T-lymphocytes (Paczesny et al. 2003). The proliferation of specific $CD4^+$ T-lymphocytes induces the differentiation and proliferation of B-lymphocytes to antitumor antibody-producing plasma cells. The activation and proliferation of $CD8^+$ T-lymphocytes induces direct cellular immunity.

Also, $CD8^+$T lymphocytes are frequently used for cell-based tumor therapy. Tumor-infiltrating T-lymphocytes are isolated from the blood, from subcutaneous or from visceral lesions (Takusaburo et al. 2001; Parmiani et al. 2003). Alternatively, lymphocytes can be generated from lymph nodes after vaccination against tumor antigens (Takusaburo et al. 2001). The lymphocytes are subsequently cultured in vitro and clonally expanded in the presence of high levels of IL-2. Finally, they are retransferred to the patient. In advanced cancer patients with different tumor entities, it was shown that these treatments can have life-prolonging effects (Takusaburo et al. 2001), and in patients with renal cancer a response to the T-cell therapy went along with a decrease in tumor load and increased survival.

Cell-based therapy approaches are also used to regenerate stable tissues. These tissues contain cells that have lost their ability to proliferate, which means that damage to these tissues is irreversible. Theoretically, multipotent stem cells have the capacity to differentiate in any tissue. Progenitor cells are usually predifferentiated and can only form a certain type of tissue, e.g., hematopoietic cells, mesenchymal cells or some types of epithelial cells.

In Parkinson's disease, dopaminergic neurons in the substantia nigra degenerate due to unknown reasons. Stiffness, motionless and tremor are typical clinical symptoms. Clinical studies have shown that the intrastriatal transplantation of dopamineric neurons, which can for example derive from embryonic mesencephalic tissue, can result in clinical improvement in some patients (Lindvall and Bjoerklund 2004). Unfortunately, overall symptomatic relief during two years after transplantation has been reported to be lower than 40% (Lindvall and Bjoerklund 2004) and does not exceed those from subthalamic deep brain stimulation (Lindvall and Hagell 2002). There is evidence, however, that re-innervation of the transplanted neurons can significantly be improved by carefully choosing the location for the graft placement, which raises the demand for dedicated noninvasive imaging strategies. Stem-cell transplantation is also under evaluation as cell therapy in cerebral stroke (Lindvall and Kokaia 2004). In this context, it was shown that neural regeneration can occur from the patient's own brain stem cells and that transplanted stem cells migrate to ischemic lesions (Arvidsson et al. 2002). However, many basic issues have still to be elucidated. In particular, most transplanted stem cells differentiate to glial cells and do not form functional neurons, as desired. A precise knowledge of stem cell biology will help to find suited stem-cell populations for transplantation and the required tissue factors to induce the neural differentiation.

The use of progenitor cells for the repair of cardiac infarctions is controversial. Several studies showed that progenitor cells migrate to cardiac infarctions; however, their role in remodelling of the infracted tissue remains uncertain. In particular, their differentiation to functional cardiomyocytes has not been proved so far. On the other hand, clinical studies indicated that transplantation of progenitor cells into the myocardium can improve regional and global contractibility as well as the end systolic volume (Dimmeler et al. 2005). One reason for this may be the differentiation of progenitor cells to endothelial cells, which support neovascularisation of the infracted area.

Beside the therapy strategies in cardiac infarctions, the differentiation of transplanted peripheral blood-derived progenitor cells to endothelial cells has also be shown to improve neovascularization in arterial occlusive disease (Losordo and Dimmeler 2004).

These examples indicate that there is a broad range of potential clinical applications for cell-based therapies. However, most of these treatments are still in an experimental or early clinical state and there are many open questions on the underlying mechanism, which have to be clarified. In order to elucidate the triggers for cell recruitment and differentiation, it is desirable to noninvasively assess cell migration, to prove correct transplantation and to monitor the presence and organization of the transplanted cells in the tissue. Several imaging modalities, such as nuclear medicine techniques, optical imaging and MRI, are basically suited for cell-tracking approaches. In the following, an overview is given on the current status of noninvasive cell-tracking approaches and its contribution to basic and preclinical research.

2 Noninvasive Cell Trafficking

2.1 Nuclear Medicine

From all imaging techniques available, those using radiotracers have the highest sensitivity and are mostly quantitative. On the other hand, nuclear medicine modalities like scintigraphy, SPECT and PET are limited in their spatial resolution and, also, the tissue contrast is low. This often makes matching with other noninvasive imaging modalities necessary to provide detailed anatomical information, such as obtained from PET-CT.

Scintigraphy is a standard nuclear medicine approach and clinically established to characterize lesions in the thyroid, to detect metastases in bone and to assess renal function. In addition, scintigraphy with radiolabeled leukocytes was the first noninvasive imaging modality used for cell tracking and the first cell-tracking approach which entered clinical evaluation.

Leukocyte scintigraphy is performed to localize occult inflammation foci in patients by visualizing the accumulation of the radiolabeled leukocytes (McAfee et al. 1984; Hughes 2003). In this, the leukocytes are removed from the peripheral blood of the patients, labeled in vitro with radiotracers, and subsequently retransferred into the patients by intraveneous injection (Fig. 1). The distribution of labelled leucocytes and their accumulation in the inflammation is then monitored using planar imaging with a gamma-camera or by SPECT.

As radiotracers ^{111}In-oxine or ^{111}In-tropolonate are broadly used. ^{111}In emits gamma rays at 173 and 247 keV and has a half-life of about 67 h, which gives a suitable time window for noninvasive imaging. During labeling, ^{111}In diffuses through the plasma membrane, is then separated from the hydrophobic complex, and binds irreversibly to cytoplasmatic and nuclear cell components.

^{99m}Tc-Hexamethylpropylenamine-oxine (^{99}Tc-HMPAO) is also used for cell labeling and clinical leukocyte scintigraphy. At 6 h, the half-life of ^{99}Tc is shorter than that of ^{111}In. The emitted gamma rays have a lower energy of 140 keV and minimal cell toxicity has been described using ^{99}Tc-HMPAO for cell labeling. ^{99}Tc-HMPAO also diffuses into the cytoplasm of the cells, there losing its hydrophobic properties.

Isolation of leucocytes from the blood

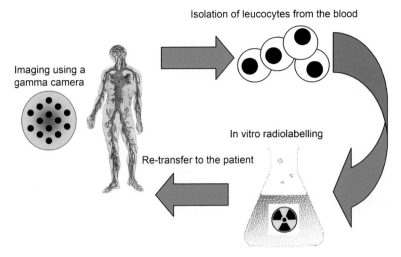

Imaging using a
gamma camera

In vitro radiolabelling

Re-transfer to the patient

Fig. 1 Sketch illustrating the principle performance of clinical leukocyte scintigraphy. Leukocytes are removed from the blood of the patient, radiolabeled and subsequently retransferred. Imaging is usually performed using a two-dimensional gamma-camera 1–4 h and 16–30 h after intraveneous retransfusion of the labeled leukocytes

As a consequence, most of the ^{99}Tc-HMPAO is trapped inside the cells. However, due to limited bio-stability of the complex, there is a relevant amount of the ^{99}Tc, which slowly leaves the cells.

Alternatively, cells can be assigned with ^{99}Tc-labelled colloids, which are phagocyted by the cells. These are casually used for leukocyte scintigraphy and experimental cell-labeling approaches (McAfee et al. 1984).

In basic research on cell migration, radiolabeling of cells is regularly performed alone or in combination with labels for other noninvasive imaging modalities, like MRI or optical imaging, and provides a quantitative reference method and a favorable "gold standard". In these approaches, however, radiolabeling is less important for the in-vivo detection of the cells than for the quantification of cell accumulation in the organs and tumors of the animals used by gamma-counting. Beside gamma-counting, the distribution of radiolabeled cells can also be visualized on histological sections using microradiographs, as demonstrated for ^{111}In-labelled T-lymphocytes in a cell-based antitumor therapy (Kircher et al. 2003).

In particular, when studying the migration of progenitor cells, the distribution of the cells within the entire animal is important to know and can point to different cell differentiation routes. In this context, it was shown in mice with myocardial infarctions that the number of progenitor cells that accumulate in the heart rose significantly if there is an infarction but that the overall distribution of the progenitor cells in the other organs of the animals was hardly affected (Brenner et al. 2004). This is due to the fact that after intraveneous injection most transplanted progenitor cells were localized in liver, spleen, kidney and bone marrow and only a small proportion entered the healthy or infracted heart.

2.2 Optical Imaging

In principal, optical imaging methods have a comparably high sensitivity for contrast agents as the techniques from nuclear medicine. In addition, optical imaging can be performed at high spatial and temporal resolution. Unfortunately, in-vivo imaging by light is limited by the scattering of photons in the tissue and depends on the tissue itself and the emission wavelength of the photons. In general, optical imaging can be performed for structures which are less than 1 mm to several centimeters deep in the tissue. In this context, optimal tissue penetration can be achieved in the near infrared range between 700 and 1,000 nm (Weissleder and Ntziachristos 2003).

In contrast to the nuclear medicine techniques, which usually are highly quantitative, the quantification of optical signals originating from deep within an object is difficult. Attempts have been done to quantify the optical signals in phantoms, e.g., by using optical tomography; however, accurate quantification in vivo is still a challenge (Schulz et al. 2004).

Two principle strategies are usually performed to label cells in vivo: the first is to mark cells with external dyes and the second is to use transgenic cells which express heterologous fluorescent proteins or enzymes that digest and, thus, activate a fluorescent probe. Direct labeling with dyes can be performed more easily and several kits are commercially available for this purpose.

It is a disadvantage of the method that in case of proliferating cells a dilution of the dyes occurs and that after several cell doublings no sufficient signal can be received from the cells any more.

While previous approaches have mostly been done with cyanine dyes or other fluorochromes, semi-inductive, inorganic nanocrystals — so-called quantum dots — are a novel group of markers whose emission spectra can be tuned to any desired wavelength (Voura et al. 2004). It is a further advantage of quantum dots that they can be excited by a large spectrum of single and multiphoton excitation light. Unfortunately, there are reports of a considerably high toxicity of quantum dots on cells, which make further biocompatibility analysis necessary (Derfus et al. 2004).

Using quantum dots, it was shown that after intraveneous injection into mice the migration of labeled metastatic tumor cells to lung, liver and spleen and the accumulation of AC133$^+$ progenitor cells nearby tumor vessels could be assessed when analyzing the totally removed organs or histological sections (Fig. 2).

In-vivo imaging after subcutaneous implantation of quantum-dot-labeled tumor cells in mice indicated that a subcutaneous deposit of less than 1,000 cells can be visualized, which in this experiment was not feasible for green fluorescent protein (GFP)-positive cells (Gao et al. 2004). However, further studies still have to prove whether movements and accumulation of quantum-dot-labeled cells can reliably be visualized transcutaneously and followed longitudinally.

Heterologuous expression of GFP, cloned from bioluminescent jellyfish, is an excellent tool to label proliferating or transdifferentiating cells (Mothe et al. 2005; Shichinohe et al. 2004; Yamauchi et al. 2005; Yamamoto et al. 2004). This is particularly true if the transplanted cells derive from transgenic animals, because after

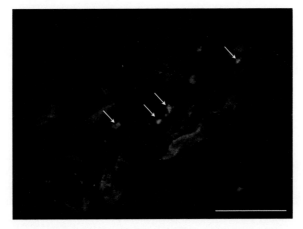

Fig. 2 Immunofluorescence image of a squamous cell carcinoma xenograft of a nude mouse after injection of quantum-dot-labeled AC133$^+$ progenitor cells. The labeled progenitor cells (*arrows*) can easily be localized nearby tumor vessels, which are labeled with an anti-CD31 antibody and an AMCA-labeled secondary antibody. *Bar*: 100 μm

in-vitro transfection of cells the expression of GFP is often downregulated over time (Onifer et al. 2003; Vroemen et al. 2003). Unfortunately, due to the limited tissue penetration of green light, imaging in the intact organism using GFP is restricted to superficial tissues. Skin flaps may allow deeper organs in the living animals to be investigated (Yamauchi et al. 2005); however, in most studies GFP is used to analyse tissue specimens or removed organs.

Red fluorescent protein (RFP) from *Discosoma* coral has a longer wavelength emission, with consequently deeper tissue penetration. It is also suited to single-cell labeling, or in combination with GFP can be used for double-labeling of different cellular components (Yamamoto et al. 2004). In this context, dual-labeled tumor cells, with GFP expression in the cytoplasm and RFP expression in the nuclei proved to be an interesting tool to study the migration and extravasation of tumor cells. In-vivo tracking of these cells was successful in the ear and in the skin flaps of living mice. In this experiment, double-labeling of these cells allowed studying mitosis and apoptosis as well as the deformation of cells and cytoplasm during migration through the vasculature (Yamauchi et al. 2005).

Alternative heterologeous cell labels are the enzymes β-galactosidase (encoded by the *Escherichia coli lacZ* gene) and human placental alkaline phosphatase (hPAP). Using progenitor cells from transgenic rats expressing *lacZ*, for example, enabled these cells to be tracked into cardiac infarctions (Takahashi et al. 2003; Inoue et al. 2005) and, in another approach, transgenic tumor cells expressing this enzyme allowed micrometastases to be detected in mice (Lin et al. 1990). For visualization of these labels, however, fixation of the tissue and substrates which undergo chromogenic enzyme-based activation are required. As a consequence, analysis of these labels can only succeed postmortem.

Transgenic expression of luciferase can be used to visualize transgenic cells in vivo and has been frequently used to depict tumor growth and spread in rodents (Contag et al. 2000). However, in-vivo imaging with luciferase only works reliably if sufficient delivery of the luciferin substrate can be guaranteed.

3 MRI

3.1 Cell Labelling for MRI

Superparamagnetic iron oxide particles (SPIO) with aggregated iron oxide cores and dextrane coating layers were suggested as potential liver-specific MR contrast agents as early as the mid 1980s. After intravenous injection, the particles are rapidly phagocyted by liver macrophageous and produce a drop of signal intensity in normal liver tissue. As a consequence, hepatocellular carcinomas or metastases become visible due to the negative contrast of the normal liver tissue. In addition, high uptake of SPIO is observed in spleen, bone marrow and lymph nodes as a consequence of phagocytosis of the particles by cells of the reticuloendothelial system (RES).

Approaches were performed using the uptake of SPIO in lymph nodes to delineate and detect lymph node metastases of prostate cancers, which proved to be promising in early clinical trials (Harisinghani et al. 2003). SPIO were also injected intraveneously to label macrophages, which infiltrated kidney grafts in rats (Beckmann et al. 2003), brain infarctions (Kleinschnitz et al. 2003) and cardiac infarction in vivo (Chapon et al. 2003). Thus, these particles offer new ways to perform a labelling of macrophages in vivo.

In-vitro studies showed that SPIO are also phagocytosed by leukocytes, fibroblasts mesenchymal progenitors and other cells to a different degree (Fig. 3).

While most clinically used SPIO have mean particle diameters of more than approximately 50 nm, dextran-coated ultrasmall SPIO (USPIO) — which were first described by Weissleder et al. (1990) — are less than 50 nm in diameter. Even smaller particles, described as "very small superparamagnetic iron oxide particles (VSOP)," which were coated with citrate and had diameters between 2 and 10 nm have been reported by Taupitz et al. (2003).

An overview on cell labeling approaches using SPIO is given in Table 1. In this context, it was shown that uptake of the particles depends on the particle size, surface charge and is variable for different cell types. In general, phagocytosis is more intense for larger particles (Sun et al. 2005) and particles with a negative surface charge (Fleige et al. 2002). Higher uptake usually also occurs for particles with a positive surface charge compared with particles with a neutral surface charge. While phagocytosis is the dominant uptake mechanism for the larger particles, pinocytosis becomes more important for small USPIO and VSOP.

However, there are cells, which hardly show any phagocytosis, such as pluripotent progenitor cells, but which are highly relevant for cell-tracking approaches.

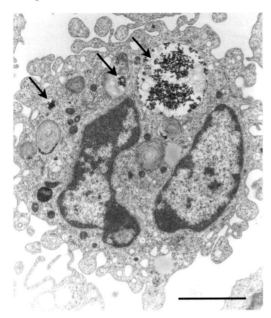

Fig. 3 Transmission electron microscopy (TEM) image of a human leukocyte after incubation with dextran-coated SPIO for 3 h. The particles are internalized and accumulated in large lysosomes in the cell (*arrows*). *N* nucleus. *Bar*: 2 μm

Thus, to improve labeling efficiency for nonphagocytic cells, monoclonal antibodies were covalently bonded to USPIO in order to induce receptor-mediated endocytosis (RME). For example, the mouse anti-Tfr monoclonal antibody OX-26 has been conjugated to dextran-coated monocrystalline iron oxide to magnetically label oligodendrocyte progenitors and neural precursor cells (Bulte et al. 1999, 2003). To further increase cellular uptake and specificity of iron oxide, human immunodeficiency virus transactivator transcription (HIV-Tat) protein, which contains a membrane translocating signal, was also coupled to iron oxide nanoparticles to facilitate incorporation into cell (Kircher et al. 2003; Lewin et al. 2000).

The disadvantage of using biomolecules to improve cell labeling is that active peptides and antibodies have the capability to induce apoptosis, as is known from HIV-Tat for neural cells, or that they may alter the biological function of the cells in an uncontrolled fashion. Another way to improve labeling efficacy of cells is the use of transfection agents, which mostly means that the SPIO are incorporated into liposomal structures that have the potential to cross the plasma membrane and release the particles intracellularly (Frank et al. 2002).

Imaging of cells labeled with SPIO is performed using T2-weighted and T2*-weighted MR sequences, where the labeled cells appear as black spots in the tissue. The detection limits are dependent on the intracellular iron concentrations achieved, the field strength of the MRI scanner, and the weighting and spatial resolution of the MR sequence. While it has been shown in vitro that in homogeneous media

Table 1 Overview on iron oxide particle type, size and coating, and on the cells which are used for MR cell-labeling experiments. *MSC* mesenchymal stem cell, *HeLa* human cervical carcinoma cell line

Particles	Size	Coating	Cell type	References
MPIO	0.9–5.8 μm	Divinyl benzene/styrene	Hepatocytes, embryonic fibroblasts, MSC	Shapiro et al. (2005)
Feridex (SPIO)	~150 nm	Dextran	Monocytes	Zelivyanskaya et al. (2003)
Ferumoxidesand MION-46L	~150 nm, 8–20 nm	Dextran	Lymphocytes, MSC, CG-4 cells, cervix cancer cells	Frank et al. (2003)
SHU 555aSHU 555c	45–65 nm, <40 nm	Dextran	progenitor cells, fibroblasts, hepatocarcinoma cells	Sun et al. (2005)
Magneticpoly-saccharides	~50 nm	Dextran	hematopoietic progenitor cells, dendritic cells	Daldrup-Link et al. (2003); Ahrens et al. (2003)
CLIO	~45 nm	Dextran	Lymphocytes, CD34[+] prog. cells	Josephson et al. (1999); Lewin et al. (2000)
Anionic maghemite nanoparticles	~35 nm	DMSA	Macrophages, HeLa	Billotey et al. (2003); Wilhelm et al. (2003)
Ferumoxtran	~35 nm	Dextran	Embryonic stem cells, muscle stem cells, MSC	Hoehn et al. (2002); Cahill et al. (2003); Kraitchman et al. (2003)
AquaMag-100BMS180549	~35 nm	Dextran	T-cells	Yeh et al. (1993)
MION-46L	8–20 nm	Dextran	Oligodendrocytes, neural precursor cells, T-cells	Bulte et al. (1999), (2003); Anderson et al. (2004)
MION	8–20 nm	Dextran	C6 tumor cell	Weissleder et al. (1997)
MION	12–14 nm	PEG-phospholipid	Fibroblasts, macrophages	Nitin et al. (2004); Moore et al. (1997)
VSOP-C125	~8 nm	Citrate	Macrophages	Fleige et al. (2002)
MD-100	7–8 nm	Dendrimers	Stem cells, neural progenitor cells, olfactory ensheathing glia, muscle stem cells	Bulte et al. (2001a), (2001b), (2001c); Hakumaki et al. (2001); Lee et al. (2004); Walter et al. (2004)

it is feasible to visualize single cells even at 1.5 T (Foster-Gareau et al. 2003), it becomes problematic in vivo when basic tissue heterogeneity makes higher contrast of labeled cells necessary. Furthermore, the scan times which can be applied in vivo have to be made shorter in order to be tolerated by the animal. "Off resonance imaging" may be a promising tool to switch the negative signal of iron oxides to a positive one and to suppress the endogenous tissue contrast, thus increasing the detection specificity for iron-loaded cells. While initial results using this method are promising, its value for in-vivo imaging has to be evaluated in ongoing studies.

All these imaging methods benefit from higher magnetic fields and, therefore, it is plausible that most applications on cell tracking are performed with high-field MR scanners (>4.7 T), which allow scanning with higher spatial resolution and provide an enhanced T2*-contrast.

Attempts have been done to image cells at positive contrast. For this purpose, usually the paramagnetic effects of gadolinium and manganese ions are used. The contrast is generated by a decrease of the T1-relaxation time due to an interaction of the paramagnetic ions with the surrounding protons. A cellular uptake often reduces the interaction of the contrast material with protons due to compartmentalization and thus decreases the achieved intracellular contrast. Thus, higher load with paramagnetic substances does not automatically provide a more efficient label, which makes these imaging strategies difficult. The use of higher magnetic field does not necessarily also improve sensitivity, because the T1-relaxation time increases at higher field strength.

However, beside these limitations it was shown that labeling of cells with liposomes containing paramagnetic and fluorescent metalloporphyrins (Daldrup-Link et al. 2004) or Gd-containing lipophilic nanoparticles (Vuu et al. 2005) allows an efficient label in vitro. Our own observations showed that a high labeling efficacy of cells can also be achieved with manganese chloride, which enters the cells via the calcium transporters. Unfortunately, in immortalized stem cells high cell toxicity was observed for manganese chloride, which makes this method questionable for this purpose.

Recently, promising first results were presented using ^{19}F MRI for the detection of dendritic cells in mice which were labeled with perfluoropolyether (PFPE) (Ahrens et al. 2005). In this study, fusion MR images were presented, in which the normal anatomy of the animal was assessed with proton MRI and the signal of the PFPE-labeled cells was captured with ^{19}F MRI at 11.7 T (Ahrens et al. 2005). An advantage of this method is the high specificity of ^{19}F MRI for the PFPE-labeled cells due to the low fluor content of normal tissue. A limitation may be that MR scanners with high magnetic fields may be required to reach a sufficient sensitivity for the detection of labeled cells.

3.2 In-vivo Detection of Cell Migration by MRI

If cell-tracking approaches are compared with those using specific USPIO-based contrast agents that bind to cellular targets, the following statements can be made. In the case of cell tracking, in-vitro cell labeling provides an optimal label for a small number of cells that have to be detected in vivo after transplantation. As a consequence, cell tracking approaches benefit from small voxel sizes in order to detect the one or few cells in a voxel which are highly loaded with iron oxide particles. In contrast, imaging with specific contrast agents, which label more cells in a voxel but to a less intense degree, may gain from higher signal-to-noise ratio MR sequences of lower spatial resolution.

Table 2 Summary of important in-vivo cell tracking studies, including the particle types, tracked cells and target organs used. *MSC* mesenchymal stem cells

Particles	Cells	Trafficking to	References
Feridex (SPIO)	Human monocytes	Brain	Zelivyanskaya et al. (2003)
SPIO	Oligodendrocytes	Brain	Franklin et al. (1999)
MD-100	Oligodendroglial progenitor cells	Brain	Bulte et al. (2001)
MION (USPIO)	Neural percusor cells	Brain	Bulte et al. (2003)
Ferumotran (USPIO)	Embryonic stem cells	Brain	Hoehn et al. (2002)
Ferumotran (USPIO)	T-cells	Spinal cord	Anderson et al. (2004)
MION (USPIO)	Oligodendrocyte progenitor cells	Spinal cord	Bulte et al. (1999)
MD-100	Embryonic stem cells	Spinal cord	Bulte et al. (2001)
	Olfactory ensheathing glia cells	Spinal cord	Lee et al. (2004)
MD-100	Muscle stem cells	Muscle	Walter et al. (2004)
Ferumoxide (SPIO)	Muscle stem cells	Muscle	Cahill et al. (2003)
Ferumoxide (SPIO)	MSC	Myocardial infarction	Kraitchman et al. (2003)
Sinerem (USPIO)	Embryonic ventricular cardiomyocytes	Myocardial infarction	Kuestermann et al. (2005)
Iron fluorophore particles (IFP)	MSC	Myocardial infarction	Hill et al. 2003
CLIO-Tat	T-cells	Tumors	Kircher et al. (2003)
Ferumoxide-protamine sulfate (FePro) complexes	Progenitor cells	Tumors	Arbab et al. (2006)
Ferridex	Dendritic cells	Lymph nodes	de Vries et al. (2005)
PFPE	Dendritic cells	Lymph nodes	Ahrens et al. (2005)

As a consequence, except in the case where high amounts of cells migrate to the target tissue, in-vivo cell tracking requires small voxel sizes and can hardly be performed on MR scanners with less than 3 T.

In line with the most common clinical indications for cellular therapies, MR cell tracking studies also frequently focus on the imaging of labeled cytotoxic immuno-cells to tumors and the visualization of labeled progenitor cells during tissue regeneration and repair (Table 2).

Initial studies with labeled progenitor cells were performed by Lewin et al. (2000), who demonstrated that even single Clio-Tat-USPIO-labeled progenitor cells can be detected in excised bone marrow specimens of mice at high MR field. An even more important result was that Clio-Tat-USPIO labeling did not affect the intracorporal distribution of the labeled cells in mice after intraveneous injection. Clio-Tat-USPIOs were also used to label cytotoxic T-cells, which were specifically activated to induce lysis of ovalbumin-expressing tumor cells. Using MRI, the migration of these T-cells into tumors expressing ovalbumin was successfully tracked, while no relevant accumulation occurred in nontransfected tumors. Subsequently, only transfected tumors responded to the T-cell therapy (Kircher et al. 2003).

MRI was also used to investigate the migration of AC133$^+$ endothelial progenitor cells (EPCs) into tumors, where they differentiated into vascular cells, thereby contributing to tumor angiogenesis (Arbab et al. 2006). Using SPIO-labeled EPCs, their accumulation in the tumors could be assessed using a 7-T MRI scanner and histology proved the accumulation of these cells at highly vascularized tumor borders. Our own observations using SPIO, ^{111}In and quantum dot triple-labeled AC133[+] progenitor cells found that only a small proportion of the injected progenitor cells finally entered the tumors and that their differentiation occurred to a higher degree into smooth muscle actin-positive pericytes than into CD31-expressing endothelial cells. However, progenitor cell differentiation and migration to the tumors may vary between different tumor models.

Magnetically labeled stem cells have also been used in cardiac research. In initial studies these cells were injected into cardiac infarctions in pigs, which were induced by trans-catheter occlusion of the left anterior descending artery or by temporal occlusion of this vessel using an angioplasty balloon (Hill et al. 2003; Kraitchman et al. 2003). The labeled stem cells were clearly visualized in the myocardium and the infracted area. In a healthy mouse heart, highly resolved MR imaging at 7 T indicated that embryonic cardiomyocytes injected into the myocardium organize along myocardial fibers, which was validated by histology. In ischemic lesions, MRI and Prussian Blue detection of iron-loaded cells showed that these cells transmigrate and integrate at the border of the fibrotic tissue (Kuestermann et al. 2005).

The migration of embryonic stem cells to ischemic lesions was also shown for rats with strokes that were induced by temporal occlusion of the middle cerebral artery (Hoehn et al. 2002). The embryonic stem cells labeled with SPIO by lipofection were injected into the healthy hemisphere. During the following days, MR imaging was capable of tracking migration of the labeled cells from the injection site to the ischemic lesion (Fig. 4), and histological evaluation indicated that these cells developed a neuron-like shape with long dendritic or axon-like extensions.

4 Future and Perspectives of Noninvasive Cell Tracking

Cell tracking has already become an important tool for biomedical imaging in preclinical research. It is favorably suited to studying the mechanisms of tumor spread and the interaction of tumor cells with stroma, endothelium and circulating cells. Noninvasive cell tracking has also shown potential as a valuable tool to monitor cell-based tumor defense.

In preclinical research, cell tracking gives new insights into progenitor cell biology, which is relevant for many diseases that go along with the regression of stable tissues. Using high-field MRI, the correct implantation of progenitor cells can be proved, and even the migration of a single or a few labeled cells and their integration into the target tissue can be monitored.

The broad clinical translation of cell tracking approaches, however, has only been done for the leukocyte scintigraphy so far, with the aim of detecting occult inflammations.

A clinical implementation of cell-tracking methods using MRI may be considered to prove the correct transplantation of high numbers of labeled cells, e.g.,

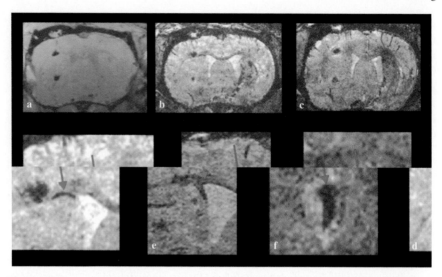

Fig. 4 a–f Coronal section through a rat brain at various times after implantation of embryonic stem cells into the hemisphere contralateral to the induced transient 60-min focal ischemia. Three-dimensional data sets were recorded at the day of implantation (**a**) and at 6 (**b**) and 8 (**c**) days after implantation. For orientation, the necrotic tissue area is outlined on **c**. Note, at 6 days (**b**) the discrete dark line (*arrow* in **d**, with higher magnification) along the corpus callosum between the cortical implantation site and the ventricular wall showing cells migrating toward the lesioned hemisphere. At 8 days (**c**), a dark region becomes visible in the dorsal part of the lesioned territory reflecting first arrival of USPIO-labeled cells. At higher magnification (**d**), the migration along the corpus callosum becomes more pronounced and is clearly visible. Taken from another animal example, the lining along the ventricular wall (**e**) and the accumulation of labeled stem cells on the choroid plexus (**f**) are also presented with high magnification. (From Hoehn et al. 2002)

of dendritic cells in immune therapy of melanomas (de Vries et al. 2005), in Parkinson's disease, liver cell therapy in cirrhosis or in myocardial infarctions. However, whether these methods will work reliably at MR fields of 3 T or below is still questionable. In addition, ex-vivo cell labeling requires dedicated sterile laboratories, which makes the performance complicated and cost intensive.

Thus, to date cell tracking using radio-, optically or magnetically labeled cells can be considered to be mostly a valuable tool for preclinical and basic research, with a certain potential for clinical translation.

References

Ahrens ET, Feili-Hariri M, Xu H et al (2003) Receptor-mediated endocytosis of iron-oxide particles provides efficient labeling of dendritic cells for in vivo MR imaging. Magn Reson Med 49:1006–1013
Ahrens ET, Flores R, Xu H et al (2005) In vivo imaging platform for tracking immunotherapeutic cells. Nat Biotechnol 23:983–987

Anderson SA, Shukaliak-Quandt J, Jordan EK et al (2004) Magnetic resonance imaging of labeled T-cells in a mouse model of multiple sclerosis. Ann Neurol 55:654–659

Arbab AS, Pandit SD, Anderson SA et al (2006) MRI and confocal microscopy studies of magnetically labeled endothelial progenitor cells trafficking to sites of tumor angiogenesis. Stem Cells 24:671–678

Arvidsson A, Collin T, Kirik D et al (2002) Neuronal replacement from endogenous precursors in the adult brain after stroke. Nat Med 8:963–970

Beckmann N, Cannet C, Fringeli-Tanner M et al (2003) Macrophage labeling by SPIO as an early marker of allograft chronic rejection in a rat model of kidney transplantation. Magn Reson Med 49:459–467

Billotey C, Wilhelm C, Devaud M et al (2003) Cell internalization of anionic maghemite nanoparticles: quantitative effect on magnetic resonance imaging. Magn Reson Med 49:646–654

Bulte JWM, Zhang S, van Gelderen P et al (1999) Neurotransplantation of magnetically labeled oligodendrocytes progenitors: MR tracking of cell migration and myelination. Proc Natl Acad Sci U S A 96:15256–15261

Bulte JWM, Douglas T, van Gelderen P et al (2001a). Cellular imaging using magnetodendrimers: application to human stem cells and neoplastic cells in vivo. Proc Int Soc Magn Reson Med 9:52

Bulte JWM, Lu J, Zywicke H et al (2001b) 3D MR tracking of magnetically labeled embryonic stem cells transplanted in the contusion injured rat spinal cord. Proc Int Soc Magn Reson Med 9:130

Bulte JWM, Douglas T, Witwer B et al (2001c) Magnetodendrimers allow endosomal magnetic labeling and in vivo tracking of stem cells. Nat Biotechnol 19:1141–1147

Bulte JWM, Ben-Hur T, Miller BR et al (2003) MR microscopy of magnetically labeled neurospheres transplanted into the Lewis EAE rat brain. Magn Reson Med 50:201–205

Brenner W, Aicher A, Eckey T et al (2004) ^{111}In-labeled CD34+ hematopoietic progenitor cells in a rat myocardial infarction model. J Nucl Med 45:512–518

Cahill KS, Silver X, Gaidosh G et al (2003) Noninvasive monitoring and tracking of muscle stem cells. Proc Int Soc Magn Reson Med 11:368

Chapon C, Franconi F, Lemaire L et al (2003) High field magnetic resonance imaging evaluation of superparamagnetic iron oxide nanoparticles in a permanent rat myocardial infarction. Invest Radiol 38:141–146

Contag CH, Jenkins D, Contag PR et al (2000) Use of reporter genes for optical measurements of neoplastic disease in vivo. Neoplasia 2:41–52

Daldrup-Link HE, Rudelius M, Oostendorp RAJ et al (2003) Targeting of hematopoietic progenitor cells with MR contrast agents. Radiology 228:760–767

Daldrup-Link HE, Rudelius M, Metz S et al (2004) Cell tracking with gadophrin-2: a bifunctional contrast agent for MR imaging, optical imaging, and fluorescence microscopy. Eur J Nucl Med Mol Imaging 31:1312–1321

De Vries IJ, Lesterhuis WJ, Barentsz JO et al (2005) Magnetic resonance tracking of dendritic cells in melanoma patients for monitoring cellular therapy. Nat Biotechnol 23:1407–1413

Derfus AM, Chan WCW, Bhatia SN (2004) Probing the cytotoxicity of semiconductor quantum dots. Nano Letters 4:11–18

Dimmeler S, Zeiher AM, Schneider MD (2005) Unchain my heart: the scientific foundations of cardiac repair. J Clin Invest 115:572–583

Foster-Gareau P, Heyn C, Alejski A et al (2003) Imaging single mammalian cells with a 1.5 T clinical MRI scanner. Magn Reson Med 49:968–971

Frank JA, Zywicke H, Jordan EK, et al. (2002). Magnetic intracellular labeling of mammalian cells by combining (FDA-approved) superparamagnetic iron oxide MR contrast agents and commonly used transfection agents. Acad Radiol 9 Suppl 2:484–487

Frank JA, Miller BR, Arbab AS et al (2003) Clinically applicable labeling of mammalian and stem cells by combining superparamagnetic iron oxides and transfection agents. Radiology 228:480–487

Franklin RJ, Blaschuk KL, Bearchell MC et al (1999) Magnetic resonance imaging of transplanted oligodendrocyte precursors in the rat brain. Neuroreport 10:3961–3965

Fleige G, Seeberger F, Laux D et al (2002) In vitro characterization of two different ultrasmall iron oxide particles for magnetic resonance cell tracking. Invest Radiol 37:482–488

Gao X, Cui Y, Levenson RM et al (2004) In vivo cancer targeting and imaging with semiconductor quantum dots. Nat Biotechnol 22:969–976

Hakumaki JM, Savitt JM, Gearhart JD et al (2001) MRI detection of labeled neural progenitor cells in a mouse model of Parkinson's disease. Dev Brain Res 132:43–44

Harisinghani MG, Barentsz J, Hahn PF et al (2003) Noninvasive detection of clinically occult lymph-node metastases in prostate cancer. N Engl J Med 348:2491–2499

Hill JM, Dick AJ, Raman VK et al (2005) Serial cardiac magnetic resonance imaging of injected mesenchymal stem cells. Circulation 108:1009–1014

Hoehn M, Kuestermann E, Blunk J et al (2002) Monitoring of implanted stem cell migration in vivo: a highly resolved in vivo magnetic resonance imaging investigation of experimental stroke in rat. Proc Natl Acad Sci U S A 99:16267–16272

Hughes DK (2003) Nuclear medicine and infection detection: the relative effectiveness of imaging with ^{111}In-oxine-, ^{99m}Tc-HMPAO-, and ^{99m}Tc-stannous fluoride colloid-labelled leucocytes and with ^{67}Ga-citrate. J Nucl Med Technol 31:196–201

Inoue H, Ohsawa I, Murakami T et al (2005). Development of new inbred transgenic strains of rats with LacZ or GFP. Biochem Biophys Res Commun 329:288–295

Josephson L, Tung CH, Moore A et al (1999) High-efficiency intracellular magnetic labeling with novel superparamagnetic-Tat peptide conjugates. Bioconjug Chem 10:186–191

Kircher MF, Allport JR, Graves EE et al (2003) In vivo high resolution three-dimensional imaging of antigen-specific cytotoxic T-lymphocyte trafficking to tumors. Cancer Res 63:6838–6846

Kleinschnitz C, Bendszus M, Frank M (2003) In vivo monitoring of macrophage infiltration in experimental ischemic brain lesions by magnetic resonance imaging. J Cereb Blood Flow Metab 23:1356–1361

Kuestermann E, Roell W, Breitbach M et al (2005) Stem cell implantation in ischemic mouse heart: a high-resolution magnetic resonance imaging investigation. NMR Biomed 18:362–370

Kraitchman DL, Heldman AW, Atalar E et al (2003) In vivo magnetic resonance imaging of mesenchymal stem cells in myocardial infarction. Circulation 107:2290–2293

Lee I-H, Bulte JWM, Schweinhardt P et al (2004). In vivo magnetic resonance tracking of olfactory ensheathing glia grafted into the rat spinal cord. Exp Neurol 187:509–516

Lin WC, Pretlow TP, Pretlow TG et al (1990) Bacterial lacZ gene as a highly sensitive marker to detect micrometastasis formation during tumor progression. Cancer Res 50:2808–2817

Lindvall O, Hagell P (2000) Clinical observation after neural transplantation in Parkinson's disease. Prog Brain Res 127:299–320

Lindvall O, Bjoerklund A (2004) Cell Therapy in Parkinson's Disease. NeuroRx 1:382–393

Lindvall O, Kokaia Z (2004) Recovery and rehabilitation in stroke: stem cells. Stroke 35: 2691–2694

Lewin M, Carlesso N, Tung CH, Tang XW, Cory D, Scadden DT, Weissleder R (2000) Tat peptide-derivatized magnetic nanoparticles allow in vivo tracking and recovery of progenitor cells. Nat Biotechnol 18:410–414

Losordo DW, Dimmeler S (2004) Therapeutic angiogenesis and vasculogenesis for ischemic disease: part II: cell based therapies. Circulation 109:2692–2697

McAfee JG, Subramanian G, Gagne G (1984) Techniques of leukocyte harvesting and labelling: problems and perspectives. Semin Nucl Med 2:83–106

Mothe AJ, Kulbatski I, van Bendegem RL et al (2005). Analysis of green fluorescent protein expression in transgenic rats for tracking transplanted neural stem/progenitor cells. J Histochem Cytochem 53:1215–1226

Moore A, Weissleder R, Bogdanov A Jr (1997) Uptake of dextrancoated monocrystalline iron oxides in tumor cells and macrophages. J Magn Reson Imaging 7:1140–1145

Nitin N, LaConte LEW, Zurkiya O et al (2004) Functionalization and peptide-based delivery of magnetic nanoparticles as an intracellular MRI contrast agent J Biol Inorg Chem 9:706–712

Onifer SM, White LA, Whitenmore SR et al (1993) In vitro labeling strategies for identifying primary neural tissue and a neuronal cell line after transplantation in the CNS. Cell Transplant 2:131–149

Paczesny S, Ueno H, Fay J et al (2003) Dendritic cells as vectors for immunotherapy of cancer. Semin Cancer Biol 13:439–447

Parmiami G, Castelli C, Rivoltini L et al (2003) Immunotherapy of melanoma. Semin Cancer Biol 13:391–400

Schulz RB, Ripoll J, Ntziachristos V (2004). Experimental fluorescence tomography of tissues with noncontact measurements. IEEE Transact Med Imaging 23:492–500

Shapiro EM, Skrtic S, Koretsky A P (2005) Sizing it up: cellular MRI using micro-sized iron oxide particles. Magn Reson Med 53:329–338

Shichinohe H, Kuroda S, Lee JB (2004) In vivo tracking of bone marrow stromal cells transplanted into mice cerebral infarct by fluorescence optical imaging. Brain Res Prot 13:166–175

Sun R, Dittrich J, Le-Huu M et al (2005) Physical and biological characterization of superparamagnetic iron oxide- and ultrasmall superparamagnetic iron oxide-labeled cells: a comparison. Invest Radiol 40:504–513

Takahashi M, Hakamata Y, Murakami T et al (2003) Establishment of lacZ-transgenic rats: a tool for regenerative research in myocardium. Biochem Biophys Res Commun 305:904–908

Takusaburo E, Ogama N, Shimanuki H et al (2001) Effector mechanism and clinical response of BAK (BRM-activated killer) immuno-cell therapy for maintaining satisfactory QOL of advanced cancer patients utilizing CD56-positive NIE (neuro-immune-endocrine) cells. Microbiol Immunol 45:403–411

Taupitz M, Schmitz S, Hamm B (2003) Superparamagnetic iron oxide particles: current state and future development. Rofo 175:752–765

Voura EB, Jaiswal JK, Mattoussi H et al (2004) Tracking metastatic tumor cell extravasation with quantum dot nanocrystals and fluorescence emission-scanning microscopy. Nat Med 10: 993–998

Vroemen M, Aigner L, Winkler J et al (2003) Adult neural progenitor cell grafts survive after acute spinal cord injury and integrate along axonal pathways. Eur J Neurosci 18:743–751

Vuu K, Xie J, McDonald MA et al (2005) Gadolinium-rhodamine nanoparticles for cell labeling and tracking via magnetic resonance and optical imaging. Bioconjug Chem 16:995–999

Walter GA, Cahill KS, Huard J et al (2004) Noninvasive monitoring of stem cell transfer for muscle disorders. Magn Reson Med 51:273–277

Weissleder R, Ntziachristos (2003) Shedding light onto live molecular targets. Nat Med 9:123–128

Weissleder R, Elizondo G, Wittenberg J et al (1990) Ultrasmall superparamagnetic iron oxide: characterization of a new class of contrast agents for MR imaging. Radiology 175:489–493

Weissleder R, Cheng HC, Bogdanova A et al (1997) Magnetically labeled cells can be detected by MR imaging. J Magn Reson Imaging 7:258–263

Yamamoto N, Jiang P, Yang M, et al. (2004). Cellular dynamics visualized in live cells in vitro and in vivo by differential dual-color nuclear-cytoplasic fluorescent-protein expression. Cancer Res 64:4251–4256

Wilhelm C, Billotey C, Roger J et al (2003) Intracellular uptake of anionic superparamagnetic nanoparticles as a function of their surface coating. Biomaterials 24:1001–1011

Yamauchi K, Yang M, Jiang P et al (2005) Real-time in vivo dual-color imaging of intracapillary cancer cell and nucleus deformation and migration. Cancer Res 65:4246–4252

Yeh TC, Zhang W, Ildstad ST et al (1993) Intracellular labeling of T-cells with superparamagnetic contrast agents. Magn Reson Med 30:617–625

Zelivyanskaya ML, Nelson JA, Poluektova L et al (2003) Tracking superparamagnetic iron oxide labeled monocytes in brain by high-field magnetic resonance imaging. J Neurosci Res 73: 284–295

Noninvasive Tracer Techniques to Characterize Angiogenesis

Roland Haubner

Abstract Great efforts are being made to develop antiangiogenesis drugs for treatment of cancer as well as other diseases. Some of the compounds are already in clinical trials. Imaging techniques allowing noninvasive monitoring of corresponding molecular processes can provide helpful information for planning and controlling corresponding therapeutic approaches but will also be of interest for basic science. Current nuclear medicine techniques focus on the development of tracer targeting the vascular endothelial growth factor (VEGF) system, matrix metalloproteinases (MMP), the ED-B domain of a fibronectin isoform, and the integrin $\alpha v \beta 3$. In this chapter, the recent tracer developments as well as the preclinical and the clinical evaluations are summarized and the potential of the different approaches to characterize angiogenesis are discussed.

1 Biological Background

Angiogenesis, the formation of new vessels out of the existing vasculature, is involved in numerous biological processes, such as embryogenesis, wound healing,

Roland Haubner
Universitätsklinik für Nuklearmedizin, Medizinische Universität Innsbruck, Anichstrasse 35, 6020 Innsbruck, Austria
roland.haubner@i-med.ac.at

W. Semmler and M. Schwaiger (eds.), *Molecular Imaging II.*
Handbook of Experimental Pharmacology 185/II.
323

tissue remodeling and female reproductive cycle. Also, numerous disorders are characterized by either an excess or an insufficient number of blood vessels. Best known disorders are rheumatoid arthritis (Storgard et al. 1999), psoriasis (Creamer et al. 2002), restenosis (Bishop et al. 2001), diabetic retinopathy (Chavakis et al. 2002) and tumor growth (Folkman 2002).

Angiogenesis is a multistep process, which is regulated by a balance between pro- and antiangiogenic factors (Ellis et al. 2002; Kuwano et al. 2001). The angiogenic switch is often triggered by an insufficient nutrient supply, resulting in hypoxic cells (Carmeliet and Jain 2000). Binding of the hypoxia inducible factor to the hypoxia response element activates expression of vascular endothelial growth factor (VEGF), a key player in vessel growth and maturation. Other stimuli include mechanical and metabolic stress, genetic mutations, and immune/inflammatory response. Additional regulating factors [e.g., basic and acid fibroblast growth factor (bFGF, aFGF), platelet-derived endothelial cell growth factor (PDGF)] are locally secreted by a variety of cells, but can also emanate from blood and the extracellular matrix (Hagedorn and Bikfalvi 2000; Kuwano et al. 2001).

After activation, the endothelial cells excrete proteolytic enzymes [e.g., matrix metalloproteinases (MMPs)], to degrade the basement membrane and the extracellular matrix (ECM) (Rundhaug 2005; Vihinen and Kahari 2002). Beside the proteolytic activity, MMPs have a proangiogenic role, by, for example, releasing matrix-bound proangiogenic factors, but can also play an antiangiogenic role, by, for example, cleaving matrix components into antiangiogenic factors [for details see (Rundhaug 2005)].

One receptor class playing a key role during migration of endothelial cells in the basement membrane are the integrins (Eliceiri and Cheresh 2000; Hynes et al. 1999). But these receptors are not only involved in endothelial cell adhesion, they are also important regulators of endothelial cell growth, survival and differentiation. It has been demonstrated that antibodies as well as low-molecular-weight antagonists recognizing the integrins $\alpha v \beta 3$ and $\alpha v \beta 5$, block angiogenesis in murine tumor models and in retinal angiogenesis (Brooks et al. 1994, 1995; Hammes et al. 1996). However, based on several knock-out experiments, there is evidence that $\alpha v \beta 3$ and $\alpha v \beta 5$ are rather antiangiogenic or negative regulators of angiogenesis than proangiogenic (Hynes 2002).

In further steps, extracellular matrix proteins such as tenascin, laminin, or collagen type IV are produced to provide new ECM components. By forming tight junctions, the endothelial cells reorganize, leading to newly built tubes. These new tubes connect with the microcirculation resulting in an operational new vasculature.

2 Molecular Targets for Imaging Angiogenesis

As described, angiogenesis is a multistep process which offers a variety of targets for therapeutic interventions (Hagedorn and Bikfalvi 2000). Thus, great efforts are being made to develop corresponding drugs. These developments are focused on growth receptor antagonists, metalloproteinase inhibitors, adhesion antagonists, and antagonists blocking endothelial cell function (e.g., angiostatin).

In preclinical studies, successful effects on tumor growth and metastasis formation could be demonstrated for a variety of different compounds. Those encouraging experimental studies have already led to initial clinical trials (Gasparini et al. 2005; Rosen 2000). However, currently available imaging techniques are limited in monitoring treatment using this class of drugs. Antitumor activity is generally assessed by determining the percentage of patients in whom a significant reduction of the tumor size is achieved during a relatively short period of therapy ("response rate"). Thus, this method may not be applicable for a form of therapy that is aimed at disease stabilization and prevention of metastases. Therefore, new methods are needed for planning and monitoring of treatments targeting the angiogenic process.

There are different approaches currently being studied, including magnetic resonance imaging, Doppler ultrasound and scintigraphic techniques. This chapter is focused on nuclear medicine tracer techniques for angiogenesis imaging.

Several potential targets for the design of radiolabelled compounds for monitoring of angiogenesis are conceivable. At the moment, most of the work is concentrated on the development of radiolabelled $\alpha v\beta3$-antagonists and MMP inhibitors. Another approach focuses on a single-chain Fv antibody fragment selectively binding to a particular fibronectin isoform and on antibodies/proteins targeting the VEGF system. All these approaches will be discussed here.

2.1 Radiolabelled Antibody Fragments Against the ED-B Domain of Fibronectin

Fibronectin exists in several isoforms (e.g., III CS, ED-A, ED-B) (Hynes 1985). These isoforms are involved in a variety of processes, including cell migration, wound healing, and oncogenic transformation. It has been shown that the isoform containing the ED-B domain is important in vascular proliferation and is widely expressed in fetal and neoplastic tissue. In contrast, it shows a highly restricted distribution in normal adult tissue (Castellani et al. 2000). Neri et al. (1997) demonstrated that the fluorescence-labelled anti-ED-B single-chain Fv antibody fragment selectively accumulates around blood vessels in tumor tissue in a murine tumor model. Based on these results, a radioiodinated anti-ED-B antibody fragment with affinities in the picomolar range has been synthesized. The selectively binding radiolabelled single-chain fragment scFv(L19) showed high accumulation in different animal/tumor models (Tarli et al. 1999). In addition, microautoradiography and immunohistochemistry demonstrated selective accumulation in tumor vessels. In contrast, no activity accumulation was found in vessels of other organs.

In an initial clinical study (Santimaria et al. 2003), including patients with lung, colorectal, or brain cancer, in 16 of 20 patients injected with the ^{123}I-labelled dimeric single-chain fragment L19(scFv)$_2$ different levels of tracer accumulation were found either in the primary tumor or metastases 6 h post injection. These data indicate that radiolabelled antibody fragments against the ED-B domain of fibronectin are potential new tracers for noninvasive angiogenesis monitoring. Moreover, modification resulting in a trimethyl-stannyl benzoate bifunctional derivative allows labelling with ^{211}At and offers a new approach for radioimmunotherapy (Demartis et al. 2001).

Meanwhile, a variety of different formats have been tested to identify the best-suited radioimmunoconjugate (Berndorff et al. 2005; Borsi et al. 2002). These studies include the complete human IgG1 L19-IgG1 ($\sim$150kDa), the "small immunoprotein" L19-SIP ($\sim$80kDa), and the single-chain fragment scFv(L19) ($\sim$50kDa). The fastest clearance, but also the lowest stability, was found for scFv(L19). The most favorable therapeutic index in a murine tumor model was found for ^{131}I-labelled L19-SIP, resulting in significant tumor growth delay and prolonged survival after a single injection in a F9 murine teratocarcinoma model. In a further study (Tijink et al. 2006), the potential of radioimmunotherapy with ^{131}I-L19-SIP, either alone or in combination with cetuximab, for treatment of head and neck squamous cell carcinoma has been evaluated. A significant tumor growth delay and improved survival in murine FaDu as well as HNX-OE models have been found. The best survival and cure rates were obtained, however, when radioimmunotherapy and cetuximab were combined. Altogether, these data indicate that ED-B fibronectin-targeted radioimmunotherapy could be a new approach to treat solid tumors.

2.2 Tracer for Imaging VEGF or the VEGF Receptor

VEGF, a central cytokine in the angiogenic process, plays an important role in the development of new vasculature (e.g., during embryogenesis and tumorgenesis). There are some isoforms which are freely diffusible (e.g., VEGF$_{165}$, VEGF$_{145}$, VEGF$_{121}$) but also isoforms which remain cell-associated (e.g., VEGF$_{206}$, VEGF$_{189}$) (Cross and Claesson-Welsh 2001). The major isoform found in tumors is VEGF$_{165}$, which can associate with cells via a heparin-binding domain (Neufeld et al. 1996). The VEGF receptor family consists of VEGFR-1 (or flt-1), VEGFR-2 (or KDR/flk-1), and VEGFR-3. The first two are found on vascular endothelial cells, whereas the latter is expressed on lymphatic endothelial cells (Cross and Claesson-Welsh 2001). Both the receptors and the ligands are targets for developing tracer for monitoring angiogensesis.

2.2.1 Radiolabelled VEGF Derivatives

Li et al. (2001) carried out direct labelling of VEGF$_{165}$ and VEGF$_{121}$ with ^{123}I-iodine and found that labelling does not influence the functional properties of both proteins. This was recently confirmed for VEGF$_{165}$ by Cornelissen et al. (2005). In addition, it was found that [^{123}I]VEGF$_{165}$ binds to a higher number of different tumor cell types as $[^{123}I]VEGF_{121}$. Thus, for a first patient study including 18 patients with gastrointestinal tumors $[^{123}I]VEGF_{165}$ uptake was determined. An overall VEGF receptor sensitivity of 58% was found, varying from 78% for primary pancreatic cancers to 33% for lung metastasis (Li et al. 2003). A safety and radiation dosimetry study including data from nine patients with pancreatic carcinoma showed favorable dosimetry with the highest absorbed organ dose in thyroid indicating some deiodination of the tracer (Li et al. 2004). However, no detailed analysis of tumor tissue has been carried out to identify correlation of tracer uptake with receptor expression or vessel density.

Another strategy uses the interactions between two fragments of the ribonuclease I known as HuS and Hu-tag (Blankenberg et al. 2004). The $[^{99m}Tc]HYNIC$-HuS binds to the Hu-tag conjugated to $VEGF_{121}$ forming the radiolabelled protein complex. This approach may avoid loss of targeting activity which can occur by direct labelling of proteins. Indeed they found a marked decreased ability of the HYNIC-VEGF to stimulate the VEGFR-2 compared with native VEGF or HuS/Hu-VEGF. The authors emphasize that they can image tumor vasculature even in very small tumors. However, owing to the increased dissociation of injected complexes in the larger blood pool in humans compared with mice, this adapter/docking tag system may be much less effective for clinical imaging. Thus, the same group developed a cysteine-containing peptide tag (C-tag) (Blankenberg et al. 2006). The corresponding fusion proteins can be conjugated with a bifunctional chelator (here HYNIC-maleimide). $[^{99m}Tc]HYNIC$-C-tagged VEGF allows visualization of the tumor in Balb/c mice with 4T1 murine mammary carcinoma. Moreover, uptake decreased in mice treated with different dose regimens using cyclophosphamide. Based on these preclinical data, the authors concluded that $[^{99m}Tc]HYNIC$-C-tagged VEGF can be rapidly prepared for imaging of tumors and its response to chemotherapy. However, biodistribution data also showed a comparable or even higher activity concentration in many organs, including lungs, spleen, liver and kidneys.

2.2.2 Anti-VEGF Antibodies

In addition to the approaches with radiolabelled VEGF derivatives, a monoclonal antibody (VG76e) recognizing human $VEGF_{121}$, $VEGF_{165}$, and $VEGF_{189}$ has been used (Collingridge et al. 2002). In this study different radioiodine labelling strategies — including direct labelling via the IodoGen method and indirect labelling via the Bolton-Hunter reagent or m-N-succiniimidyl iodobenzoic acid — have been compared. Great differences in immunoreactivity and binding affinities have been found for the antibodies labelled via the different strategies, with the best results obtained using the Bolton-Hunter method. Here, the direct-labelling strategy resulted in a loss of immunoreactivity. In-vivo evaluation of the best derivative showed a slow and time-dependent activity accumulation in the tumor tissue, reaching peak levels not before 24 h after tracer injection. At this time point, most of the normal tissue showed a lower activity concentration than the tumor. Thus, further studies in patients are planned to evaluate the potential of this tracer.

2.3 Radiolabelled MMP Inhibitors

Matrix metalloproteinases are capable of degrading proteins of the extracellular matrix (Curran and Murray 2000). The MMP family is divided into five classes: collagenases (MMP-1, MMP-8, MMP-13), gelatinases (MMP-2, MMP-9), stromolysins (MMP-3, MMP-7, MMP-10, MMP-11, MMP-12), membrane type (MT)-MMPs (MMP-14, MMP-15, MMP-16, MMP-17) and nonclassified MMPs (MMP-18, MMP-19, MMP-20, MMP-23, MMP-24) (Hidalgo and Eckhardt 2001). MMP activity is controlled by a balance between expression of endogenous MMP inhibitors and proenzyme synthesis (Gomez et al. 1997). An increased proenzyme production results in degradation of the basement membrane and the extracelluar matrix (Foda and Zucker 2001). The gelatinases MMP-2 and MMP-9 are most consistently detected in malignant tissue (Iwata et al. 1996; Nguyen et al. 2001). Their overexpression correlates with tumor aggressiveness and metastatic potential. Due to their important role in tumor-induced angiogenesis and metastasis, MMPs are potential targets for therapeutic interventions (Matter 2001; Vihinen and Kahari 2002). Thus, great efforts are being made to develop MMP inhibitors. Many of them are in preclinical or already in clinical studies.

2.3.1 Peptide Based Inhibitors

Using phage display libraries a disulfide bridged decapeptide (CTTHWGFTLC) was found which selectively inhibits MMP-2 and MMP-9 (Koivunen et al. 1999). This peptide suppressed migration of endothelial and tumor cells in vitro and mediated homing of phages in the tumor vasculature. Based on these results, yCT-THWGFTLC was synthesized, radioiodinated and evaluated (Kuhnast et al. 2004). In-vitro data showed that the modified peptide has similar inhibitory capacities for MMP-2 as found for the parent peptide and that the tracer was not degraded by activated MMP-2 and MMP-9. However, in-vivo studies revealed low metabolic stability and high lipophilicity, resulting in moderate uptake in the tumor but high activity concentration in liver and kidneys, indicating that further improvements concerning metabolic stability as well as pharmacokinetic behavior have to be carried out to make this compound suitable for imaging angiogensis.

2.3.2 Small Molecular Mass Inhibitors

Due to the importance of MMPs during tumor-induced angiogenesis and tumor metastasis, numerous peptidomimetic and nonpeptidic inhibitors are currently being investigated. Detailed structure activity investigations (Aranapakam et al. 2003; Kiyama et al. 1999; Levy et al. 1998; Pelmenschikov and Siegbahn 2002) showed that some of the most important characteristics for high-affinity binding are a coordination site binding to the catalytic zinc ion, a lipophilic site interacting with a hydrophobic cleft, and hydrophobic interactions between the sulfonylamide substituent of the corresponding ligand and the binding pocket.

Starting from different D-amino acid scaffolds, ^{18}F-labelled MMP-2 inhibitors have been synthesized (Furumoto et al. 2002). In-vitro assays demonstrated micromolar inhibitory activities. Based on an other N-sulfonylamino acid derivative, a ^{11}C-labelled analogue was synthesized, which showed strong inhibitory effectiveness for the gelatinases MMP-2 and MMP-9 (Kuhnast et al. 2003). A broad range MMP inhibitor belonging again to the N-sulfonylamino acid family was used as a further lead structure for the synthesis of [11]C- and ^{18}F-labelled derivatives (Fei et al. 2002, 2003a; Zheng et al. 2002, 2003). They were either labelled at the phenyl group or at the hydroxamic acid function. Some of the described radiolabelled compounds have comparable inhibitory effectiveness on MMP-1 as found for the parent structure CGS 27023A. Recently, radiolabelled biphenylsulfonamide-based MMP inhibitors have been developed (Fei et al. 2003b), which showed high inhibitory effectiveness on MMP-13. Oltenfreiter et al. (2004, 2005a) labelled hydroxamic and carboxylic acid-containing MMP inhibitors also based on amino acid scaffolds. Labelling was carried out via an electrophilic aromatic substitution using ^{123}I-iodine. Again these compounds showed high inhibitory capacities on gelatinases.

However, in contrast to the promising in-vitro data, the data resulting from the in-vivo evaluations, carried out yet, are not very promising. For some tracers, biodistribution data in normal mice indicate favorable pharmacokinetics (Kuhnast et al. 2003; Oltenfreiter et al. 2004, 2005a) and metabolic stability (Kuhnast et al. 2003). However, the biodistribution studies as well as micro-PET images using murine tumor models demonstrated low tracer accumulation in the corresponding tumors (Oltenfreiter et al. 2005b; Zheng et al. 2003, 2004). Altogether, a variety of radiolabelled compounds have been introduced which showed in-vitro assays with promising results. But, at the moment, corresponding in-vivo data do not confirm that this class of tracer allows monitoring of angiogenesis. Thus, before further compounds are introduced, a detailed verification of the corresponding animal models may be of great importance.

2.4 Radiolabelled Integrin Antagonists

The integrin αvβ3 is involved in mediating the migration of endothelial cells during blood vessel formation. Moreover, it plays an important role in a diversity of pathological dysfunctions, including osteoporosis, restenosis, inflammatory processes, and tumor metastasis, making it an interesting target for drug development. A unique binding epitope found in several extracellular matrix proteins is the amino acid sequence arginine-glycine-aspartic acid (RGD, amino acid single letter code) (Ruoslahti and Pierschbacher 1987). Thus, a variety of linear as well as cyclic peptide antagonists, including the RGD-sequence, have been developed. Intensive structure/activity relationship studies resulted in the cyclic pentapeptide cyclo(-Arg-Gly-Asp-DPhe-Val-), which showed high affinity and selectivity for αvβ3 [for a review, see Haubner et al. (1997)]. This peptide has been used as a lead structure for the development of radiotracers for the noninvasive determination of the $\alpha v\beta 3$ integrin status using nuclear medicine tracer techniques (Haubner 2006; Haubner and Wester 2004). The first evaluation of this approach has been carried out using the radioiodinated peptides 3-[*I]Iodo-DTyr[4]-cyclo(-Arg-Gly-Asp-DTyr-Val-) and 3-[*I]Iodo-Tyr[5]-cyclo(-Arg-Gly-Asp-DPhe-Tyr-) (Haubner et al. 1999). These compounds showed comparable affinity and selectivity as the lead structure and receptor-specific accumulation in the tumor. However, the predominantly hepatobiliary elimination resulted in unfavorable activity concentration in the liver and intestine. Thus, different strategies to improve the pharmacokinetic behavior of these radiolabelled peptides have been studied. They include conjugation with sugar moieties, hydrophilic amino acids and polyethylene glycol.

2.4.1 Optimization of Pharmacokinetics

The glycosylation approach (Haubner et al. 2001a, 2001b) is based on the introduction of sugar amino acids (SAA), which were conjugated to the pentapeptide via the ε-amino function of the corresponding lysine. In biodistribution studies, the resulting glycosylated peptides ([*I]Gluco-RGD (Haubner et al. 2001a) and [18F]Galacto-RGD (Haubner et al. 2001b, 2004b)) showed a clearly reduced activity concentration in liver and an increased activity uptake and retention in the tumor compared with the first-generation peptides. Currently, [18F]Galacto-RGD is being evaluated in a clinical study, in which it has demonstrated high metabolic stability and rapid predominant renal excretion, resulting in good tumor/background ratios (Beer et al. 2005, 2006; Haubner et al. 2005). In addition, this initial study indicates that tracer accumulation correlates with $\alpha v\beta 3$ expression on blood vessels in the tumor lesions. Moreover, great inter- and intraindividual variation in tracer accumulation was found, indicating great differences in receptor expression and demonstrating the importance of these techniques for the planning and controlling of corresponding anti-$\alpha v\beta 3$-directed therapies.

Tetrapeptides containing hydrophobic D-amino acids were also used to improve the pharmacokinetics of peptide-based tracer (Haubner et al. 2002). D-Amino acids were used to guarantee metabolic stability of the compounds. The [18F]-labelled peptides showed high $\alpha v\beta 3$ selectivity and receptor-specific accumulation. However, tracer uptake in the M21 melanoma was lower compared with the glycosylated RGD-peptides. Nevertheless, due to the rapid predominantly renal elimination of [18F]DAsp$_3$-RGD tumor/background ratios calculated from small animal PET images were comparable with [18F]Galacto-RGD.

The third strategy uses polyethylene glycol (PEG) conjugation, which can improve several properties of peptides and proteins, including immunogenicity, plasma stability, and pharmacokinetics (Harris and Chess 2003; Harris et al. 2001). Thus, a 2-kDa PEG moiety was attached to the ε-amino function of cyclo(-Arg-Gly-Asp-DTyr-Lys-) (Chen et al. 2004d). The [125I]-labeled PEGylated derivative ([125I]-RGD-PEG) was compared with the radioiodinated cyclo(-Arg-Gly-Asp-DTyr-Lys-) ([125I]-RGD). The PEGylated derivative showed a more rapid blood clearance, a decreased activity concentration in the kidneys and a slightly increased activity retention in the tumor. However, tumor uptake for ^{125}I-RGD-PEG was lower and activity retention in liver and intestine was higher, as found for ^{125}I-RGD. In another study, $[^{18}F]$FB-RGD, a $[^{18}F]$fluorobenzoyl-labelled RGD peptide, and the PE-Gylated analogue $[^{18}F]$FB-PEG-RGD were compared (Chen et al. 2004c). Again, activity retention of the PEGylated peptide in the tumor was improved compared with the lead structure. But initial elimination from blood was slower and the activity concentration in the liver and kidneys was higher, as for $[^{18}F]$FB-RGD. $[^{18}F]$FB-RGD was used to image brain-tumor growth in a murine tumor model (Chen et al. 2005). In this model, longitudinal microPET imaging allowed visualization and quantification of anatomical variations during brain tumor growth and angiogenesis. In addition, the effect of PEGylation was studied by comparing ^{64}Cu-DOTA-RGD and ^{64}Cu-DOTA-PEG-RGD (Chen et al. 2004a). In this case, PEGylation reduced activity concentration in the liver and small intestine, and resulted in a faster blood clearance, while the tumor uptake as well as retention was not affected. In summary, these studies revealed very different effects of PEGylation on the pharmacokinetics and tumor uptake of RGD-peptides, which seem to strongly depend on the nature of the lead structure.

2.4.2 Radiometalated Derivatives

In addition to the radiohalogenated peptides, a variety of peptides labelled with ^{99m}Tc-technitium, ^{111}In-indium, ^{64}Cu-copper, ^{90}Y-yttrium and ^{188}Re-rhenium have been introduced. In most cases, the corresponding chelator system is conjugated via the ε-amino function of the lysine of cyclo(-Arg-Gly-Asp-DPhe/Tyr-Lys-). Van Hagen et al. (2000) demonstrated αvβ3 selective binding of DTPA-RGD on blood vessels of human tumor-tissue sections using receptor autoradiography and immunohistochemistry. Recently, DTPA-RGD-peptides have been synthesized using a solid-phase system (Wang et al. 2005). The authors suggest that this approach may allow construction of DTPA-containing peptide libraries for high throughput screening.

Conjugation of the tetrapeptide sequence H-Asp-Lys-Cys-Lys-OH with the cyclic pentapeptide and subsequent ^{99m}Tc-labelling resulted in $[^{99m}Tc]$DKCK-RGD (Haubner et al. 2004a). Gamma-camera images 4 h p.i. showed a clearly contrasting tumor but also high activity concentration in the kidneys, which may be due to the lysine-containing chelating sequence. Thus, further optimization concerning metabolic stability and pharmacokinetic behavior seems to be recommended. Most recently, cyclo(-Arg-Gly-Asp-DTyr-Lys-) was conjugated with different chelator systems, including HYNIC, a pyrazolyl-derivative, an isonitril-conjugate and a Cys-moiety (Decristoforo et al. 2006, 2007). The compounds could be labelled with high specific activities in high radiochemical yields. In-vitro stability was high for all compounds, but plasma protein binding and lipophilicity varied considerably between different radiolabelled conjugates, resulting in significant differences concerning pharmacokinetic behaviour as well as tumour uptake (0.2–2.7% ID/g). The highest specific tumour uptake and tumour/background ratios were found for ^{99m}Tc-EDDA/HYNIC-cyclo(-Arg-Gly-Asp-DTyr-Lys-), which are comparable with $[^{18}F]$-Galacto-RGD.

A DOTA conjugated RGD-peptide was labelled with ^{64}Cu-copper and compared with the radioiodinated cyclo(-Arg-Gly-Asp-DTyr-Lys-) (Chen et al. 2004e). In a murine orthotopic human breast cancer model, the ^{64}Cu-labelled peptide showed lower tumor uptake and retention and unfavorable activity retention in liver and kidneys. The authors argue that the high liver uptake could be due to ^{64}Cu-transchelation to superoxide dismutase and/or the persistent localization of the possible metabolite ^{64}Cu-DOTA-Lys-OH in this tissue. However, good tumor/blood and tumor/muscle ratios 1 h p.i. allowed clear delineation of the tumor. Nevertheless, the highest activity concentration was found in liver, intestine and bladder, indicating that further optimization of the tracer is needed. One approach using PEGylated RGD-peptides resulting in decreased activity concentration in liver and small intestine has already been discussed above (Chen et al. 2004a).

The disulfide-bridged undecapeptide RGD-4C (Cys^2-Cys^{10}, Cys^4-Cys^8) H-Ala-Cys-Asp-Cys-Arg-Gly-Asp-Cys-Phe-Cys-Gly-OH has also been used as an alternative lead structure. RGD-4C binds with high affinity ($K_D \sim 100$ nM) to both integrin $\alpha v \beta 3$ and $\alpha v \beta 5$ (Assa-Munt et al. 2001). The derivative (Cys^1-Cys^9, Cys^3-Cys^7)H-Cys-Asp-Cys-Arg-Gly-Asp-Cys-Phe-Cys-OH was conjugated with HYNIC and labelled using ^{99m}Tc (Su et al. 2002, 2003). However, in murine tumor models only marginal tumor uptake was found, which can be explained by the low association constant of this ^{99m}Tc-labelled RGD-4C derivative for $\alpha v \beta 3$ (7×10^6 M^{-1}). Thus, either the deletion of the terminal amino acids, the conjugation with HYNIC, and/or the labelling with ^{99m}Tc-technetium impairs the affinity, resulting in a peptide that appears unsuitable for in-vivo imaging of $\alpha v \beta 3$ expression.

2.4.3 The "Multimerization" Approach

In addition to the monomeric RGD peptides, multimeric compounds presenting more than one RGD site have also been introduced. The most obvious advantage of this "multimerization" concept is that multimeric tracers should show higher uptake at the target site due to an increased apparent ligand concentration. Janssen et al. (2002a, 2002b) conjugated two cyclo(-Arg-Gly-Asp-DPhe-Lys-) peptides via a glutamic acid linker. DOTA or HYNIC were used as chelator moieties and coupled to the free amino function of the linker. The dimeric ^{99m}Tc-HYNIC-Glu-[cyclo(-Arg-Gly-Asp-DPhe-Lys-)]$_2$ showed a tenfold higher affinity for $\alpha v \beta 3$ and a better retention as the monomeric ^{99m}Tc-HYNIC-cyclo(-Arg-Gly-Asp-DPhe-Lys-). However, activity retention of ^{99m}Tc-HYNIC-Glu-[cyclo(-Arg-Gly-Asp-DPhe-Lys-)]$_2$ in kidneys was also high.

In a systematic study on the influence of mulitmerization on receptor affinity and tumor uptake, a series of monomeric, dimeric, tetrameric and octameric RGD peptides have been synthesized (Poethko et al. 2004a, 2004b; Thumshirn et al. 2003).

The multimers were produced by conjugating the monomeric peptide cyclo(-Arg-Gly-Asp-DPhe-Glu-) via corresponding PEG linker and lysine moieties. Labelling is based on the chemoselective oxime formation. Therefore, the linker was modified via an aminooxo function. As a prosthetic group an ^{18}F-labelled aldehyde has been used. In in-vitro assays, an increasing binding affinity in the series monomer, dimer, tetramer and octamer has been found. Initial PET images resulting from a clinical scanner confirm these findings. Images of mice bearing the $\alpha v\beta 3$-positive melanoma on the right flank and the $\alpha v\beta 3$-negative melanoma on the left flank showed an increasing activity accumulation in the receptor-positive tumor in the series monomer, dimer and tetramer.

In another study, the dimeric peptide Glu-[cyclo(-Arg-Gly-Asp-DTyr-Lys-)]$_2$ was labelled by conjugating 4-[^{18}F]fluorobenzoic acid to the N^{α}-amino function of the glutamate (Chen et al. 2004f; Zhang et al. 2006). This dimer demonstrated significantly higher tumor uptake and extended tumor retention in comparison with the monomeric [^{18}F]FB-cyclo(-Arg-Gly-Asp-DTyr-Lys-). Moreover, the dimeric RGD peptide showed predominant renal excretion, whereas the monomeric peptide was excreted primarily via the biliary route. Hence, the authors conclude that the synergistic effect of polyvalency and improved pharmacokinetics may be responsible for the superior imaging characteristics. Comparable effects have been found for dimeric ^{64}Cu-labelled peptides (Chen et al. 2004b). In addition, the tetrameric [^{64}Cu]DOTA-Glu-{Glu-[cyclo(-Arg-Gly-Asp-DPhe-Lys-)]$_2$}$_2$ (Wu et al. 2005) showed significantly higher integrin binding affinity than the corresponding monomeric and dimeric RGD peptides, most likely due to a polyvalence effect. Once more, tumor uptake was rapid and high, and the tumor washout was slow.

3 Summary and Conclusion

Noninvasive monitoring of the angiogenic process would be of great interest for clinicians as well as basic science. Several approaches, including nuclear medicine tracer techniques, are currently being studied. In nuclear medicine, development is focused on radiolabelled tracer allowing the noninvasive determination of the ED-B domain of fibronectin, the expression of VEGF and the VEGF receptor, matrix metalloproteinases or the $\alpha v\beta 3$ integrin.

The ^{123}I-labeled antibody fragment against the ED-B domain of a fibronectin isoform widely expressed on neoplastic tissue was studied in 20 patients. In 16 patients, different levels of tracer accumulation were found.

Immunohistochemical staining of tumor tissue using an antibody against the ED-B domain has shown that the protein is expressed in the tumor vasculature. In further studies, it has to be demonstrated that the signal correlates with protein expression in corresponding patients. Moreover, a preclinical study with a ^{131}I-labelled analogue indicates that fibronectin ED-B-domain-targeted radioimmunotherapy may be a new approach to treat tumors.

To determine growth receptor expression, VEGF as well as anti-VEGF antibodies have been studied. In a preliminary study injecting $[^{123}I]VEGF_{165}$ into 18 patients with gastrointestinal tumors, an overall sensitivity of 58% was found. However, further studies — e.g., correlating the signal with VEGF receptor expression — have to demonstrate the potential of this strategy.

A variety of different MMP inhibitors have been studied for noninvasive determination of MMP activity. In contrast to the promising in-vitro data, corresponding in-vivo evaluation of some of those derivatives have not yet assessed the potential of this class of tracer to monitor angiogenesis.

Most work is focused on the development of tracers monitoring $\alpha v \beta 3$ integrin expression. The commonly used lead structure is the cyclic pentapeptide cyclo(-Arg-Gly-Asp-DPhe-Val-). Most detailed evaluation was carried out using the glycosylated derivative $[^{18}F]$Galacto-RGD. Preclinical as well as the first clinical studies, including more than 60 patients, strongly indicated that tracer uptake correlates with $\alpha v \beta 3$ integrin expression. Moreover, it was demonstrated that introduction of PEG and, especially, carbohydrates improved pharmacokinetic properties. In addition, it has been shown that derivatives containing two to eight RGD moieties in one compound resulted in an improved binding affinity in vitro and in an increased and prolonged uptake in vivo. A disadvantage concerning monitoring of tumor-induced angiogenesis is that this integrin is not only expressed on endothelial cells but can also be found on tumor cells. Thus, in oncological settings it will be problematic to clearly correlate the resulting signal with neovascularization but, nevertheless, $\alpha v \beta 3$ imaging will give helpful information for planning and controlling corresponding $\alpha v \beta 3$-targeted therapies. Concerning other pathological processes, the signal will exclusively originate from the activated endothelial cells and, consequently, may allow monitoring of the angiogenic process noninvasively.

In conclusion, great efforts are made to develop tracers for monitoring angiogenesis. At the moment, the most promising approach is based on the noninvasive determination of the $\alpha v \beta 3$ expression, where the most intensive biological evaluation has been carried out. However, for all approaches further pre- and clinical studies have to follow to allow final prediction about the potential of the different approaches in monitoring angiogenesis.

References

Aranapakam V, Davis JM, Grosu GT, Baker J, Ellingboe J, Zask A, Levin JI, Sandanayaka VP, Du M, Skotnicki JS, DiJoseph JF, Sung A, Sharr MA, Killar LM, Walter T, Jin G, Cowling R, Tillett J, Zhao W, McDevitt J, Xu ZB (2003) Synthesis and structure-activity relationship of N-substituted 4-arylsulfonylpiperidine-4-hydroxamic acids as novel, orally active matrix metalloproteinase inhibitors for the treatment of osteoarthritis. J Med Chem 46:2376–2396

Assa-Munt N, Jia X, Laakkonen P, Ruoslahti E (2001) Solution structures and integrin binding activities of an RGD peptide with two isomers. Biochemistry 40:2373–2378

Beer AJ, Haubner R, Goebel M, Luderschmidt S, Spilker ME, Wester HJ, Weber WA, Schwaiger M (2005) Biodistribution and pharmacokinetics of the alphavbeta3-selective tracer ^{18}F-Galacto-RGD in cancer patients. J Nucl Med 46:1333–1341

Beer AJ, Haubner R, Sarbia M, Goebel M, Luderschmidt S, Grosu AL, Schnell O, Niemeyer M, Kessler H, Wester HJ, Weber WA, Schwaiger M (2006) Positron emission tomography using [18F]Galacto-RGD identifies the level of integrin αvβ3 expression in man. Clin Cancer Res 12:3942–3949

Berndorff D, Borkowski S, Sieger S, Rother A, Friebe M, Viti F, Hilger CS, Cyr JE, Dinkelborg LM (2005) Radioimmunotherapy of solid tumors by targeting extra domain B fibronectin: identification of the best-suited radioimmunoconjugate. Clin Cancer Res 11:7053s–7063s

Bishop GG, McPherson JA, Sanders JM, Hesselbacher SE, Feldman MJ, McNamara CA, Gimple LW, Powers ER, Mousa SA, Sarembock IJ (2001) Selective αvβ3-receptor blockade reduces macrophage infiltration and restenosis after balloon angioplasty in the atherosclerotic rabbit. Circulation 103:1906–1911

Blankenberg FG, Mandl S, Cao YA, O'Connell-Rodwell C, Contag C, Mari C, Gaynutdinov TI, Vanderheyden JL, Backer MV, Backer JM (2004) Tumor imaging using a standardized radiolabeled adapter protein docked to vascular endothelial growth factor. J Nucl Med 45:1373–1380

Blankenberg FG, Backer MV, Levashova Z, Patel V, Backer JM (2006) In vivo tumor angiogenesis imaging with site-specific labeled 99mTc-HYNIC-VEGF. Eur J Nucl Med Mol Imaging 33: 841–848

Borsi L, Balza E, Bestagno M, Castellani P, Carnemolla B, Biro A, Leprini A, Sepulveda J, Burrone O, Neri D, Zardi L (2002) Selective targeting of tumoral vasculature: comparison of different formats of an antibody (L19) to the ED-B domain of fibronectin. Int J Cancer 102: 75–85

Brooks PC, Montgomery AM, Rosenfeld M, Reisfeld RA, Hu T, Klier G, Cheresh DA (1994) Integrin αvβ3 antagonists promote tumor regression by inducing apoptosis of angiogenic blood vessels. Cell 79:1157–1164

Brooks PC, Stromblad S, Klemke R, Visscher D, Sarkar FH, Cheresh DA (1995) Antiintegrin αvβ3 blocks human breast cancer growth and angiogenesis in human skin. J Clin Invest 96: 1815–1822

Carmeliet P, Jain RK (2000) Angiogenesis in cancer and other diseases. Nature 407:249–257

Castellani P, Dorcaratto A, Pau A, Nicola M, Siri A, Gasparetto B, Zardi L, Viale G (2000) The angiogenesis marker ED-B+ fibronectin isoform in intracranial meningiomas. Acta Neurochir 142:277–282

Chavakis E, Riecke B, Lin J, Linn T, Bretzel RG, Preissner KT, Brownlee M, Hammes HP (2002) Kinetics of integrin expression in the mouse model of proliferative retinopathy and success of secondary intervention with cyclic RGD peptides. Diabetologia 45:262–267

Chen X, Hou Y, Tohme M, Park R, Khankaldyyan V, Gonzales-Gomez I, Bading JR, Laug WE, Conti PS (2004a) Pegylated Arg-Gly-Asp peptide: 64Cu labeling and PET imaging of brain tumor αvβ3-integrin expression. J Nucl Med 45:1776–1783

Chen X, Liu S, Hou Y, Tohme M, Park R, Bading JR, Conti PS (2004b) MicroPET imaging of breast cancer αv-integrin expression with 64Cu-labeled dimeric RGD peptides. Mol Imaging Biol 6:350–359

Chen X, Park R, Hou Y, Khankaldyyan V, Gonzales-Gomez I, Tohme M, Bading JR, Laug WE, Conti PS (2004c) MicroPET imaging of brain tumor angiogenesis with 18F-labeled PEGylated RGD peptide. Eur J Nucl Med Mol Imaging 31:1081–1089

xChen X, Park R, Shahinian AH, Bading JR, Conti PS (2004d) Pharmacokinetics and tumor retention of 125I-labeled RGD peptide are improved by PEGylation. Nucl Med Biol 31:11–19

Chen X, Park R, Tohme M, Shahinian AH, Bading JR, Conti PS (2004e) MicroPET and autoradiographic imaging of breast cancer alpha v-integrin expression using 18F- and 64Cu-labeled RGD peptide. Bioconjug Chem 15:41–49

Chen X, Tohme M, Park R, Hou Y, Bading JR, Conti PS (2004f) Micro-PET imaging of alphavbeta3-integrin expression with 18F-labeled dimeric RGD peptide. Mol Imaging 3: 96–104

Chen X, Park R, Khankaldyyan V, Gonzales-Gomez I, Tohme M, Moats RA, Bading JR, Laug WE, Conti PS (2005) Longitudinal MicroPET Imaging of Brain Tumor Growth with F-18-labeled RGD peptide. Mol Imaging Biol 29:1–7

Collingridge DR, Carroll VA, Glaser M, Aboagye EO, Osman S, Hutchinson OC, Barthel H, Luthra SK, Brady F, Bicknell R, Price P, Harris AL (2002) The development of [^{124}I]iodinated-VG76e: a novel tracer for imaging vascular endothelial growth factor in vivo using positron emission tomography. Cancer Res 62:5912–5919

Cornelissen B, Oltenfreiter R, Kersemans V, Staelens L, Frankenne F, Foidart JM, Slegers G (2005) In vitro and in vivo evaluation of [^{123}I]-VEGF165 as a potential tumor marker. Nucl Med Biol 32:431–436

Creamer D, Sullivan D, Bicknell R, Barker J (2002) Angiogenesis in psoriasis. Angiogenesis 5:231–236

Cross MJ, Claesson-Welsh L (2001) FGF and VEGF function in angiogenesis: signalling pathways, biological responses and therapeutic inhibition. Trends Pharmacol Sci 22:201–207

Curran S, Murray GI (2000) Matrix metalloproteinases: molecular aspects of their roles in tumour invasion and metastasis. Eur J Cancer 36:1621–1630

Decristoforo C, Faintuch-Linkowski B, Rey A, von Guggenberg E, Rupprich M, Hernandez-Gonzales I, Rodrigo T, Haubner R (2006) [^{99m}Tc]HYNIC-RGD for imaging integrin αvβ3 expression. Nucl Med Biol 33:945–952

Decristoforo C, Santos I, Pietzsch HJ, Duatti A, Smith CJ, Rey A, Alberto R, von Guggenberg E, Haubner R (2007) Comparision of in vitro and in vivo properties of ^{99m}Tc-cRGD peptides labelled using different novel Tc-cores. Q J Nucl Med Mol Imaging 51:33–41

Demartis S, Tarli L, Borsi L, Zardi L, Neri D (2001) Selective targeting of tumour neovasculature by a radiohalogenated human antibody fragment specific for the ED-B domain of fibronectin. Eur J Nucl Med 28:534–539

Eliceiri BP, Cheresh DA (2000) Role of αv integrins during angiogenesis. Cancer J Sci Am 6:S245–S249

Ellis LM, Liu W, Fan F, Jung YD, Reinmuth N, Stoeltzing O, Takeda A, Akagi M, Parikh AA, Ahmad S (2002) Synopsis of angiogenesis inhibitors in oncology. Oncology 16:14–22

Fei X, Zheng QH, Hutchins GD, Liu X, Stone KL, Carlson KA, Mock BH, Winkle WL, Glick-Wilson BE, Miller KD, Fife RS, Sledge GW, Sun HB, Carr RE (2002) Synthesis of MMP inhibitor radiotracers [^{11}C]methyl-CGS 27023A and its analogs, new potential PET breast cancer imaging agents. J Label Compd Radiopharm 45:449–470

Fei X, Zheng Q-H, Liu X, Wang J-Q, Stone KL, Miller KD, Sledge GW, Hutchins GD (2003a) Synthesis of MMP inhibitor radiotracer [^{11}C]CGS 25966, a new potential PET tumor imaging agent. J Label Compd Radiopharm 46:343–351

Fei X, Zheng QH, Liu X, Wang JQ, Sun HB, Mock BH, Stone KL, Miller KD, Sledge GW, Hutchins GD (2003b) Synthesis of radiolabeled biphenylsulfonamide matrix metalloproteinase inhibitors as new potential PET cancer imaging agents. Bioorg Med Chem Lett 13:2217–2222

Foda HD, Zucker S (2001) Matrix metalloproteinases in cancer invasion, metastasis and angiogenesis. Drug Discov Today 6:478–482

Folkman J (2002) Role of angiogenesis in tumor growth and metastasis. Semin Oncol 29:15–18

Furumoto S, Iwata R, Ido T (2002) Design and synthesis of fluorine-18 labeled matrix metalloproteinase inhibitors for cancer imaging. J Label Compd Radiopharm 45:975–986

Gasparini G, Longo R, Toi M, Ferrara N (2005) Angiogenic inhibitors: a new therapeutic strategy in oncology. Nat Clin Pract Oncol 2:562–577

Gomez DE, Alonso DF, Yoshiji H, Thorgeirsson UP (1997) Tissue inhibitors of metalloproteinases: structure, regulation and biological functions. Eur J Cell Biol 74:111–122

Hagedorn M, Bikfalvi A (2000) Target molecules for anti-angiogenic therapy: from basic research to clinical trials. Crit Rev Oncol Hematol 34:89–110

Hammes HP, Brownlee M, Jonczyk A, Sutter A, Preissner KT (1996) Subcutaneous injection of a cyclic peptide antagonist of vitronectin receptor-type integrins inhibits retinal neovascularization. Nat Med 2:529–533

Harris JM, Chess RB (2003) Effect of pegylation on pharmaceuticals. Nat Rev Drug Discov 2: 214–221

Harris JM, Martin NE, Modi M (2001) Pegylation: a novel process for modifying pharmacokinetics. Clin Pharmacokinet 40:539–551

Haubner R (2006) $\alpha v \beta 3$-integrin imaging: a new approach to characterise angiogenesis? Eur J Nucl Med Mol Imaging 13:54–63

Haubner R, Wester HJ (2004) Radiolabeled tracers for imaging of tumor angiogenesis and evaluation of anti-angiogenic therapies. Curr Pharm Des 10:1439–1455

Haubner R, Finsinger D, Kessler H (1997) Stereoisomeric Peptide Libraries and Peptidomimetics for Designing Selective Inhibitors of the $\alpha v \beta 3$ Integrin for a New Cancer Therapy. Angew Chem Int Ed Engl 36:1374–1389

Haubner R, Wester HJ, Reuning U, Senekowitsch-Schmidtke R, Diefenbach B, Kessler H, Stocklin G, Schwaiger M (1999) Radiolabeled $\alpha v \beta 3$ integrin antagonists: a new class of tracers for tumor targeting. J Nucl Med 40:1061–1071

Haubner R, Wester HJ, Burkhart F, Senekowitsch-Schmidtke R, Weber W, Goodman SL, Kessler H, Schwaiger M (2001a) Glycosylated RGD-containing peptides: tracer for tumor targeting and angiogenesis imaging with improved biokinetics. J Nucl Med 42:326–336

Haubner R, Wester HJ, Weber WA, Mang C, Ziegler SI, Goodman SL, Senekowitsch-Schmidtke R, Kessler H, Schwaiger M (2001b) Noninvasive imaging of $\alpha v \beta 3$ integrin expression using ^{18}F-labeled RGD-containing glycopeptide and positron emission tomography. Cancer Res 61:1781–1785

Haubner R, Kuhnast B, Wester HJ, Weber WA, Huber R, Senekowitsch-Schmidtke R, Ziegler SI, Goodman SL, Kessler H, Schwaiger M (2002) [F-18]-RGD-Peptides Conjugated with Hydrophilic Tetrapeptides for the Noninvasive Determination of the $\alpha v \beta 3$ Integrin. J Nucl Med 43 (Suppl):89P

Haubner R, Bruchertseifer F, Bock M, Kessler H, Schwaiger M, Wester HJ (2004a) Synthesis and biological evaluation of a ^{99m}Tc-labelled cyclic RGD peptide for imaging the alphavbeta3 expression. Nuklearmedizin 43:26–32

Haubner R, Kuhnast B, Mang C, Weber WA, Kessler H, Wester HJ, Schwaiger M (2004b) ^{18}F]Galacto-RGD: synthesis, radiolabeling, metabolic stability, and radiation dose estimates. Bioconjug Chem 15:61–69

Haubner R, Weber WA, Beer AJ, Vabuliene E, Reim D, Sarbia M, Becker KF, Goebel M, Hein R, Wester HJ, Kessler H, Schwaiger M (2005) Noninvasive visualization of the activated alphavbeta3 integrin in cancer patients by positron emission tomography and ^{18}F]Galacto-RGD. PLoS Med 2:29

Hidalgo M, Eckhardt SG (2001) Development of matrix metalloproteinase inhibitors in cancer therapy. J Natl Cancer Inst 93:178–93

Hynes R (1985) Molecular biology of fibronectin. Annu Rev Cell Biol 1:67–90

Hynes RO (2002) A reevaluation of integrins as regulators of angiogenesis. Nat Med 8:918–921

Hynes RO, Bader BL, Hodivala-Dilke K (1999) Integrins in vascular development. Braz J Med Biol Res 32:501–510

Iwata H, Kobayashi S, Iwase H, Masaoka A, Fujimoto N, Okada Y (1996) Production of matrix metalloproteinases and tissue inhibitors of metalloproteinases in human breast carcinomas. Jpn J Cancer Res 87:602–611

Janssen ML, Oyen WJ, Dijkgraaf I, Massuger LF, Frielink C, Edwards DS, Rajopadhye M, Boonstra H, Corstens FH, Boerman OC (2002a) Tumor targeting with radiolabeled $\alpha v \beta 3$ integrin binding peptides in a nude mouse model. Cancer Res 62:6146–6151

Janssen MLH, Oyen WJG, Massuger LFAG, Frielink C, Dijkgraaf I, Edwards DS, Rajopadhye WJ, Corstens FHM, Boerman OC (2002b) Comparison of a monomeric and dimeric radiolabeled RGD-peptide for tumor imaging. Cancer Biother Radiopharm 17:641–646

Kiyama R, Tamura Y, Watanabe F, Tsuzuki H, Ohtani M, Yodo M (1999) Homology modeling of gelatinase catalytic domains and docking simulations of novel sulfonamide inhibitors. J Med Chem 42:1723–1738

Koivunen E, Arap W, Valtanen H, Rainisalo A, Medina OP, Heikkila P, Kantor C, Gahmberg CG, Salo T, Konttinen YT, Sorsa T, Ruoslahti E, Pasqualini R (1999) Tumor targeting with a selective gelatinase inhibitor. Nat Biotechnol 17:768–774

Kuhnast B, Bodenstein C, Wester HJ, Weber WA (2003) Carbon-11 labeling of a N-sulfonylamino acid derivative: a potential tracer for MMP-2 and MMP-9 imaging. J Label Compd Radiopharm 46:1093–1103

Kuhnast B, Bodenstein C, Haubner R, Wester HJ, Senekowitsch-Schmidtke R, Schwaiger M, Weber WA (2004) Targeting of gelatinase activity with a radiolabeled cyclic HWGF peptide. Nucl Med Biol 31:337–344

Kuwano M, Fukushi J, Okamoto M, Nishie A, Goto H, Ishibashi T, Ono M (2001) Angiogenesis factors. Intern Med 40:565–572

Levy DE, Lapierre F, Liang W, Ye W, Lange CW, Li X, Grobelny D, Casabonne M, Tyrrell D, Holme K, Nadzan A, Galardy RE (1998) Matrix metalloproteinase inhibitors: a structure-activity study. J Med Chem 41:199–223

Li S, Peck-Radosavljevic M, Koller E, Koller F, Kaserer K, Kreil A, Kapiotis S, Hamwi A, Weich HA, Valent P, Angelberger P, Dudczak R, Virgolini I (2001) Characterization of ^{123}I-vascular endothelial growth factor-binding sites expressed on human tumour cells: possible implication for tumour scintigraphy. Int J Cancer 91:789–796

Li S, Peck-Radosavljevic M, Kienast O, Preitfellner J, Hamilton G, Kurtaran A, Pirich C, Angelberger P, Dudczak R (2003) Imaging gastrointestinal tumours using vascular endothelial growth factor-165 (VEGF165) receptor scintigraphy. Ann Oncol 14:1274–1277

Li S, Peck-Radosavljevic M, Kienast O, Preitfellner J, Havlik E, Schima W, Traub-Weidinger T, Graf S, Beheshti M, Schmid M, Angelberger P, Dudczak R (2004) Iodine-123-vascular endothelial growth factor-165 (^{123}I-VEGF165). Biodistribution, safety and radiation dosimetry in patients with pancreatic carcinoma. Q J Nucl Med Mol Imaging 48:198–206

Matter A (2001) Tumor angiogenesis as a therapeutic target. Drug Discov Today 6:1005–1024

Neri D, Carnemolla B, Nissim A, Leprini A, Querze G, Balza E, Pini A, Tarli L, Halin C, Neri P, Zardi L, Winter G (1997) Targeting by affinity-matured recombinant antibody fragments of an angiogenesis associated fibronectin isoform. Nat Biotechnol 15:1271–1275

Neufeld G, Cohen T, Gitay-Goren H, Poltorak Z, Tessler S, Sharon R, Gengrinovitch S, Levi BZ (1996) Similarities and differences between the vascular endothelial growth factor (VEGF) splice variants. Cancer Metastasis Rev 15:153–158

Nguyen M, Arkell J, Jackson CJ (2001) Human endothelial gelatinases and angiogenesis. Int J Biochem Cell Biol 33:960–970

Oltenfreiter R, Staelens L, Lejeune A, Dumont F, Frankenne F, Foidart JM, Slegers G (2004) New radioiodinated carboxylic and hydroxamic matrix metalloproteinase inhibitor tracers as potential tumor imaging agents. Nucl Med Biol 31:459–468

Oltenfreiter R, Staelens L, Hillaert U, Heremans A, Noel A, Frankenne F, Slegers G (2005a) Synthesis, radiosynthesis, in vitro and preliminary in vivo evaluation of biphenyl carboxylic and hydroxamic matrix metalloproteinase (MMP) inhibitors as potential tumor imaging agents. Appl Radiat Isot 62:903–913

Oltenfreiter R, Staelens L, Labied S, Kersemans V, Frankenne F, Noel A, Van de Wiele C, Slegers G (2005b) Tryptophane-based biphenylsulfonamide matrix metalloproteinase inhibitors as tumor imaging agents. Cancer Biother Radiopharm 20:639–647

Pelmenschikov V, Siegbahn PE (2002) Catalytic mechanism of matrix metalloproteinases: two-layered ONIOM study. Inorg Chem 41:5659–5666

Poethko T, Schottelius M, Thumshirn G, Hersel U, Herz M, Henriksen G, Kessler H, Schwaiger M, Wester HJ (2004a) Two-step methodology for high-yield routine radiohalogenation of peptides: ^{18}F-labeled RGD and octreotide analogs. J Nucl Med 45:892–902

Poethko T, Schottelius M, Thumshirn G, Herz M, Haubner R, Henriksen G, Kessler H, Schwaiger M, Wester HJ (2004b) Chemoselective pre-conjugate radiohalogenation of unprotected mono- and multimeric peptides via oxime formation. Radiochimica Acta 92:317–327

Rosen L (2000) Antiangiogenic strategies and agents in clinical trials. Oncologist 1:20–27

Rundhaug JE (2005) Matrix metalloproteinases and angiogenesis. J Cell Mol Med 9:267–285

Ruoslahti E, Pierschbacher MD (1987) New perspectives in cell adhesion: RGD and integrins. Science 238:491–497

Santimaria M, Moscatelli G, Viale GL, Giovannoni L, Neri G, Viti F, Leprini A, Borsi L, Castellani P, Zardi L, Neri D, Riva P (2003) Immunoscintigraphic detection of the ED-B domain of fibronectin, a marker of angiogenesis, in patients with cancer. Clin Cancer Res 9: 571–579

Storgard CM, Stupack DG, Jonczyk A, Goodman SL, Fox RI, Cheresh DA (1999) Decreased angiogenesis and arthritic disease in rabbits treated with an $\alpha v\beta 3$ antagonist. J Clin Invest 103:47–54

Su ZF, Liu G, Gupta S, Zhu Z, Rusckowski M, Hnatowich DJ (2002) In vitro and in vivo evaluation of a Technetium-99m-labeled cyclic RGD peptide as a specific marker of $\alpha v\beta 3$ integrin for tumor imaging. Bioconjug Chem 13:561–570

Su ZF, He J, Rusckowski M, Hnatowich DJ (2003) In vitro cell studies of technetium-99m labeled RGD-HYNIC peptide, a comparison of tricine and EDDA as co-ligands. Nucl Med Biol 30:141–149

Tarli L, Balza E, Viti F, Borsi L, Castellani P, Berndorff D, Dinkelborg L, Neri D, Zardi L (1999) A high-affinity human antibody that targets tumoral blood vessels. Blood 94:192–198

Thumshirn G, Hersel U, Goodman SL, Kessler H (2003) Multimeric cyclic RGD peptides as potential tools for tumor targeting: solid-phase peptide synthesis and chemoselective oxime ligation. Chemistry 9:2717–2725

Tijink BM, Neri D, Leemans CR, Budde M, Dinkelborg LM, Stigter-van Walsum M, Zardi L, van Dongen GA (2006) Radioimmunotherapy of head and neck cancer xenografts using ^{131}I-labeled antibody L19-SIP for selective targeting of tumor vasculature. J Nucl Med 47: 1127–1135

van Hagen PM, Breeman WA, Bernard HF, Schaar M, Mooij CM, Srinivasan A, Schmidt MA, Krenning EP, de Jong M (2000) Evaluation of a radiolabelled cyclic DTPA-RGD analogue for tumour imaging and radionuclide therapy. Int J Cancer 90:186–198

Vihinen P, Kahari VM (2002) Matrix metalloproteinases in cancer: prognostic markers and therapeutic targets. Int J Cancer 99:157–166

Wang W, McMurray JS, Wu Q, Campbell ML, Li C (2005) Convenient solid-phase synthesis of diethylenetriaminepenta-acetic acid (DTPA)- conjugated cyclic RGD peptide analogues. Cancer Biother Radiopharm 20:547–556

Wu Y, Zhang X, Xiong Z, Cheng Z, Fisher DR, Liu S, Gambhir SS, Chen X (2005) microPET imaging of glioma integrin $\alpha v\beta 3$ expression using ^{64}Cu-labeled tetrameric RGD peptide. J Nucl Med 46:1707–1718

Zhang X, Xiong Z, Wu Y, Cai W, Tseng JR, Gambhir SS, Chen X (2006) Quantitative PET Imaging of Tumor Integrin $\alpha v\beta 3$ Expression with ^{18}F-FRGD2. J Nucl Med 47:113–121

Zheng QH, Fei X, Liu X, Wang JQ, Bin Sun H, Mock BH, Lee Stone K, Martinez TD, Miller KD, Sledge GW, Hutchins GD (2002) Synthesis and preliminary biological evaluation of MMP inhibitor radiotracers [11C]methyl-halo-CGS 27023A analogs, new potential PET breast cancer imaging agents. Nucl Med Biol 29:761–770

Zheng QH, Fei X, DeGrado TR, Wang JQ, Lee Stone K, Martinez TD, Gay DJ, Baity WL, Mock BH, Glick-Wilson BE, Sullivan ML, Miller KD, Sledge GW, Hutchins GD (2003) Synthesis, biodistribution and micro-PET imaging of a potential cancer biomarker carbon-11 labeled MMP inhibitor (2R)-2-[[4-(6-fluorohex-1-ynyl)phenyl]sulfonylamino]-3-methylbutyric acid [(11)C]methyl ester. Nucl Med Biol 30:753–760

Zheng QH, Fei X, Liu X, Wang JQ, Stone KL, Martinez TD, Gay DJ, Baity WL, Miller KD, Sledge GW, Hutchins GD (2004) Comparative studies of potential cancer biomarkers carbon-11 labeled MMP inhibitors (S)-2-(4'-[11C]methoxybiphenyl-4-sulfonylamino)-3-methylbutyric acid and N-hydroxy-(R)-2-[[(4'-[11C]methoxyphenyl)sulfonyl]benzylamino]-3-methylbut anamide. Nucl Med Biol 31:77–85

Molecular Imaging-guided Gene Therapy of Gliomas

Maria A. Rueger, Alexandra Winkeler, Anne V. Thomas, Lutz W. Kracht, and Andreas H. Jacobs(✉)

Abstract Gene therapy of patients with glioblastoma using viral and non-viral vectors, which are applied by direct injection or convection-enhanced delivery (CED), appear to be satisfactorily safe. Up to date, only single patients show a significant therapeutic benefit as deduced from single long-term survivors. Non-invasive imaging by PET for the identification of viable target tissue and for assessment of transduction efficiency shall help to identify patients which might benefit from gene therapy, while non-invasive follow-up on treatment responses allows early and dynamic adaptations of treatment options. Therefore, molecular imaging has a critical impact on the development of standardised gene therapy protocols and on efficient and safe vector applications in humans.

1 Introduction

Gliomas are the most common primary intracranial neoplasms. They can be divided into astrocytomas, oligodendrogliomas, and mixed gliomas or oligo-astrocytomas, respectively. Grading is performed according to the World Health Organization

Andreas H. Jacobs

Laboratory for Gene Therapy and Molecular Imaging at the Max-Planck Institute for Neurological Research with Klaus-Joachim-Zülch-Laboratories of the Max Planck Society and the Faculty of Medicine of the University of Cologne, Center for Molecular Medicine (CMMC), Departments of Neurology at the University of Cologne and Klinikum Fulda, Germany
andreas.jacobs@nf.mpg.de

W. Semmler and M. Schwaiger (eds.), *Molecular Imaging II*.
Handbook of Experimental Pharmacology 185/II.
© Springer-Verlag Berlin Heidelberg 2008

(WHO), taking into account the presence of nuclear changes (WHO Grade I), mitotic activity (WHO Grade II), the presence of endothelial proliferation (WHO Grade III), and necrosis (WHO Grade IV) (Kleihues and Cavenee 2000). Glioblastoma, corresponding to WHO Grade IV, is the most fatal and most common primary brain neoplasm with an incidence of three to six in 100,000. Approximately 50% of all gliomas and 20% of all primary intracranial tumours are glioblastomas (Preston-Martin 1999). Together with all intracranial neoplasms, glioblastoma is the second most common cause of death due to an intracranial disease after stroke. In view of the high incidence and poor prognosis of malignant brain tumours treated by conventional therapies, research focusing on alternative therapies, such as gene therapy, and improved diagnostic approaches seems to be of utmost importance.

2 Gene Therapy of Patients with Gliomas

Gene therapy is based on the transduction of therapeutic genes into diseased target tissue to induce a therapeutically valuable alteration of tissue phenotype. The design of effective gene therapy strategies relies on concerted research to define alterations in tumour genetics and tumour biology, as well as to develop safe and efficient vectors and application systems to achieve efficient, targeted and regulated alteration of specific gene expression. In terms of gene therapy of malignant brain tumours, transduction of tumour cells with "therapeutic" genes may influence their biological properties by (1) rendering them sensitive to pro-drugs, (2) altering the expression of cell-cycle regulating proteins, (3) inhibiting angiogenesis, (4) stimulating the immune response, or (5) introducing selectively replicating viral vector particles (VPs). For gene therapy of glioblastomas to be successful, a multimodal approach has to be developed combining the synergism between various pro-drug activating systems (Aghi et al. 1999; Rogulski et al. 2000) with immunomodulation (Toda et al. 1998; Todo et al. 1999) mediated by selectively replicating viral vectors (Jacobs et al. 1999a, 1999b). Originally, the concept of gene therapy for glioblastoma was to transplant fibroblasts genetically engineered to secrete retroviral vectors carrying a pro-drug activating enzyme gene (Culver et al. 1992). As retroviruses would only be able to integrate their genetic material into dividing cells, this concept seemed to be safe for the selective transduction of highly proliferating tumour cells. Clinical studies revealed that suicide gene therapy based on the retrovirus vector-mediated expression of herpes simplex virus type 1 thymidine kinase (HSV-1-tk) and subsequent ganciclovir (GCV) application as an adjuvant to the surgical resection of recurrent high grade gliomas can be performed safely, although clinical responses were observed in only a few patients with small brain tumours (Ram et al. 1997; Klatzmann et al. 1998; Rainov et al. 2000). The lack of therapeutic efficiency of replication-deficient retrovirus vector systems in clinical settings may be due to (1) the inability to distribute vector-producer cells (VPCs) throughout the tumour, (2) VPC instability, (3) the low transduction efficiency of retrovirions, and (4) the heterogeneity of glioma tissue. Out of those explanations, probably the most important limitation of gene therapy for glioblastoma is the heterogeneity of the tumour tissue, with highly proliferative tumour areas alongside areas of necrosis and non-dividing tumour cells migrating into the surrounding edema. Therefore, further development of gene therapy for glioblastoma will need to concentrate on: (1) the combination of different therapeutic genes to achieve a synergistic action; (2) the combination with new or improved pro-drug suicide-gene systems (Aghi et al. 1999; Rogulski et al. 2000); (3) the combination of gene- and immunotherapy; (4) the use of replication-competent oncolytic viral vectors (Markert et al. 2000; Rampling et al. 2000); (5) the combination with genetic approaches to target vascular- and growth-factor receptors; and (6) improved methods of vector application based on convection-enhanced delivery (CED) (Voges et al. 2003).

3 Molecular Imaging of Gliomas

The discrepancy between successful experimental gene therapy protocols and the limited efficiency in their clinical application highlights the importance of developing imaging assays to (1) non-invasively determine viable target tissue which might benefit from a biological treatment paradigm, (2) assess the location, magnitude and duration of vector-mediated (exogenous) gene expression in patients in vivo, and (3) monitor therapeutic response (e.g. imaging endogenous gene expression) during and after gene therapy. The clinical gene therapy trials for glioblastoma performed so far have all suffered from a lack of ability to investigate the magnitude and extent of transduced therapeutic gene expression in vivo, the only qualitative information being obtained from biopsied tissue samples (Palu et al. 1999; Harsh et al. 2000; Papanastassiou et al. 2002). Recently, gene therapy protocols have been established employing molecular imaging technology, including metabolic imaging of target tissue (Jacobs et al. 2005a) and non-invasive monitoring of the assessment of the transduced 'tissue dose' of vector-mediated gene expression in vivo (Figs. 1 and 2) (Jacobs et al. 2001; Voges et al. 2003), which are important issues for making gene therapy widely applicable to humans. This is in line with the Recombinant DNA Advisory Committee (RAC) of the NIH, which, as a reflection of the first gene therapy death, called for better assays for measuring transgene expression in cells and tissues (Hollon 2000).

4 Assessment of Vector-mediated Gene Expression

Non-invasive monitoring and localisation of exogenous genes by molecular imaging relies on the transduction of "reporter genes" encoding enzymes (Tjuvajev et al. 1995; Contag et al. 1998; Gambhir et al. 1998) or receptors (MacLaren et al. 1999; Weissleder et al. 2000). Those reporter genes can either additionally function as therapeutic genes themselves [e.g. HSV-1-*tk* (Tjuvajev et al. 1995)] or they can be

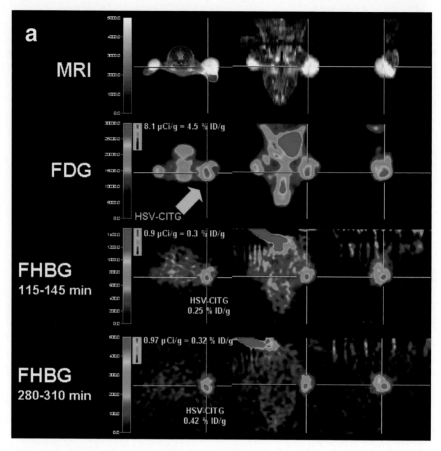

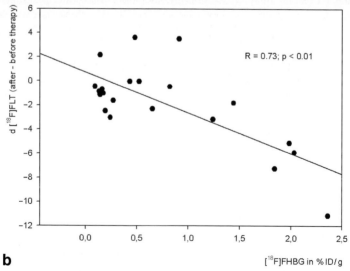

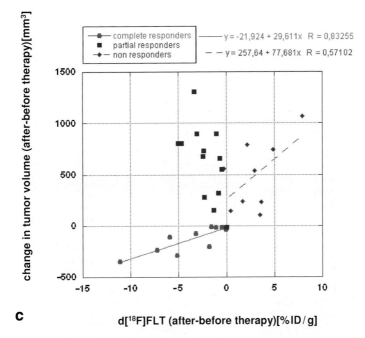

c   d[^{18}F]FLT (after-before therapy)[%ID/g]

Fig. 1 a Experimental protocol for identification of viable target tissue and assessment of vector-mediated gene expression in vivo in a mouse model with three subcutaneous gliomas. *Row 1*: localisation of tumors is displayed by MRI. *Row 2*: the viable target tissue is displayed by [^{18}F]FDG-PET; note the signs of necrosis in the lateral portion of the left-sided tumour (*arrow*). *Rows 3, 4*: following vector-application into the medial viable portion of the tumour (*arrow*) the tissue dose of vector-mediated gene expression is quantified by [^{18}F]FHBG-PET. *Row 3* shows an image acquired early after tracer injection, which is used for coregistration; *row 4* displays a late image with specific tracer accumulation in the tumor that is used for quantification. **b** Response to gene therapy correlates to therapeutic gene expression. The intensity of *cd*IRES*tk39gfp* expression, which is equivalent to transduction efficiency and tissue-dose of vector-mediated therapeutic gene expression, is measured by [^{18}F]FHBG-PET (in % ID/g), and the induced therapeutic effect is measured by [^{18}F]FLT-PET ($r = 0.73$, $P < 0.01$). Therapeutic effect ([^{18}F]FLT) was calculated as difference between [^{18}F]FLT accumulation after and before therapy. **c** Relation between changes in volumetry and [^{18}F]FLT uptake. Changes in tumour volume and [^{18}F]FLT uptake were plotted for tumours grown in 11 nude mice. There is a strong correlation between volumetry and change in FLT uptake ($r = 0.83$) for those tumours responding to therapy (*complete responders*) and a weaker correlation ($r = 0.57$) for those tumours not responding to therapy (*non-responders*). No correlation was found for those tumors where focal alterations of [^{18}F]FLT uptake occurred which did not lead to a reduction in overall tumour volume (*partial responders*). (Adapted from Jacobs et al. 2007, with permission)

transduced into the tumour cells along with any therapeutic gene of interest using gene fusion constructs [e.g. TKGFP (Jacobs et al. 1999c)] or genetic linkers such as an internal ribosome entry site [IRES (Tjuvajev et al. 1999)]. Expression of the reporter enzymes or receptors leads to a regional accumulation of trapped radiolabelled or paramagnetic "marker substrates" or receptor-binding compounds,

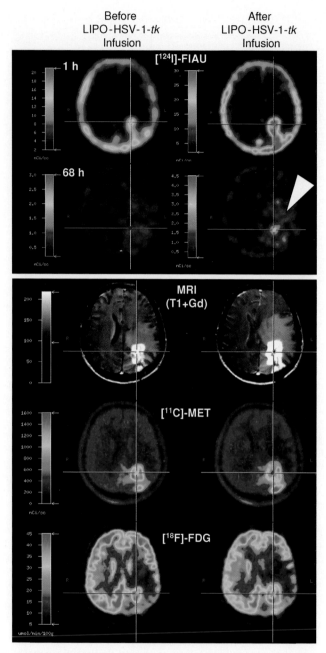

Fig. 2 Multimodal imaging for the establishment of imaging-guided gene therapy. Co-registration of [124I]FIAU, [11C]MET, [18F]FDG PET and MRI before (*left column*) and after (*right column*) targeted application (stereotactic infusion) of a gene therapy vector. The region of specific [124I]FIAU retention (68 h) within the tumour after LIPO-HSV-1-*tk* transduction (*white arrow*) resembles the proposed tissue dose of vector-mediated gene expression and shows signs of necrosis (*cross, right column*; reduced methionine uptake [MET] and glucose metabolism [FDG]) after ganciclovir treatment. (Adapted from Jacobs et al. 2001, with permission)

which can be detected by positron emission tomography (PET) or magnetic resonance imaging (MRI). The most extensively used system utilises the PET reporter gene HSV-1-*tk* (Tjuvajev et al. 1995, 1996, 1998; Gambhir et al. 1998). The reporter gene product, HSV-1-tk, selectively phosphorylates radiolabelled nucleoside analogues, rendering them incapable of exiting the cell and thus trapping them inside the cell, allowing for the visualisation by PET. Radiolabelled 2′-fluoro-2′-deoxy-1-β-D-arabinofuranosyl-5-[124]I-iodo-uracil ([124]I]FIAU) as well as other specific substrates for HSV-1-tk {e.g. 9-[4-^{18}F-fluoro-3-(hydroxymethyl)butyl]guanine (^{18}F]FHBG) or 9-[(3-^{18}F-fluoro-1-hydroxy-2-propoxy)methyl]guanine (^{18}F] FHPG)} have been successfully used for the non-invasive PET monitoring of retroviral, adenoviral, and herpes viral vector-mediated HSV-1-*tk* gene expression in various experimental rodent models (Fig. 1; Jacobs et al. 2001; reviewed by Jacobs et al. 2002; Gambhir et al. 2000; Wiebe and Knaus 2001; Blasberg and Gelovani 2002; de Vries and Vaalburg 2002). This method has been used in a phase I HSV-1-*tk* gene therapy trial investigating the safety and potential therapeutic action of intratumourally infused liposome-plasmid DNA complex followed by GCV administration (Jacobs et al. 2001; Voges et al. 2003). After identification of biologically active target tissue by multi-tracer PET, one or two catheters were stereotactically placed within the tumour and subcutaneously connected to a port. This allowed targeted intratumoural infusion of the cationic liposomal vector (Voges et al. 2003) containing an HSV-1-*tk*-carrying plasmid. A dynamic [124]I]FIAU-PET series acquired over 3 days was performed before gene transduction to evaluate the basal state of [124]I]FIAU accumulation in and wash-out from the tumour, and an identical [124]I]FIAU PET series was performed after vector application to dynamically investigate whether specific [124]I]FIAU accumulation did occur. GCV treatment was carried out starting 4 days after vector infusion. Identification of target tissue before catheter placement and treatment response were recorded by repeated MRI as well as by 2-^{18}F]fluoro-2-deoxy-D-glucose (^{18}F]FDG) and methyl-^{11}C]-L-methionine (^{11}C]MET)-PET (Fig. 2). After vector administration, in one out of eight patients, specific [124]I]FIAU-derived radioactivity was observed within the vector-infused tumour. Specific radioactivity was localised at the infusion site within the centre of the tumour and demonstrated a significant increase in the accumulation rate, K_i, of [124]I]FIAU, from 0.000047 at baseline to 0.000096 ml/min/g after vector administration (two-compartment model), and an increase in tissue/plasma radioactivity ratios over time (Patlak analysis) – both of these parameters being indicators for specific radiotracer trapping and, hence, HSV-1-*tk* expression. After GCV treatment, ^{18}F]FDG and ^{11}C]MET-PET demonstrated signs of necrosis within the volume of specific [124]I]FIAU trapping, this being indicative of the HSV-1-tk-mediated therapeutic response. The overall therapeutic effect was apparently limited to a portion of the tumour. In the seven other patients, no specific FIAU accumulation was observed. In contrast to the patient with specific [124]I]FIAU accumulation, histology in these patients exhibited a significantly lower number of proliferating tumour cells per voxel; this indicates that the threshold of PET detection is set by a certain critical number of *tk*-gene-transduced tumour cells per voxel, so that *tk*-gene-related accumulation of [124]I]FIAU can be measured and detected by PET. Current research on imaging HSV-1-*tk* gene expression is focusing on: (1) methods for exact quantification of HSV-1-tk expression (Green et al. 2004); (2) improved HSV-1-tk probes for PET (Alauddin et al. 2004a, 2004b; Kang et al. 2005) and SPECT (Choi et al. 2005); (3) translation of this imaging paradigm into other vector systems (Soghomonyan et al. 2005); (4) imaging follow-up in cancer therapy strategies (Hackman et al. 2002; Deng et al. 2004; Yaghoubi et al. 2005); (5) imaging transcriptional activation (Wen et al. 2004; Serganova et al. 2004; Sundaresan et al. 2004); (6) multimodal imaging by fusing the HSV-1-*tk* gene with further imaging genes (Jacobs et al. 1999c, 2003b; Ray et al. 2004).

5 Characterisation of Target Tissue and Assessment of Therapeutic Effect

When translating experimental gene therapy protocols into clinical application, it is mandatory to use reliable methods to follow-up on the achieved therapeutic effects. Molecular imaging methods can be used to non-invasively monitor these effects repetitively over time and are therefore an important read-out that facilitates the introduction of novel therapies. Therefore, all imaging methods that are sensitive and specific enough to monitor disease progression can serve as a read-out for gene therapy effects. Both MRI and PET aim towards (1) an exact localisation of the tumour and its relation to surrounding tissue and function; (2) the identification of biological activity (malignancy); (3) the grading of response to therapy; (4) the identification of early indicators for recurrent tumour growth. Figure 3 summarises the most important variables, which can be non-invasively assessed in patients with a suspected glioma by MR and PET imaging.

MRI with and without contrast media is widely used for primary diagnosis of brain tumours. Standard T1- and T2-weighted MRI detects brain tumours with high sensitivity. Beside primary information on the size and localisation of the tumour, MRI provides additional information about secondary phenomena, such as mass effect, edema, hemorrhage, necrosis, and signs of increased intracranial pressure at high spatial resolution and with high tissue contrast. A set of various MRI acquisition parameters, like T1-, T2-, proton-, diffusion-, and perfusion-weighted images as well as fluid attenuated inversion recovery (FLAIR) sequences give a characteristic pattern of each tumour depending on tumour type and grade. Most brain tumours are hypointense on T1-weighted images and hyperintense on FLAIR, T2-, and proton-weighted images. Tumours with high proliferative activity, such as glioblastomas, lead to a destruction of the blood-brain barrier (BBB) with subsequent leakage of the contrast medium which is being used for diagnostic purpose in T1-weighted MRI. In contrast, low-grade tumours usually have no or minimal enhancement. The contrast-enhancing lesion (T1 + Gd) corresponds histologically to a hypercellular region with neovascularization, while the central hypointense area (T1) is mainly caused by tumour necrosis. The tumour volume measured as the volume of T2 hyperintensity is the strongest predictor of overall survival in patients

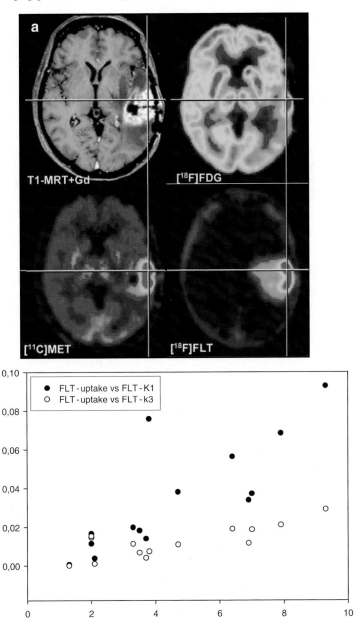

Fig. 3 a Parameters of interest in the non-invasive description of gliomas. MRI detects alteration of the blood-brain barrier and extent of peritumoral edema. Signs of increased cell proliferation can be observed by means of multi-tracer PET imaging using [^{18}F]FDG, [^{11}C]MET, and [^{18}F]FLT as specific tracers for glucose consumption, amino acid transport, and DNA synthesis, respectively (*Gd* gadolinium). (Adapted from Jacobs et al. 2002, with permission). **b** The metabolic rate constants, K1 and k3, correlate with the [^{18}F]FLT uptake ratio, indicating the relevance of increased transport and net influx of [^{18}F]FLT into tumor tissue (K1: $r = 0.85$, $P = 0.001$; k3: $r = 0.65$, $P = 0.011$; Spearman rank correlation coefficients). (Adapted from Jacobs et al. 2005b, with permission)

with supratentorial diffuse astrocytoma WHO°II, and the only predictor of malignant progression (Mariani et al. 2004). To monitor therapeutic responses, conventional contrast-enhanced MRI has the major disadvantage that residual tumour and post-surgical changes can both result in abnormal enhancement. Moreover, conventional MRI techniques usually fail to detect early treatment effects because effects are only visible after more than 12 months (Kumar et al. 2000; de Wit et al. 2004) with a substantial inter-observer variability in the assessment of treatment response (Vos et al. 2003). Especially after the application of biologically active agents such as gene therapy vectors, the value of conventional MRI to detect therapy-specific changes of tumour viability is limited, as reviewed previously (Jacobs et al. 2003a). In contrast, dynamic contrast-enhanced MRI (DCE-MRI) is a valuable tool to measure the exposure-dependent effects of drugs targeting the tumour vasculature occurring before tumour shrinkage. Tumour vasculature presents an important target for therapeutic development, with agents acting on the vascular endothelium (antivascular therapies) or the process of neoangiogenesis (antiangiogenic therapies). Antivascular and antiangiogenic therapies in different tumour types have been successfully monitored using DCE-MRI (Galbraith et al. 2003; Morgan et al. 2003). This method can also be used to characterise human gliomas (Ludemann et al. 2000), and treatment monitoring with DCE-MRI was successfully used in a xenograft model of glioblastoma in rats, and demonstrated the antiangiogenic effects of anti-VEGF antibody therapy (Gossmann et al. 2002). Diffusion-weighted MRI (DWI) detects therapy-induced water diffusion changes and is able to characterise morphological features, including edema, necrosis, and viable tumour tissue, by measuring differences in the apparent diffusion coefficient (ADC). DWI might be able to detect areas of tumour infiltration which are not visible on other MRI sequences (Provenzale et al. 2004). Diffusion-weighted MRI has been suggested to provide an early surrogate marker for quantification of treatment response (Chenevert et al. 2000). It was found that low values for the ADC, indicating high tissue viability, imply better response to radiotherapy, whereas high ADC values indicating necrosis correlate with poorer response (Mardor et al. 2004). Assessment of ADC ratios from tumour and contralateral control regions were also useful in the differentiation of radiation effects (high ADC ratios) from tumour recurrence or progression (low ADC ratios) (Hein et al. 2004). However, it should be kept in mind that dexamethasone treatment significantly reduces the diffusivity of edematous brain, thus confounding the interpretation of DWI-MRI (Sinha et al. 2004). Another important application for diffusion-weighted MRI in neuro-oncology is to monitor tumour response to convection-enhanced delivery (CED) of various drugs (Mardor et al. 2001). In trials employing CED to test local chemotherapeutics or gene therapy, DWI is being used to continuously monitor the progression of the convection process as well as its effect on the treated tissue (Lidar et al. 2004).

Because intratumoural heterogeneity of brain tumours is not adequately reflected in MRI, MRS is performed to gain additional information on metabolic and molecular tumour markers. MRS gives additional information on the real extent of the tumour and on tissue metabolites, such as N-acetylaspartate (NAA), creatine, choline, and lactate (Meyerand et al. 1999). The concentration of choline-containing compounds is a biomarker for altered membrane-phospholipid metabolism, which is a hallmark of all types of cancers (Aboagye and Bhujwalla 1999; Herminghaus et al. 2002). The increase of choline-containing compounds and of NAA appears to correlate best with the degree of tumour infiltration (Croteau et al. 2001). The appearance of creatine differentiates gliomas from metastasis, which generally lack creatine (Pirzkall et al. 2001). Because MRS can reliably differentiate pure tumour, pure necrosis, and normal tissue, specific changes in tumour metabolite levels as detected by MRS can be predictive for the effectiveness of experimental treatment strategies (Ross et al. 1995). Studies have correlated MRS variables, therapeutic response, and brain tumour survival (Herminghaus et al. 2002; Nelson et al. 2004). Progression from low-grade to high-grade gliomas leads to a characteristically increased concentration of choline and a reduced NAA peak with high diagnostic accuracy (Lehnhardt et al. 2005). MRS is also able to produce biochemical information about apoptosis of cancer cells in vivo. Accumulation of lipids can be utilised as a marker for growth arrest and can be detected by MRS, reflecting cell damage as early as 2–4 days after ganciclovir treatment in gene therapy of experimental gliomas (Hakumaki et al. 1999).

PET reveals highly specific quantitative information on the metabolic state of gliomas (Herholz et al. 1990; Jacobs et al. 2002), and allows the quantitative localisation of gene expression coding for enzymes or receptors by measuring the accumulation or binding of the respective enzyme substrates or receptor-binding compounds (Sokoloff et al. 1977; Heiss et al. 1984; Phelps 2000). Depending on the radiotracer, various molecular processes can be visualised by PET, most of them relating to an increased cell proliferation within gliomas (Fig. 3). [^{18}F]FDG is taken up by proliferating gliomas as a reflection of increased activity of membrane transporters for glucose and hexokinase gene activity. [^{18}F]FDG PET has been used to detect the metabolic differences between normal brain tissue, low-grade and high-grade gliomas, and radionecrosis (Heiss et al. 1990; Herholz et al. 1992, 1993). Increased intratumoural glucose consumption correlates with tumour grade, cell density, biological aggressiveness, and survival of patients in both primary and recurrent gliomas (Herholz et al. 1993; Goldman et al. 1996; Barker et al. 1997). In general, low-grade tumours have a metabolic activity similar to white matter, while the metabolic activity of higher-grade tumours is more similar to gray matter. However, due to the relatively high cortical background activity, [^{18}F]FDG PET is not suited to detect residual tumour after therapy (Kim et al. 1992; Wurker et al. 1996). Similar to structural imaging, the effects of radio- and chemotherapy can be visualised by [^{18}F]FDG PET only after several weeks (Brock et al. 2000). At further follow-up, however, recurrent tumour and progression from low-grade to high-grade glioma can be visualised by a newly appearing hypermetabolism (De Witte et al. 1996; Glantz et al. 1991). After radiation therapy, the co-registration with MRI improves the sensitivity of [^{18}F]FDG PET for the detection of recurrent tumour (Chao et al. 2001). However, changes in [^{18}F]FDG-uptake do not seem to be predictive of response to chemotherapy, time to progression or survival (Vlassenko et al. 2000). It should also be noted that in patients receiving corticosteroids as symptomatic treatment, evaluation of [^{18}F]FDG PET may be hampered by a reduced cortex-to-white matter ratio (Fulham et al. 1995). For these reasons, [^{18}F]FDG PET does not play a major role in the development of novel therapies for gliomas.

The radiolabelled amino acids methyl-[^{11}C]-L-methionine ([^{11}C]MET), O-(2-[^{18}F]fluoroethyl)-L-tyrosine ([^{18}F]FET), [^{11}C]tyrosine, and [^{18}F]fluorotyrosine have been shown to be more specific tracers for tumour detection and tumour delineation due to their low uptake in normal brain (Herholz et al. 1998; Kaschten et al. 1998; Chung et al. 2002; Pauleit et al. 2004). The increased methionine uptake (factor of 1.3–3.5 in comparison with a contralateral control region) is related to increased transport mediated by type L amino acid carriers (Langen et al. 2000). [^{11}C]MET-uptake correlates to cell proliferation in vitro, the expression of Ki-67 and proliferating cell nuclear antigen, as well as to microvessel density, explaining its role as a marker for active tumour proliferation (Chung et al. 2002; Kracht et al. 2003). In 80% of gliomas WHO °II [^{11}C]MET-uptake is greater than 1.5-fold of the normal brain tissue (Herholz et al. 1998), whereas glucose metabolism is reduced compared with gray matter. Most studies indicated that [^{11}C]MET-uptake is inversely correlated to prognosis (De Witte et al. 2001; Ribom et al. 2001), but due to significant [^{11}C]MET-uptake also in most low-grade gliomas this relation is less close than with [^{18}F]FDG. [^{11}C]MET PET is well suited to follow the effects of radiation therapy as a reduction of relative methionine uptake (Wurker et al. 1996). Most importantly, [^{11}C]MET PET is a useful tool to evaluate responses of gliomas to chemotherapy with procarbazine, CCNU and vincristine (PCV) (Herholz et al. 2003; Tang et al. 2005), and temozolomide (TMZ) (Galldiks et al. 2006) revealing tumour responses already after three cycles of TMZ chemotherapy. Therefore, PET imaging using [^{11}C]MET is a very useful tool in evaluating novel treatments like gene therapy. Similar results have been obtained with other tracers for amino acid transport, such as [^{18}F]FET with a reliable differentiation between post-therapeutic benign lesions and tumour recurrence after treatment of low- and high-grade tumours (Popperl et al. 2004). [^{18}F]FET PET has also been shown to be a valuable tool to monitor the effects of CED of paclitaxel in patients with recurrent glioblastoma (Popperl et al. 2005). The third parameter which can be non-invasively assessed by PET is the incorporation of nucleosides into DNA in proliferating cells. The evaluation of tumour proliferation primarily in extra-cranial tissues has been achieved using 3-deoxy-3-[^{18}F]fluoro-L-thymidine ([^{18}F]FLT), which is stable in vivo. A recent study in patients with gliomas proposes [^{18}F]FLT to be a promising tracer to study glioma proliferation, especially in areas with high [^{18}F]FDG background (Jacobs et al. 2005b). Sensitivity for the detection of gliomas was lower for [^{18}F]FLT than for [^{11}C]MET (78.3 vs 91.3%), especially for low-grade astrocytomas. Uptake ratios of [^{18}F]FLT were significantly higher than uptake ratios of [^{11}C]MET. Uptake ratios of [^{18}F]FLT in glioblastomas were significantly higher than in astrocytomas. Absolute radiotracer uptake of [^{18}F]FLT was low and significantly lower than of [^{11}C]MET (SUV 1.3 ± 0.7 vs 3.1 ± 1.0). There were tumour regions only detected by either [^{18}F]FLT or [^{11}C]MET in seven and 13 patients, respectively. Kinetic modelling revealed that [^{18}F]FLT uptake in tumour tissue seems to be predominantly due to elevated transport and net influx. However, there was also a moderate correlation between uptake ratio and phosphorylation rate k3 ($r = 0.65$, $P = 0.01$, grade II-IV gliomas;

$r = 0.76$, $P < 0.01$, grade III-IV tumours; Fig. 3b). These data indicate that $[^{18}F]FLT$ is a promising tracer for the detection and characterisation of primary CNS tumours and might help to differentiate between low- and high-grade gliomas. $[^{18}F]FLT$ uptake is mainly due to increased transport, but irreversible incorporation by phosphorylation might also contribute to its uptake. In some tumours and tumour areas, $[^{18}F]FLT$ uptake is not related to $[^{11}C]MET$ uptake. In view of the high sensitivity and specificity of $[^{11}C]MET$-PET for imaging of gliomas, it cannot be excluded that $[^{18}F]FLT$-PET was false-positive in these areas. However, the discrepancies observed for the various imaging modalities ($[^{18}F]FLT$- and $[^{11}C]MET$-PET as well as Gd-enhanced MRI) yield complementary information on the activity and the extent of gliomas and might improve early evaluation of treatment effects, especially in patients with high-grade gliomas (Shields et al. 1998; Mankoff et al. 2000). Unpublished data suggest that $[^{18}F]FLT$ can be used to monitor the therapeutic response to gene therapy in an experimental glioma model as early as 3 days after initiation of therapy.

6 Future Perspective

It should be pointed out that the presented imaging modalities are not competing with each other but give complementary information on various parameters of interest in neuro-oncology. Therefore, it is most important for the development and assessment of novel experimental therapies, like gene therapy, to combine the multimodal imaging procedures. In neuro-oncology, multimodal imaging can (1) reveal the best set of anatomical, biochemical and molecular information on a specific tumour and, hence, non-invasively determine the best target tissue for vector application in gene therapy, (2) quantify vector-mediated gene expression, and (3) assess therapeutic effects.

References

Aboagye EO, Bhujwalla ZM (1999) Malignant transformation alters membrane choline phospholipid metabolism of human mammary epithelial cells. Cancer Res 59:80–84

Aghi M, Chou TC, Suling K, Breakefield XO, Chiocca A (1999) Multimodal cancer treatment mediated by replicating oncolytic virus that delivers the oxazaphosphorine/rat cytochrome P450 2B1 and ganciclovir/herpes simplex virus thymidine kinase gene therapies. Cancer Res 59:3861–3865

Alauddin MM, Shahinian A, Gordon EM, Conti PS (2004a) Direct comparison of radiolabeled probes FMAU, FHBG, and FHPG as PET imaging agents for HSV1-tk expression in a human breast cancer model. Mol Imaging 3:76–84

Alauddin MM, Shahinian A, Park R, Tohme M, Fissekis JD, Conti PS (2004b) Synthesis and evaluation of 2′-deoxy-2′-18F-fluoro-5-fluoro-1-beta-D-arabinofuranosyluracil as a potential PET imaging agent for suicide gene expression. J Nucl Med 45:2063–2069

Barker FG, Chang SM, Valk PE, Pounds TR, Prados MD (1997) 18-Fluorodeoxyglucose uptake and survival of patients with suspected recurrent malignant glioma. Cancer 79:115–126

Blasberg RG, Gelovani J (2002) Molecular-genetic imaging: a nuclear medicine-based perspective. Mol Imaging 1:280–300

Brock CS, Young H, O'Reilly SM et al (2000) Early evaluation of tumour metabolic response using [18F]fluorodeoxyglucose and positron emission tomography: a pilot study following the phase II chemotherapy schedule for temozolomide in recurrent high-grade gliomas. Br J Cancer 82:608–615

Chao ST, Suh JH, Raja S, Lee SY, Barnett G (2001) The sensitivity and specificity of FDG PET in distinguishing recurrent brain tumor from radionecrosis in patients treated with stereotactic radiosurgery. Int J Cancer 96:191–197

Chenevert TL, Stegman LD, Taylor JM et al (2000) Diffusion magnetic resonance imaging: an early surrogate marker of therapeutic efficacy in brain tumors. J Natl Cancer Inst 92: 2029–2036

Choi SR, Zhuang ZP, Chacko AM et al (2005) SPECT imaging of herpes simplex virus type1 thymidine kinase gene expression by [(123)I]FIAU(1). Acad Radiol 12:798–805

Chung JK, Kim K, Kim SK et al (2002) Usefulness of 11C-methionine PET in the evaluation of brain lesions that are hypo- or isometabolic on 18F-FDG PET. Eur J Nucl Med Mol Imaging 29:176–182

Contag PR, Olomu IN, Stevenson DK, Contag CH (1998) Bioluminescent indicators in living mammals. Nat Med 4:245–247

Croteau D, Scarpace L, Hearshen D et al (2001) Correlation between magnetic resonance spectroscopy imaging and image-guided biopsies: semiquantitative and qualitative histopathological analyses of patients with untreated glioma. Neurosurgery 49:823–829

Culver KW, Ram Z, Wallbridge S, Ishii H, Oldfield EH, Blaese RM (1992) In vivo gene transfer with retroviral vector-producer cells for treatment of experimental brain tumors. Science 256:1550–1552

de Vries EF, Vaalburg W (2002) Positron emission tomography: measurement of transgene expression. Methods 27:234–241

de Wit MC, de Bruin HG, Eijkenboom W, Sillevis Smitt PA, van den Bent MJ (2004) Immediate post-radiotherapy changes in malignant glioma can mimic tumor progression. Neurology 63:535–537

De Witte O, Levivier M, Violon P et al (1996) Prognostic value positron emission tomography with [18F]fluoro-2-deoxy-D-glucose in the low-grade glioma. Neurosurgery 39:470–476

De Witte O, Goldberg I, Wikler D et al (2001) Positron emission tomography with injection of methionine as a prognostic factor in glioma. J Neurosurg 95:746–750

Deng WP, Yang WK, Lai WF et al (2004) Non-invasive in vivo imaging with radiolabelled FIAU for monitoring cancer gene therapy using herpes simplex virus type 1 thymidine kinase and ganciclovir. Eur J Nucl Med Mol Imaging 31:99–109

Fulham MJ, Brunetti A, Aloj L, Raman R, Dwyer AJ, Di Chiro G (1995) Decreased cerebral glucose metabolism in patients with brain tumors: an effect of corticosteroids. J Neurosurg 83:657–664

Galbraith SM, Maxwell RJ, Lodge MA et al (2003) Combretastatin A4 phosphate has tumor antivascular activity in rat and man as demonstrated by dynamic magnetic resonance imaging. J Clin Oncol 21:2831–2842

Galldiks N, Kracht LW, Burghaus L et al (2006) Use of (11)C-methionine PET to monitor the effects of temozolomide chemotherapy in malignant gliomas. Eur J Nucl Med Mol Imaging 33:516–524

Gambhir SS, Barrio JR, Wu L et al (1998) Imaging of adenoviral-directed herpes simplex virus type 1 thymidine kinase reporter gene expression in mice with radiolabeled ganciclovir. J Nucl Med 39:2003–2011

Gambhir SS, Herschman HR, Cherry SR et al (2000) Imaging transgene expression with radionuclide imaging technologies. Neoplasia 2:118–138

Glantz MJ, Hoffman JM, Coleman RE et al (1991) Identification of early recurrence of primary central nervous system tumors by [18F]fluorodeoxyglucose positron emission tomography. Ann Neurol 29:347–355

Goldman S, Levivier M, Pirotte B et al (1996) Regional glucose metabolism and histopathology of gliomas. A study based on positron emission tomography-guided stereotactic biopsy. Cancer 78:1098–1106

Gossmann A, Helbich TH, Kuriyama N et al (2002) Dynamic contrast-enhanced magnetic resonance imaging as a surrogate marker of tumor response to anti-angiogenic therapy in a xenograft model of glioblastoma multiforme. J Magn Reson Imaging 15:233–240

Green LA, Nguyen K, Berenji B et al (2004) A tracer kinetic model for 18F-FHBG for quantitating herpes simplex virus type 1 thymidine kinase reporter gene expression in living animals using PET. J Nucl Med 45:1560–1570

Hackman T, Doubrovin M, Balatoni J et al (2002) Imaging expression of cytosine deaminase-herpes virus thymidine kinase fusion gene (CD/TK) expression with [124I]FIAU and PET. Mol Imaging 1:36–42

Hakumaki JM, Poptani H, Sandmair AM, Yla-Herttuala S, Kauppinen RA (1999) 1H MRS detects polyunsaturated fatty acid accumulation during gene therapy of glioma: implications for the in vivo detection of apoptosis. Nat Med 5:1323–1327

Harsh GR, Deisboeck TS, Louis DN et al (2000) Thymidine kinase activation of ganciclovir in recurrent malignant gliomas: a gene-marking and neuropathological study. J Neurosurg 92:804–811

Hein PA, Eskey CJ, Dunn JF, Hug EB (2004) Diffusion-weighted imaging in the follow-up of treated high-grade gliomas: tumor recurrence versus radiation injury. AJNR Am J Neuroradiol 25:201–209

Heiss WD, Pawlik G, Herholz K, Wagner R, Goldner H, Wienhard K (1984) Regional kinetic constants and cerebral metabolic rate for glucose in normal human volunteers determined by dynamic positron emission tomography of [18F]-2-fluoro-2-deoxy-D-glucose. J Cereb Blood Flow Metab 4:212–223

Heiss WD, Heindel W, Herholz K et al (1990) Positron emission tomography of fluorine-18-deoxyglucose and image-guided phosphorus-31 magnetic resonance spectroscopy in brain tumors. J Nucl Med 31:302–310

Herholz K, Wienhard K, Heiss WD (1990) Validity of PET studies in brain tumors. Cerebrovasc Brain Metab Rev 2:240–265

Herholz K, Heindel W, Luyten PR et al (1992) In vivo imaging of glucose consumption and lactate concentration in human gliomas. Ann Neurol 31:319–327

Herholz K, Pietrzyk U, Voges J et al (1993) Correlation of glucose consumption and tumor cell density in astrocytomas. A stereotactic PET study. J Neurosurg 79:853–858

Herholz K, Holzer T, Bauer B et al (1998) 11C-methionine PET for differential diagnosis of low-grade gliomas. Neurology 50:1316–1322

Herholz K, Kracht LW, Heiss WD (2003) Monitoring the effect of chemotherapy in a mixed glioma by C-11-methionine PET. J Neuroimaging 13:269–271

Herminghaus S, Pilatus U, Moller-Hartmann W et al (2002) Increased choline levels coincide with enhanced proliferative activity of human neuroepithelial brain tumors. NMR Biomed 15:385–392

Hollon T (2000) Researchers and regulators reflect on first gene therapy death. Nat Med 6:6

Jacobs AH, Breakefield XO, Fraefel C (1999a) HSV-1-based vectors for gene therapy of neurological diseases and brain tumors: Part I. HSV-1 structure, replication and pathogenesis. Neoplasia 1:387–401

Jacobs AH, Breakefield XO, Fraefel C (1999b) HSV-1-based vectors for gene therapy of neurological diseases and brain tumors: Part II. Vector systems and applications. Neoplasia 1:402–416

Jacobs AH, Dubrovin M, Hewett J et al (1999c) Functional coexpression of HSV-1 thymidine kinase and green fluorescent protein: implications for noninvasive imaging of transgene expression. Neoplasia 1:154–161

Jacobs AH, Voges J, Reszka R et al (2001) Positron-emission tomography of vector-mediated gene expression in gene therapy for gliomas. Lancet 358:727–729

Jacobs AH, Dittmar C, Winkeler A, Garlip G, Heiss WD (2002) Molecular imaging of gliomas. Mol Imaging 1:309–335

Jacobs AH, Voges J, Kracht LW et al (2003a) Imaging in gene therapy of patients with glioma. J Neurooncol 65:291–305

Jacobs AH, Winkeler A, Hartung M et al (2003b) Improved herpes simplex virus type 1 amplicon vectors for proportional coexpression of positron emission tomography marker and therapeutic genes. Hum Gene Ther 14:277–297

Jacobs AH, Kracht LW, Gossmann A et al (2005a) Imaging in neurooncology. NeuroRx 2:333–347

Jacobs AH, Thomas A, Kracht LW et al (2005b) 18F-fluoro-L-thymidine and 11C-methylmethionine as markers of increased transport and proliferation in brain tumors. J Nucl Med 46:1948–1958

Jacobs AH, Rueger MA, Winkeler A et al (2007) Imaging-guided gene therapy of experimental gliomas. Cancer Res 67:1706–1715

Kang KW, Min JJ, Chen X, Gambhir SS (2005) Comparison of [14C]FMAU, [3H]FEAU, [14C]FIAU, and [3H]PCV for monitoring reporter gene expression of wild type and mutant herpes simplex virus type 1 thymidine kinase in cell culture. Mol Imaging Biol 7:296–303

Kaschten B, Stevenaert A, Sadzot B et al (1998) Preoperative evaluation of 54 gliomas by PET with fluorine-18-fluorodeoxyglucose and/or carbon-11-methionine. J Nucl Med 39:778–785

Kim EE, Chung SK, Haynie TP et al (1992) Differentiation of residual or recurrent tumors from post-treatment changes with F-18 FDG PET. Radiographics 12:269–279

Kim YJ, Dubey P, Ray P, Gambhir SS, Witte ON (2004) Multimodality imaging of lymphocytic migration using lentiviral-based transduction of a tri-fusion reporter gene. Mol Imaging Biol 6:331–340

Klatzmann D, Valery CA, Bensimon G et al (1998) A phase I/II study of herpes simplex virus type 1 thymidine kinase "suicide" gene therapy for recurrent glioblastoma. Study Group on Gene Therapy for Glioblastoma. Hum Gene Ther 9: 2595–2604

Kleihues P, Cavenee W K (2000) Pathology and genetics of tumours of the nervous system (WHO). International Agency for Research on Cancer (IARC Press), Lyon

Kracht LW, Friese M, Herholz K et al (2003) Methyl-[11C]- l-methionine uptake as measured by positron emission tomography correlates to microvessel density in patients with glioma. Eur J Nucl Med Mol Imaging 30:868–873

Kumar AJ, Leeds NE, Fuller GN et al (2000) Malignant gliomas: MR imaging spectrum of radiation therapy- and chemotherapy-induced necrosis of the brain after treatment. Radiology 217:377–384

Langen KJ, Muhlensiepen H, Holschbach M, Hautzel H, Jansen P, Coenen HH (2000) Transport mechanisms of 3-[123I]iodo-alpha-methyl-L-tyrosine in a human glioma cell line: comparison with [3H]methyl]-L-methionine. J Nucl Med 41:1250–1255

Lehnhardt FG, Bock C, Rohn G, Ernestus RI, Hoehn M (2005) Metabolic differences between primary and recurrent human brain tumors: a 1H NMR spectroscopic investigation. NMR Biomed 18:371–382

Lidar Z, Mardor Y, Jonas T et al (2004) Convection-enhanced delivery of paclitaxel for the treatment of recurrent malignant glioma: a phase I/II clinical study. J Neurosurg 100:472–479

Ludemann L, Hamm B, Zimmer C (2000) Pharmacokinetic analysis of glioma compartments with dynamic Gd-DTPA-enhanced magnetic resonance imaging. Magn Reson Imaging 18: 1201–1214

MacLaren DC, Gambhir SS, Satyamurthy N et al (1999) Repetitive, non-invasive imaging of the dopamine D2 receptor as a reporter gene in living animals. Gene Ther 6:785–791

Mankoff DA, Dehdashti F, Shields AF (2000) Characterizing tumors using metabolic imaging: PET imaging of cellular proliferation and steroid receptors. Neoplasia 2:71–88

Mardor Y, Roth Y, Lidar Z et al (2001) Monitoring response to convection-enhanced taxol delivery in brain tumor patients using diffusion-weighted magnetic resonance imaging. Cancer Res 61:4971–4973

Mardor Y, Roth Y, Ochershvilli A et al (2004) Pretreatment prediction of brain tumors' response to radiation therapy using high b-value diffusion-weighted MRI. Neoplasia 6:136–142

Mariani L, Siegenthaler P, Guzman R et al (2004) The impact of tumour volume and surgery on the outcome of adults with supratentorial WHO grade II astrocytomas and oligoastrocytomas. Acta Neurochir (Wien) 146:441–448

Markert JM, Medlock MD, Rabkin SD et al (2000) Conditionally replicating herpes simplex virus mutant, G207 for the treatment of malignant glioma: results of a phase I trial. Gene Ther 7: 867–874

Meyerand ME, Pipas JM, Mamourian A, Tosteson TD, Dunn JF (1999) Classification of biopsy-confirmed brain tumors using single-voxel MR spectroscopy. AJNR Am J Neuroradiol 20: 117–123

Morgan B, Thomas AL, Drevs J et al (2003) Dynamic contrast-enhanced magnetic resonance imaging as a biomarker for the pharmacological response of PTK787/ZK 222584, an inhibitor of the vascular endothelial growth factor receptor tyrosine kinases, in patients with advanced colorectal cancer and liver metastases: results from two phase I studies. J Clin Oncol 21:3955–3964

Nelson SJ (2004) Magnetic resonance spectroscopic imaging. Evaluating responses to therapy for gliomas. IEEE Eng Med Biol Mag 23:30–39

Palu G, Cavaggioni A, Calvi P et al (1999) Gene therapy of glioblastoma multiforme via combined expression of suicide and cytokine genes: a pilot study in humans. Gene Ther 6:330–337

Papanastassiou V, Rampling R, Fraser M et al (2002) The potential for efficacy of the modified (ICP 34.5(-)) herpes simplex virus HSV1716 following intratumoural injection into human malignant glioma: a proof of principle study. Gene Ther 9:398–406

Pauleit D, Floeth F, Tellmann L et al (2004) Comparison of O-(2-18F-fluoroethyl)-L-tyrosine PET and 3-123I-iodo-alpha-methyl-L-tyrosine SPECT in brain tumors. J Nucl Med 45:374–381

Phelps ME (2000) PET: the merging of biology and imaging into molecular imaging. J Nucl Med 41:661–681

Pirzkall A, McKnight TR, Graves EE et al (2001) MR-spectroscopy guided target delineation for high-grade gliomas. Int J Radiat Oncol BiolPhys 50:915–928

Popperl G, Gotz C, Rachinger W, Gildehaus FJ, Tonn JC, Tatsch K (2004) Value of O-(2-[18F]fluoroethyl)- L-tyrosine PET for the diagnosis of recurrent glioma. Eur J Nucl Med Mol Imaging 31:1464–1470

Popperl G, Goldbrunner R, Gildehaus FJ et al (2005) O-(2-[18F]fluoroethyl)-L-tyrosine PET for monitoring the effects of convection-enhanced delivery of paclitaxel in patients with recurrent glioblastoma. Eur J Nucl Med Mol Imaging 32:1018–1025

Preston-Martin S (1999) Epidemiology. In: Berger MS, Wilson CD (eds) The gliomas. Saunders, Philadelphia, pp 2–11

Provenzale JM, McGraw P, Mhatre P, Guo AC, Delong D (2004) Peritumoral brain regions in gliomas and meningiomas: investigation with isotropic diffusion-weighted MR imaging and diffusion-tensor MR imaging. Radiology 232:451–460

Rainov NG (2000) A phase III clinical evaluation of herpes simplex virus type 1 thymidine kinase and ganciclovir gene therapy as an adjuvant to surgical resection and radiation in adults with previously untreated glioblastoma multiforme. Hum Gene Ther 11:2389–2401

Ram Z, Culver KW, Oshiro EM et al (1997) Therapy of malignant brain tumors by intratumoral implantation of retroviral vector-producing cells. Nat Med 3:1354–1361

Rampling R, Cruickshank G, Papanastassiou V et al (2000) Toxicity evaluation of replication-competent herpes simplex virus (ICP 34.5 null mutant 1716) in patients with recurrent malignant glioma. Gene Ther 7:859–866

Ray P, De A, Min JJ, Tsien RY, Gambhir SS (2004) Imaging tri-fusion multimodality reporter gene expression in living subjects. Cancer Res 64:1323–1330

Ribom D, Eriksson A, Hartman M et al (2001) Positron emission tomography (11)C-methionine and survival in patients with low-grade gliomas. Cancer 92:1541–1549

Rogulski KR, Wing MS, Paielli DL, Gilbert JD, Kim JH, Freytag SO (2000) Double suicide gene therapy augments the antitumor activity of a replication-competent lytic adenovirus through enhanced cytotoxicity and radiosensitization. Hum.Gene Ther 11:67–76

Ross BD, Kim B, Davidson BL (1995) Assessment of ganciclovir toxicity to experimental intracranial gliomas following recombinant adenoviral-mediated transfer of the herpes simplex virus thymidine kinase gene by magnetic resonance imaging and proton magnetic resonance spectroscopy. Clin Cancer Res 1:651–657

Serganova I, Doubrovin M, Vider J et al (2004) Molecular imaging of temporal dynamics and spatial heterogeneity of hypoxia-inducible factor-1 signal transduction activity in tumors in living mice. Cancer Res 64:6101–6108

Shand N, Weber F, Mariani L et al (1999) A phase 1–2 clinical trial of gene therapy for recurrent glioblastoma multiforme by tumor transduction with the herpes simplex thymidine kinase gene followed by ganciclovir. GLI328 European-Canadian Study Group. Hum Gene Ther 10: 2325–2335

Shields AF, Grierson JR, Dohmen BM et al (1998) Imaging proliferation in vivo with [F-18]FLT and positron emission tomography. Nat Med 4:1334–1336

Sinha S, Bastin ME, Wardlaw JM, Armitage PA, Whittle IR (2004) Effects of dexamethasone on peritumoural oedematous brain: a DT-MRI study. J Neurol Neurosurg Psychiatry 75: 1632–1635

Soghomonyan SA, Doubrovin M, Pike J et al (2005) Positron emission tomography (PET) imaging of tumor-localized Salmonella expressing HSV1-TK. Cancer Gene Ther 12:101–108

Sokoloff L, Reivich M, Kennedy C et al (1977) The [14C]deoxyglucose method for the measurement of local cerebral glucose utilization: theory, procedure, and normal values in the conscious and anesthetized albino rat. J Neurochem 28:897–916

Sundaresan G, Paulmurugan R, Berger F et al (2004) MicroPET imaging of Cre-loxP-mediated conditional activation of a herpes simplex virus type 1 thymidine kinase reporter gene. Gene Ther 11:609–618

Tang BN, Sadeghi N, Branle F, De Witte O, Wikler D, Goldman S (2005) Semi-quantification of methionine uptake and flair signal for the evaluation of chemotherapy in low-grade oligodendroglioma. J Neurooncol 71:161–168

Tjuvajev JG, Stockhammer G, Desai R et al (1995) Imaging the expression of transfected genes in vivo. Cancer Res 55:6126–6132

Tjuvajev JG, Finn R, Watanabe K et al (1996) Noninvasive imaging of herpes virus thymidine kinase gene transfer and expression: a potential method for monitoring clinical gene therapy. Cancer Res 56:4087–4095

Tjuvajev JG, Avril N, Oku T et al (1998) Imaging herpes virus thymidine kinase gene transfer and expression by positron emission tomography. Cancer Res 58:4333–4341

Tjuvajev JG, Joshi A, Callegari J et al (1999) A general approach to the non-invasive imaging of transgenes using cis-linked herpes simplex virus thymidine kinase. Neoplasia 1:315–320

Toda M, Rabkin SD, Martuza RL (1998) Treatment of human breast cancer in a brain metastatic model by G207, a replication-competent multimutated herpes simplex virus 1. Hum Gene Ther 9:2177–2185

Todo T, Rabkin SD, Sundaresan P et al (1999) Systemic antitumor immunity in experimental brain tumor therapy using a multimutated, replication-competent herpes simplex virus. Hum Gene Ther 10:2741–2755

Vlassenko AG, Thiessen B, Beattie BJ, Malkin MG, Blasberg RG (2000) Evaluation of early response to SU101 target-based therapy in patients with recurrent supratentorial malignant gliomas using FDG PET and Gd-DTPA MRI. J Neurooncol 46:249–259

Voges J, Reszka R, Gossmann A et al(2003) Imaging-guided convection-enhanced delivery and gene therapy of glioblastoma. Ann Neurol 54:479–487

Vos MJ, Uitdehaag BM, Barkhof F et al (2003) Interobserver variability in the radiological assessment of response to chemotherapy in glioma. Neurology 60:826–830

Weissleder R, Moore A, Mahmood U et al (2000) In vivo magnetic resonance imaging of transgene expression. Nat Med 6:351–355

Wen B, Burgman P, Zanzonico P et al (2004) A preclinical model for noninvasive imaging of hypoxia-induced gene expression; comparison with an exogenous marker of tumor hypoxia. Eur J Nucl Med Mol Imaging 31:1530–1538

Wiebe LI, Knaus EE (2001) Enzyme-targeted, nucleoside-based radiopharmaceuticals for scintigraphic monitoring of gene transfer and expression. Curr Pharm Des 7:1893–1906

Wurker M, Herholz K, Voges J et al (1996) Glucose consumption and methionine uptake in low-grade gliomas after iodine-125 brachytherapy. Eur J Nucl Med 23:583–586

Yaghoubi SS, Barrio JR, Namavari M et al (2005) Imaging progress of herpes simplex virus type 1 thymidine kinase suicide gene therapy in living subjects with positron emission tomography. Cancer Gene Ther 12:329–339

Index

Printing: Krips bv, Meppel, The Netherlands
Binding: Stürtz, Würzburg, Germany